Advance Praise for *Eat What You Love, Love What You Eat*

"*Eat What You Love, Love What You Eat* offers compelling and valuable insights into the psychology of eating . . . Navigating the shoals of nutrition doesn't have to become a compulsive obsession or failed effort . . . Reading this book reminds and reeducates us how to find pleasure in these earthly delights."
—Brian Luke Seaward, PhD, author of *Managing Stress* and *Stressed Is Desserts Spelled Backward*

"*Eat What You Love, Love What You Eat* is truly brilliant—I will definitely use it . . . to help end mindless and emotional eating. It is so easy to read that even the most tired dieter will love it!"
—Jeanne Rust, PhD, CEO and founder of Mirasol and Tranformational Living.

"*Eat What You Love, Love What You Eat* will give readers a completely new mindset around food. In place of restriction, deprivation, and misery, they'll discover flexibility, freedom, and joy."
—Sharon Salomon, MS, RD

"Dr. May offers a lifeline for anyone who suffers from disordered eating patterns. She helps us answer the question, "what am I hungry for?" with confidence! If you are ready to change the way you think and feel about food, *Eat What You Love, Love What You Eat* provides a practical road map to creating healthier attitudes about food that will enable you to live a life free of emotional eating."
—Diane E. Raymond, Personal Trainer, Founder of Blue Sky Gym and www.AnywhereWorkout.com

"Dr. May . . . truly understands . . . that for everyone who struggles with food and body image, it's not about the food. Her . . . concrete tools to help others get off the yo-yo dieting rollercoaster are a healing balm that so many of us need."
—Esther Kane, MSW, author of *It's Not About the Food: A Woman's Guide to Making Peace with Food and Our Bodies*

"Michelle May's compassion and ability to explain the concept of mindful eating comes from her personal and clinical experience . . . [She] helps the reader pause to decipher the cause of unhealthy eating behaviors to . . . create a more nourishing eating style."
—Megrette Fletcher, MEd, RD, CDE, executive director, The Center for Mindful Eating

"Working *with* our human nature instead of fighting against it, *Eat What You Love, Love What You Eat* reverses the nonstop cycle of overeating through a process that will enrich your whole life, well beyond mere weight loss."
—John Corso, MD, author of *Stupid Reasons People Die*

"Think. Nourish. Live. Eat. In four simple themes, *Eat What You Love, Love What You Eat* takes you gently through the not-so-simple task of eating when hungry, stopping when full, and loving every bite along the way . . . Rediscover one of the great pleasures of life—eating what you love without shame, guilt, or regret!"
—Elizabeth Patch, author and illustrator of *More to Love*

"Dr. May's wise advice on creating a balanced lifestyle will surely help those who've struggled with their body image to step off the self-hatred treadmill and instead do what works for them . . . I recommend it for any parent who wants to model healthy body behavior for their kids."
—Dara Chadwick, author of *You'd Be So Pretty If . . . Teaching Our Daughters to Love Their Bodies— Even When We Don't Love Our Own*

"In *Eat What you Love, Love What You Eat*, Michelle May demonstrates that living healthy *can* be fun and enjoyable."
—Connie Diekman, MEd, RD, LD, FADA, director of university nutrition at Washington University in St Louis, former president of American Dietetic Association

"*Eat What You Love, Love What You Eat* will put mindful eating at the forefront of the obesity epidemic, replacing the restriction and deprivation messages that will never work."
—Dr. Karen Wolfe, author of *Create the Body Your Soul Desires* and *The Conscious Body Method*

EAT WHAT
YOU LOVE
LOVE WHAT
YOU EAT

How to Break Your Eat-Repent-Repeat Cycle

Michelle May, M.D.
Based on the Am I Hungry?® Mindful Eating Workshops

GREENLEAF
BOOK GROUP PRESS

In view of the complex, individual nature of health and fitness issues, this book and the ideas, programs, procedures, and suggestions are not intended to replace the advice of trained medical professionals. All matters regarding one's health require medical supervision.

The author's role is strictly educational in the context of these materials. The author is not providing any medical assessment, individualized therapeutic interventions, or personal medical advice. Seek medical advice from your personal health care provider regarding your personal risks and benefits insofar as adopting the recommendations of this program.

The author disclaims any liability arising directly or indirectly from the use of this book or program.

Published by Greenleaf Book Group Press
Austin, TX
www.greenleafbookgroup.com

Distributed by Greenleaf Book Group LLC

For ordering information or special discounts for bulk purchases, please contact Greenleaf Book Group LLC at PO Box 91869, Austin, TX 78709, 512.891.6100.

Design and composition by Greenleaf Book Group LLC
Cover design by Greenleaf Book Group LLC

Am I Hungry?® is a registered trademark of Am I Hungry?, P.L.L.C.
Am I Hungry?®
P.O. Box 93686
Phoenix, AZ 85070-3686
Visit www.AmIHungry.com for more resources.

Publisher's Cataloging-In-Publication Data
(Prepared by The Donohue Group, Inc.)
May, Michelle.
    Eat what you love : love what you eat : how to break your eat-repent-repeat cycle / Michelle May. -- 1st ed.

    p. : ill. ; cm.

    "Based on Am I Hungry? Mindful Eating workshops."
    Includes bibliographical references and index.
    ISBN: 978-1-60832-003-5

1. Food habits. 2. Nutrition. 3. Health. 4. Exercise. I. Title.

RM222.2 .M3965 2010
613.2/5   2009930304

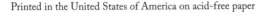

Part of the Tree Neutral™ program, which offsets the number of trees consumed in the production and printing of this book by taking proactive steps, such as planting trees in direct proportion to the number of trees used: www.treeneutral.com

Printed in the United States of America on acid-free paper

10 11 12 13 14   10 9 8 7 6 5 4 3 2

First Edition

Dedicated to Owen, Tyler, and Elyse
for your love, inspiration, and support

CONTENTS

PART 3: LIVE

PART 4: EAT

ACKNOWLEDGMENTS

Thank you.

Those two simple words represent much more than I can possibly express here. Those two words also apply to many more people than I can possibly include here. Yet, I am deeply grateful for the events and the people that have been a part of this journey.

Thank you to the thousands of individuals who have shared their secret struggles with yo-yo dieting with me. Whether during an Am I Hungry?® workshop or a conference presentation, please know that I have learned as much from you as you have from me. If you recognize your story in these pages, I am especially grateful because your words will now help others.

I am grateful for all of the voices of reason that have continued to swim against the current in this diet-crazed world. I believe the tide is finally turning. I am humbled by the many women and men who have chosen to invest their time and energy to become Am I Hungry?® facilitators in order to free their patients, their clients, and their communities from the grips of their eat-repent-repeat cycles.

This book would not have been possible without the expert guidance of many individuals. I am grateful to my early teachers, particularly Lisa Galper, Psy.D. Thank you Janet Carr, M.S., R.D. for your review and input on the Nourish chapters and Rebecca Johnson, M.S., for your fabulous review and contributions to the Live chapters. Tiffany Gray, thank you for conducting a thorough literature review and Greg Hansen for your fitness illustrations. I am also grateful to all of those who have helped me spread the word, including Melissa Sileo at Smith Publicity, and Corinne Shark who created the amazing Eat What You Love book trailer on YouTube.

It is not possible to name all of the editors, designers, and reviewers who contributed along the way, but their lovely fingerprints are all over these pages—thank you! And to Matthew Donnelley and the entire team at Greenleaf Book Group—thank you for seeing my vision. You have been fabulous to work with!

I am blessed to have been surrounded by love and light. Thank you God for giving me everything and everyone I needed to do this work. I deeply appreciate my many dear friends and colleagues who have believed in me all the way. I have also been blessed with not just two parents who love and support me, but four—George and Dixie, Bill and Janie—thank you. Thank you to my children, Tyler and Elyse, whose love and laughs mean the world to me, and to my husband, Owen who has been an incredible gift in my life.

Thank you.

INTRODUCTION

Do you love to eat? Do you feel guilty when you eat certain foods? Do you feel deprived when you don't get to eat what you want? Are you confused about what you're supposed to eat? Do you obsess about everything you eat? When you eat something you think you shouldn't, is it hard to stop? Do you think, "Oh well, I've already blown it. I might as well keep eating and restart my diet tomorrow"?

Do you say you love to eat but eat so fast that you barely notice the taste after the first few bites? Do you eat while you're doing other things, like watching TV, working, or driving? Do you feel stuffed at the end of a meal? Do you start thinking about food again soon after you're finished?

Do you eat because you're hungry? Do you even know what hunger feels like anymore? Do you eat because it's time to, because the food looks good, or because you're stressed, bored, or one of a thousand other reasons? Does eating make you feel better—but only for a little while? Does that sometimes lead to even more eating?

Do you think of exercise as a punishment for eating? Or do you exercise to earn the right to eat? Are you able to do all the things you want? What are you putting off until you lose weight? Have you forgotten that the purpose of eating is to fuel your life? Could these be a few of the reasons you continue to struggle with your weight? Could this be why diets just haven't worked for you—or most other people?

You have a choice to make. You can continue to try every diet that comes along, only to gain the weight back when you begin to feel hungry, bored, stressed, or deprived. Or you can learn how to eat what you love and love what you eat. The answers have been within your reach the whole time, but you've been reaching out instead of reaching in.

Eat What You Love, Love What You Eat will help you discover how pleasurable it is to eat mindfully, savoring every aspect of the experience. You'll *relearn* to trust your natural ability to eat just the right amount of food. And you'll meet your other needs—coping with stress or relieving boredom, for example—in more fulfilling ways. You'll learn to eat the foods you love fearlessly, without guilt or overeating. You'll find joy in movement and be amazed at your body's capacity to grow stronger and more flexible.

Eat What You Love, Love What You Eat is based on the Am I Hungry? Mindful Eating Workshops, a comprehensive program that has helped thousands of people change their fundamental relationship with food. By asking the deceptively simple question "Am I hungry?" you open the door to a much deeper awareness and understanding of yourself. Once inside, there's much to explore. You see, it's not just about *what* you eat; it's also about *why* and *how* you eat. In fact, for many of us, it's not about food at all.

This is not a diet book. You know that weight management really is more complex than simply knowing what to eat and how much to exercise. The failure of most diets proves it. My goal is to break this process into a series of manageable, sustainable steps that you can master one at a time.

This will be a very personal journey. You'll bring your own experiences, thoughts, feelings, and beliefs to the table. Every choice you make is an opportunity to experience and better understand why you do the things you do and then to choose differently the next time if it will serve you better. Let me emphasize that this will be a learning process. Perfection isn't necessary. Be kind and patient with yourself; the freedom and enjoyment you'll discover are well worth it.

Eat What You Love, Love What You Eat has four parts: Think, Nourish, Live, and Eat. The first three parts each have eight chapters.

Part 1, *Think*, teaches you to ask yourself questions to gain awareness of why, when, what, how, and how much you eat, and where you invest your energy. As you become more fully aware of what you believe, think, feel, and do, you'll better understand how to get the results you want. You'll build a powerful foundation of important life and weight management skills and fulfilling ways of nourishing your body, mind, heart, and spirit—without dieting.

Though what you'll learn in part 1 really sets this program apart from all others, nutrition and physical activity are also important for vitality and health.

Part 2, *Nourish*, is written from an all-foods-fit perspective because I believe that nutrition information should be used as a tool, not a weapon. Ultimately, every decision is yours to make and is never wrong when you're eating mindfully. This concept may seem revolutionary; you likely are governed by diet rules that are rigid, confusing, or tainted with negative messages such as "eating fat is bad" or "exercise helps burn off calories when you cheat." As you let go of those restrictive and complicated rules, you may want additional nutrition information to help you make choices.

Part 3, *Live*, shows you how to add physical activity to your life, and life to your physical activity! I strongly believe that small changes gradually integrated into your lifestyle are far more powerful than one huge temporary overhaul. These small, focused suggestions are probably very different from the "all-or-nothing" approach of your past, so please be open to giving them a try.

Part 4, *Eat*, includes great recipes for some of my family's favorite dishes. My husband, Owen, is a professional spa chef, and we have a passion for making nutritious taste delicious. I'll refer you to those recipes throughout the Nourish chapters. (All references to specific recipes are flagged with an image of a plate, as shown here.)

Am I Hungry? workshops are available nationwide and are presented by hundreds of licensed Am I Hungry? facilitators. We've worked with thousands of participants, and I've included some of their stories, either word for word, or as composites of several people with similar experiences. Most of the names have been changed.

Their stories illustrate key concepts, but more important, as you read them I hope you'll see that you're not alone and that there's hope. I also open each chapter with my own personal experiences. Let me start now by sharing how I came to do this work.

MY STORY

I was overweight from an early age. Picture a girl with red hair, lots of freckles—and chubby. My parents didn't have a lot of money, so we didn't waste food; besides, there were starving children in Africa. My athletic, skinny younger brother could, and would, eat anything that wasn't nailed down, so I made sure to get my share first. My grandmothers were both wonderful cooks, and I learned early on that food was love. My mother, on the other hand, was slender and dieted to stay that way. She was the only one in our family who never ate her baked potato. I believed that when I grew up, I wouldn't get to eat potatoes anymore either.

When my parents began having marital problems, I found comfort and security in eating. Soon after they divorced, a girl at my new dance school teased me about being fat, so I quit taking lessons and gained more weight. Through my teens I spent most of my free time hanging around with my friends at a fast-food joint or eating in front of the TV set. I still remember how embarrassed and guilty I felt when my stepdad realized that my friend and I had eaten a whole package of cookies—thirty-six to be exact.

I always put a lot of pressure on myself and then used food to relieve the stress. It usually worked—at least for a little while. In the long run, though, my main coping mechanism itself became a major source of stress for me. I was trapped in a vicious cycle.

Subtle and not-so-subtle comments and upsetting shopping trips to find clothes made it clear I had to do something. The stage was set. For the next twenty-plus years, I was on one diet after another. I had my favorite: the one that worked—as long as I stuck to it. I tried to be good, but I always ended up cheating. I discovered that exercise helped, but I used it mostly as a way of paying penance when I was bad. I was ashamed of my body, ashamed of my eating, and ashamed of my cheating. I developed features of an eating disorder that helped me cope with my painful relationship with food. Without realizing it, I was caught in another vicious cycle.

Ironically, despite the fact that I wasn't able to stick to a diet, I successfully finished college, medical school, and a family medicine residency. I eventually found myself in the position of advising my patients to lose weight. Most of them didn't seem to fare any better than I had. That was little consolation.

I felt discouraged and helpless. How could I tell someone to do something I hadn't been able to do myself? I knew it was time to try again, but it didn't seem fair; my husband and children never dieted, and they never struggled with their weight. They ate whatever they wanted, but they rarely ate more than they needed.

Did they just have a better metabolism? That was probably part of it. I knew mine was a mess after years of overeating and dieting. Did they have more willpower? No. I doubt they could follow a diet for very long either. But there was something else, something fundamentally different about the way they thought about food. I realized they didn't really think about food at all—unless they were hungry.

Could the answer really be that obvious? Could I learn to listen again to my body's innate wisdom to guide my eating? My little voice said, "I can't stand the thought of another diet. I'll try anything else."

It was surprisingly simple, but it was not always easy. After years of trying to follow other people's rules about food, ignoring hunger, and eating for all sorts of other reasons, it was difficult to trust my body and my instincts. Gradually, I developed a more mindful, satisfying way to eat and maintain a healthy weight naturally.

Something else completely unexpected happened along the way. I discovered parts of myself I had lost—or I didn't even know existed. I found peace, health, and wholeness. I also discovered a purpose for my life and a passion for helping others find wholeness, too.

Eat Mindfully, Live Vibrantly!
Michelle May, M.D.

PART 1

THINK

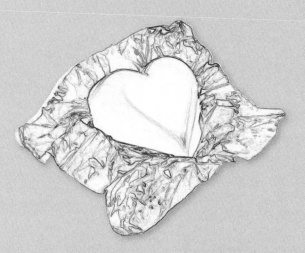

CHAPTER 1

IN CHARGE,
NOT IN CONTROL

know the feeling. "I can't take it anymore—I just have to lose this weight." Whenever my little voice told me I was too fat, I'd buy the latest diet book, join a gym, or head back to a meeting.

"Time to get back in control," my little voice said. I weighed myself and calculated how long it would take to get to my goal weight if I lost two pounds a week. I cleaned out my refrigerator, my kitchen cabinets, and my desk drawer. I threw away (or finished off) the chips and cookies and started eating celery sticks for snacks. I read every label so I'd know what I could eat and what I shouldn't. I took my lunch to work every day and tried out new healthy recipes on my family. ("Oh no, Mom's on a diet again!") I drank my eight glasses of water every day and got up early almost every morning to walk. "This feels great!" my little voice said.

The weight started to come off. I'd lose three or four pounds the first week—never mind that part of it was water or even muscle. I already felt thinner—and a little smug. As I watched everyone else in the break room scarfing down doughnuts, I'd think, "If they had self-control like me, they'd know those things are bad and they'd resist them, too." Eventually, someone would notice I'd lost weight, so I'd talk about my latest diet. They'd tell me about theirs, and everyone within earshot would chime in with their favorite diet story. Soon the conversation would drift to food and eating—our favorite topics.

Then a little while later came the inevitable weigh-in when I didn't lose as much as I thought I should. I vowed to try harder, and I did. But my little voice said, "This isn't worth it." I reminded myself about all the reasons I wanted to lose weight. When I saw someone eating ice cream, my voice said, "It's not fair." Then one morning my alarm went off for my walk, and my little voice said, "This is too hard." I turned off the alarm, rolled over, and went back to sleep.

Later that day I bought a bag of candy at the store "for the kids." I got out to the parking lot and my little voice said, "You've been so good; you can have one piece." I ate a piece and the voice continued, "You can walk a little extra tomorrow; have another one." I ate one more, then another, and by the time I got home, half the bag was gone. The voice said, "You already blew it. You might as well eat the rest so you won't be tempted when you go back on your diet tomorrow. Besides, how are you going to explain away half a bag of candy?" So I finished it off and buried the empty bag in the bottom of the garbage can.

Then the little voice changed. "I can't believe you did that after how hard you've worked! You couldn't stick to it, just like all the other times." I knew that at any given moment, I was just one piece of candy away from being right back where I'd started. The voice screamed at me, "You're so out of control. What a loser!"

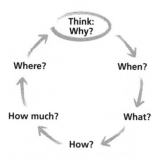

WHY DO I EAT?

Maybe you want to lose a few pounds, or maybe you need to lose a lot.

Anything might have triggered your decision to lose weight: planning a Caribbean cruise, dreading your twentieth high school reunion, or feeling winded as you try to outrun your toddler headed toward a busy street. Maybe you have nothing left in your closet that fits, or you feel uncomfortable sitting in a chair with armrests—or you can't sit in a chair with armrests anymore. Maybe your doctor told you the reason your knees hurt all the time is that they're carrying a heavier load than they were designed for and your joints are wearing out. Maybe she told you that you have high blood pressure or diabetes, or that you will if you don't do something about your weight.

Maybe you just can't stand the thought of another diet. You know that before long, whatever motivated you in the first place won't seem that important anymore. Your willpower becomes want-power, and your little voice will whisper, "Maybe next time it'll be different." You'll go back to eating like before until something happens to give you that feeling again, the one that says, "I have to do it this time."

And now that you are reading this book, your little voice might be saying, "But why should this time be any different? You know you won't be able to do it."

But you *can* do it because this book really is different. In fact, it may even seem a bit too different. Your little voice might say, "No dieting? How's that going to help? You're already out of control. What you really need is willpower and some strict rules to whip yourself into shape!"

Deep down inside, don't you believe there has to be a better way?

There is.

STRATEGIES: RECOGNIZING YOUR EATING PATTERNS

Look at the following statements to see which, if any, apply to you. (To take this quiz online and receive an assessment of your eating style, please visit www.AmIHungry.com.)

__ I am hungry all the time.

__ I am never hungry.

__ I can't tell when I'm hungry.

__ I know I'm not hungry, but I eat anyway.

__ I am starving by the time I eat, so I'll eat anything I can get my hands on.

__ I eat by the clock.

__ I think about food all the time.

__ I love food and eating too much to be at a healthy weight.

__ I think healthy food is boring.

__ I use food to cope with stress and other feelings.

__ I am an emotional eater.

__ I eat when I'm bored.

__ I eat when I'm stressed.

__ I eat when I'm nervous.

__ I eat when I'm sad.

__ I eat when I'm angry.

__ I eat when I'm lonely.

__ I eat when I'm tired.

___ I reward myself with food.

___ I comfort myself by eating.

___ I celebrate every special occasion or milestone by eating.

___ I don't know why I eat.

___ I often eat until I'm stuffed.

___ I have trouble stopping myself when I eat "bad" foods.

___ I have tried a lot of diets.

___ I am either dieting or eating too much.

___ I think thin people have more willpower than I do.

___ I think thin people have better metabolisms than I do.

___ I feel guilty about eating certain foods.

___ I have a love-hate relationship with food.

___ I sometimes ignore hunger in order to control my weight.

___ I eat on a schedule even when I'm not hungry.

___ I decide ahead of time what I'm going to eat for the entire day.

___ I avoid certain foods because they're fattening.

___ I am confused about what I should be eating.

___ I am frustrated that "experts" keep changing their minds about what we should eat.

___ I hate to exercise.

___ I don't really like exercise, but I do it so I can eat what I want.

___ I make myself do more exercise if I've eaten too much.

___ I dread the thought of going on another diet, but I just don't know what else to do.

Take this quiz again after reading this book to see how much has changed!

Hungry for Answers

Long-term weight management isn't about being *in control*. It's about being *in charge*. To understand why this distinction is so important, consider the differences between people who don't struggle with their weight, people who are overweight, and people who are always on a diet. What characteristics and traits do these people have? Why do they eat? What role does food play in their lives? Think of their eating patterns—what, how often, and how much do they eat? How physically active are they?

People generally fall into eating patterns that I call Instinctive Eating, Overeating, or Restrictive Eating. Many of us have a combination of these patterns.

Instinctive Eating

Think of someone who naturally stays within her healthy weight range. Think about a person who seems to do this effortlessly rather than someone who exerts incredible willpower and self-control. Perhaps you're thinking of your spouse, a friend, a child, or even yourself—before you began gaining weight or struggling with food. These are people who stay slim without a great deal of effort, like Tom and his wife, Angie.

I never worry about my weight; I just eat when I'm hungry and stop when I start feeling full. My wife, Angie, is the same way. We take gourmet-cooking classes together, but we really don't think or talk about food all the time like a lot of people we know. I honestly don't have a problem turning down great food if I'm not hungry; I mean, what's the point? We're both pretty high energy; we play in a softball league and love to hike on the weekends. I think we weigh about the same as when we met in college, give or take a few pounds. I've never been on a diet; they seem crazy to me. I love food and I can eat pretty much whatever I want, but I've made changes as I've gotten older and more health conscious. I wish I could tell you what I do to manage my weight, but to be honest, I just don't have to think about it all that much. Frankly, it's a little hard for me to understand why overweight people don't just stop overeating.

Overeating

Think of somebody you know who is overweight. It may be you or someone you know well. Sarah is fairly typical of a lot of people I've worked with who struggle with their weight.

> Paul and I are both overweight, so I'm starting to worry about our health. Paul has high blood pressure now, and my doctor said my blood sugar was borderline high. I just don't feel very healthy and I'm tired all the time.
>
> It seems like we're thinking and talking about food, eating, and dieting all the time. We joke that we're star members of the clean plate club; the all-you-can-eat buffet loses money on Paul. I often eat until I'm stuffed—but I always manage to find room for dessert. I guess I never thought about whether I was hungry. I don't think I actually ever get hungry, but Paul says he's hungry all the time. We just eat because it's mealtime or because something looks good—whether we're hungry or not.
>
> I guess I reward myself, comfort myself, and entertain myself by eating. I hate feeling so out of control around food. We've been on lots of different diets, but one of us always ends up cheating, so we eventually just quit. I usually gain more weight than I lost. I know we should exercise, but it's really hard; it makes me feel like I am being punished for overeating. I just wish I was one of those skinny people who has more willpower and a better metabolism than I do.

Restrictive Eating

Now think of someone you know who always seems to be on a diet. You probably know a lot of people like this: people who try to manage their weight by chronically restricting their eating and exercising almost compulsively. Here's how Karen described it.

> I know I drive my husband, Mark, crazy because I'm always trying to lose that last ten pounds. I weigh myself every morning and sometimes after I eat. Those numbers on the scale can make or break my day, but the truth is, I think I'm

too fat no matter how much I weigh. I'm always on one diet or another. I think I have every diet book ever written. I felt like I was starving on some of them, so now I eat every three hours so I don't get hungry and lose control.

The funny thing is, I think about food all the time; I worry a lot about what I should or shouldn't be eating. Mark teases me that I don't eat real food—just chemically altered diet-friendly versions of food. I sometimes secretly eat something I shouldn't then end up eating whatever I can get my hands on because I've blown it. I know I need to stay on a diet since it's the only way I can control myself around bad foods. When I cheat I have to starve myself or force myself to exercise more to make up for it. I almost never miss my daily exercise regimen because I'm too worried I'll gain weight. I just wish Mark had more self-control and would eat healthier.

Do you recognize your eating pattern in one or more of these stories? Let's take a closer look at each one, using the Eating Cycle as a way to understand how you make conscious or subconscious decisions about eating, and how each decision affects the other choices you make.

THE EATING CYCLE

The Eating Cycle consists of six stages that answer six main questions.

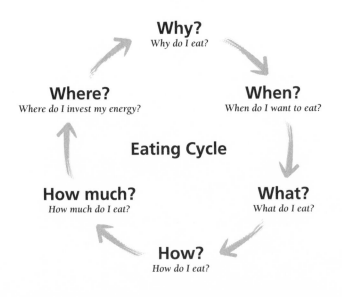

Why?
Why do I eat?

Where?
Where do I invest my energy?

When?
When do I want to eat?

Eating Cycle

How much?
How much do I eat?

What?
What do I eat?

How?
How do I eat?

WHY?	Why do I eat? In other words, what is driving my eating cycle at any given time?
WHEN?	When do I want to eat? When do I think about eating? When do I decide to eat?
WHAT?	What do I eat? What do I choose from all of the available options?
HOW?	How do I eat? How, specifically, do I get the food I've chosen into my body?
HOW MUCH?	How much do I eat? How much fuel do I consume?
WHERE?	Where do I invest my energy? That is, where does the fuel I've consumed go?

Let's apply the Eating Cycle to the three main patterns of eating to better understand what's really going on.

Instinctive Eating

Here's how someone who eats instinctively answers the six fundamental questions in the Eating Cycle.

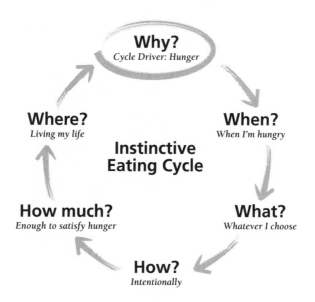

WHY?   Your cycle driver is hunger. In other words, hunger is your primary cue for eating. Hunger guides you to decide when and how much to eat.

WHEN?   When your body needs fuel, it triggers the sensations that tell you you're hungry. You decide when to eat based on how hungry you are, but you also consider other factors like convenience, social norms, and the availability of appetizing food. When you occasionally eat even though you're not hungry, you don't feel guilty, just full—so you don't eat again right away.

WHAT?   You eat whatever you want. Your choices are affected by your preferences and your awareness and degree of concern about nutrition information, as well as what foods are available. You naturally seek balance, variety, and moderation in your eating. In the Instinctive Eating Cycle, you don't use rigid rules to decide what to eat; therefore, you don't judge yourself for what you eat. Eating is usually pleasurable, but food doesn't hold any particular power over you.

HOW?   You eat intentionally and with purpose. Since you're eating to satisfy hunger and nourish your body, you pay attention to the food and your body's signals.

HOW MUCH?   You decide how much food to eat by how hungry you are, how filling the food is, how soon you'll be eating again, and other factors. When your hunger is satisfied, you usually stop eating—even if there's food left. You recognize that being too full is uncomfortable and unnecessary.

WHERE?   Your energy goes toward living your life. Your physical energy can be directed toward your activities during work, play, exercise, and even rest. Your mental energy can be focused on your daily tasks and goals. Your emotional and spiritual energy can be focused on your relationships and purpose. Any leftover fuel you consume is stored until it's needed.

Once the fuel you've consumed is depleted or stored, the signs of hunger return, triggering your desire to eat again. The Instinctive Eating Cycle repeats

> **MINDFUL MOMENT:** When you are eating instinctively, you eat what you love, but you don't obsess about food because you don't need to. Instead, you trust your body to let you know when and how much to eat.

itself, perhaps three or four times a day or every few hours, depending on what and how much you eat and how much fuel you need on a particular day.

Overeating

Here's how someone who is in a pattern of overeating answers the six fundamental questions in the Eating Cycle.

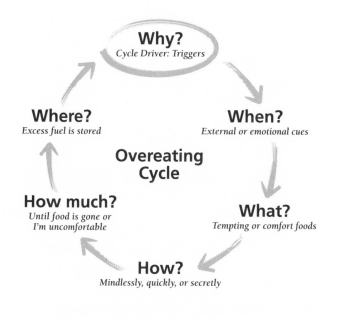

WHY?	Your cycle drivers are your triggers: that is to say, eating provides temporary distraction or pleasure. For example, if the trigger is boredom, eating distracts you and gives you something to do for a little while. If the trigger is a big tray of brownies, eating several

might be pleasurable for a few moments. The distraction or pleasure is initially satisfying and therefore drives the Overeating Cycle.

WHEN?   Your desire to eat is triggered by conscious or unconscious physical, environmental, and emotional triggers. Examples of physical triggers are thirst, fatigue, or pain. Environmental cues such as the time of day, appetizing food, or certain activities associated with food may trigger your urges to eat. Emotions such as stress, boredom, guilt, loneliness, anger, or happiness may also trigger eating. Sometimes hunger triggers the initial urge to eat, but then environmental and emotional cues lead to overeating. If you're in the habit of eating for all these reasons, when do you feel like eating? All the time!

WHAT?   The types of food you choose to eat in response to triggers other than hunger are more likely to be foods that are convenient, tempting, and comforting. For example, if you're at a ball game, you might eat a hot dog, a jumbo pretzel, or a plate of nachos even if you aren't hungry. If your trigger is stress, you might choose chocolate or potato chips. It's less likely you'll choose nutritious foods in your Overeating Cycle since you're not eating in response to your body's physical needs.

HOW?   In the Overeating Cycle, you're more likely to eat mindlessly, automatically, quickly, or secretly. You may eat, or continue to eat, whether you're hungry or not. You might unconsciously grab a handful of candy or nuts from a bowl as you pass by. You might eat while you're distracted watching TV, driving, working, or talking on the phone. You might eat secretly or quickly to finish before someone catches you. You might feel guilty about eating, and therefore you aren't able to fully enjoy it. Eating this way is not very satisfying physically or emotionally.

HOW MUCH?   If hunger doesn't tell you to start eating, what tells you to stop? In an Overeating Cycle, the amount of food you eat depends on how much food you've been served or how much is in the package. You might eat until you feel bad or until you're interrupted. All too often, you feel uncomfortably full, miserable, or even numb instead of content and satisfied after eating.

WHERE?   When you eat food your body didn't ask for, your body has no choice but to store it. The excess fuel you've consumed is saved for later in the form of body fat. You might feel self-conscious or less energetic, and as a result, you might not feel like being physically active. Perhaps you avoid certain experiences like dating, going on vacation, or buying clothes that look and feel good because you want to lose weight first. Perhaps you feel so bad about yourself for being overweight that you don't ask for that raise you deserve or you don't set appropriate limits with other people, leading to even more emotional triggers and more overeating.

When you ignore your true needs and eat instead, you feel disconnected and out of control. When you eat for reasons other than hunger, the distraction and pleasure are only temporary; consequently, you have to eat more to feel better, feeding a vicious cycle.

Restrictive Eating

Here's how someone in a restrictive eating pattern answers the six fundamental questions in the Eating Cycle.

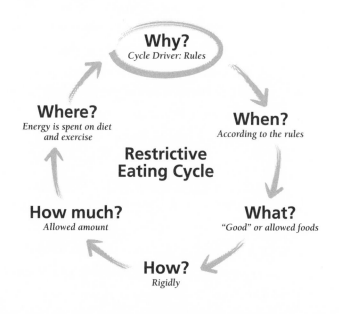

WHY?   Your cycle drivers are rules that determine when, what, and how much to eat. The rules may come from an "expert," or they may be self-imposed. Your decisions about eating are controlled rather than intuitive. When you're in a Restrictive Eating Cycle, the number on the scale or how well you've been following the rules determines how you feel about yourself on a particular day.

WHEN?   The rules determine whether or not you're allowed to eat: for example, "Eat every three hours," or "Never eat after 7:00 p.m." These rules serve the purpose of externally limiting your intake. In the first example, eating by the clock prevents you from getting hungry; theoretically, your eating should be easier to control. Prohibiting eating in the evening prevents overeating due to triggers like watching television or loneliness. However, these rules place artificial constraints on your eating that don't necessarily honor your body's natural hunger rhythms—and they don't address the real reasons you want to eat in the first place.

WHAT?   You should eat only the "good" foods that are allowed on your diet. You may have to resist your favorite "sinfully delicious" foods or avoid situations and places where your forbidden foods would tempt you. Some diets allow you to eat any food you want, but higher-calorie foods are treated as special. These powerful foods must be substituted, calculated, earned, or eaten only on "cheat days." In the Restrictive Eating Cycle, choosing the right food is very important because when your choice is good, you're good. But when your choice is bad, you're bad.

HOW?   Following the rules may require you to be very structured or even rigid in your eating. However, always having to choose "good" foods may cause you to feel deprived, while choosing "bad" foods causes you to feel guilty.

HOW MUCH?   You eat the allowed amount since the quantity of food is predetermined by the rules. This may require weighing, measuring, counting, or using some other external way to determine how much food you can have or how much food you should eat. These rules prevent you from eating too much food, or perhaps from not eating enough, based on the assumption that you don't have the ability to consume an appropriate amount of food without following a set of strict rules.

WHERE?   The Restrictive Eating Cycle requires a great deal of mental and emotional energy. As in the Instinctive Eating Cycle, your body will use whatever fuel it needs for work, play, exercise, and rest, but if you're eating more "healthy" foods than your body needs, the excess will still be stored. If you're significantly under-eating, your body may attempt to conserve as much fuel as possible by lowering your metabolism. You may spend a lot of your energy figuring out how to get the most food while still staying within the confines of your diet. Furthermore, while exercise is important for overall health and fitness, in the Restrictive Eating Cycle, exercise is sometimes used to earn the right to eat, to punish yourself for overeating, or to pay penance for eating a bad food.

While other people admire your willpower and self-control, many of your thoughts, feelings, and activities revolve around food, exercise, and weight. Although you're dependent on rules to drive your Restrictive Eating Cycle, those rules mainly focus on food and exercise without adequately addressing why you want to eat in the first place. For many people, the rules consume their energy and distract them from meeting their true needs and living their lives fully.

THE EAT-REPENT-REPEAT CYCLE

When you eat due to external or emotional triggers, the temporary distraction or pleasure you receive can act like an engine that drives your cycle. When you decide that going on a diet is the only way to regain control and stop yourself from overeating, you switch from your Overeating Cycle to your Restrictive Eating Cycle.

In your Restrictive Eating Cycle, triggers may still drive your cycle, even though you eat only those foods that are allowed on your diet. For example, when you feel stressed, you might eat a lot of veggies or popcorn instead of chips. You still aren't coping effectively with stress, and you're still overeating in response to cues other than hunger. Eventually, you begin to feel deprived, hungry, or worn out by all the time and energy it takes to follow the rules. So you cheat, feel guilty, and give up, shifting back into your Overeating Cycle, once again eating your favorite foods in response to the triggers you never dealt with in the first place.

It's common for people to shift back and forth between overeating and restrictive eating. You might switch cycles over the course of weeks or months, or you might move rapidly from one cycle to the other in the same day or even in the same meal. You start out with good intentions but quickly lose control.

This pattern is known as yo-yo dieting, but when the Overeating and Restrictive Eating Cycles are intertwined, I refer to it as the eat-repent-repeat cycle. You move wildly from one extreme to the other, feeling powerless to change without understanding why.

A Pendulum Instead of a Yo-yo

As you look at your own eating cycles, you may realize that when you're overeating, you usually feel *out of control*. When you're dieting, you finally feel *in control*—but it's usually too difficult (and boring!) to sustain permanently.

The problem is that a yo-yo is either up or down. You're either tightly wound up in rules or you're unraveling and heading toward the bottom again. Even if you decide you don't want to spend the rest of your life in one of these two extremes, there's no real in-between. The common advice to "follow a healthy lifestyle" usually means exercise and watch what you eat—not terribly helpful if you've been trying unsuccessfully to do that for years.

MINDFUL MOMENT: In the eat-repent-repeat cycle, when you eat what you want, you feel guilty; when you eat what you "should," you feel deprived. Either way, you're almost never at peace with your choices.

Instead of a yo-yo, I prefer to think of a pendulum. A pendulum, while still conjuring up images of extremes, will find a gentle arc somewhere in the middle as it loses energy. What I mean is that when you finally stop wasting so much of your energy on overeating and dieting, you'll naturally settle into a more comfortable, centered space, freeing up your energy for more enjoyable, productive, and fulfilling activities.

Freedom and Flexibility

That smaller, gentle arc of a pendulum is instinctive eating. Instead of the extremes of trying to stay in control or spinning out of control, you're *in charge*. At any given time, you have the freedom and flexibility to mindfully fuel yourself the way you want to. You were born with the natural ability to effortlessly manage your weight this way.

If you're exposed to food when you're not hungry, you may take a passing interest in it, but you probably won't eat a significant amount because you'd feel uncomfortable afterward. You can eat anything you want when you're hungry, so you don't have to spend a lot of time deciding in advance what you're going to eat. You can consciously choose to follow a healthier diet, but you don't expect yourself to be perfect. You truly enjoy food because you don't feel physically or emotionally uncomfortable during or after eating. And when you're satisfied, you go on living your life without thinking about food again until your body tells you to.

Eating instinctively doesn't mean eating perfectly. You might eat for pleasure, convenience, or a special occasion like a birthday party, even if you aren't hungry. You might choose comfort foods when you feel stressed or go out to dinner to reward yourself. You might even overeat sometimes because the food tastes so good that you decide it's worth feeling uncomfortable afterward. All these are part of eating instinctively when you're mindful and in charge of the decisions you make.

RELEARNING TO EAT INSTINCTIVELY

To resolve your weight and food issues without endless dieting you must restore your Instinctive Eating Cycle. Instead of following strict rules created by experts, *you* can become the expert on meeting your needs. I'll teach you how to use the fundamental information delivered by your hunger cues to determine when, what, and how much you need to eat. I'll also help you understand why you want to eat for reasons other than hunger. This awareness will give you the opportunity to meet your true needs more effectively.

Imagine what it will be like when you reestablish physical hunger as your primary cue for eating! You'll become mindful of your body's messages about when to eat, what kind of food satisfies you, and how much food you need. You'll have the tools to manage your weight no matter where you are or what you're doing—celebrating the holidays, doing business over lunch, or relaxing on vacation.

You'll discover that it's possible to balance eating for nourishment with eating for enjoyment. There won't be any more good or bad foods to worry about. You won't be required to count calories, exchanges, fat grams, or points. You won't be told to eliminate your favorite "fattening" foods. You won't need to tolerate tasteless food substitutes. You won't have to avoid certain restaurants or cheat on your birthday. And you won't need an endless supply of willpower and self-control. Eating will become pleasurable again, free from guilt and deprivation.

Once you relearn to recognize and respond appropriately to hunger, you'll see whether there are other needs you've been trying to satisfy by eating. You'll learn to meet those needs in positive and constructive ways so food can serve its proper function—to nourish you and fuel a fulfilling life.

When you learn to manage your eating by listening to your instincts, you'll begin to trust your ability to take charge of other areas of your life as well. When you're *in charge* instead of trying to stay *in control*, you'll feel more motivated to make certain eating and activity choices—not because you have to, but because you want to. Little by little, you'll free yourself from your focus on food and weight and discover new tools and energy for a more balanced, satisfying, and vibrant life.

With your renewed ability to eat instinctively, you won't need to be in control because you'll be in charge, like Lori explained in this e-mail.

> **MINDFUL MOMENT:** Instead of following strict rules created by so-called experts, you will become the expert on meeting your needs.

I've lost about 50 pounds so far and I feel great. I'm eating whatever I want, and I usually only eat when I'm hungry. Not everything I eat is perfect, but I eat a lot healthier now. I still have desserts and sweets when I really want them. I can't even imagine how I used to be able to eat so much and feel so full all the time. I still don't like to exercise indoors, but I'm more active now. I can't wait to get out and start hiking as soon as the weather changes. It feels so good to be able to wear clothes that I haven't been able to wear for years—and to cross my legs again! I feel like I'm back in charge of my life.

Your eating cycles provide important information about why, when, what, how, and how much you eat, and where you invest your energy. When you're in an Overeating Cycle, your triggers drive the cycle. When you're in a Restrictive Eating Cycle, your rules drive the cycle. When you're in an Instinctive Eating Cycle, your body's need for fuel drives the cycle. Each decision affects the rest of your decisions. Over the next seven chapters, we'll explore each decision and you'll relearn to eat instinctively without overeating, deprivation, or guilt.

CHAPTER 2

TRUST YOUR BODY WISDOM

woke up in the morning thinking about what I'd have for dinner before my feet even hit the floor. My little voice scolded me for the cookies I'd had before I went to bed, so I decided to skip breakfast. Besides, whenever I ate breakfast it seemed like I was hungry all day. I didn't have time anyway, so I had a couple cups of coffee instead.

All morning it seemed like everything irritated me and it was hard to stay focused. An hour before lunch, I needed a break. I came across doughnuts in the staff lounge and quickly ate one, then another. Back to work for another hour except that now I felt a little sick.

When friends asked me to join them for lunch, my little voice said, "You better, because you probably won't have another chance to eat all afternoon." There was a "meal deal" at the fast-food place. It's hard to pass up a bargain, so for only 49 cents more, I upsized everything.

The fries were cold and limp, but I ate them anyway so they wouldn't go to waste. I was stuffed by the time I was done and wished I hadn't eaten so much. I embarrassed myself by nodding off during a meeting after lunch. I drank another cup of coffee to give me more energy and somehow got through the afternoon.

By the time I got home I was famished. I had to make dinner, but first I needed a quick snack. Three handfuls of chips later I started cooking, but it felt like a chore since I wasn't hungry anymore. I ate dinner with my family anyway. It had been a rough day; when the kids were finally in bed, I sat down for my favorite TV show and some cookies.

Maybe tomorrow would be better.

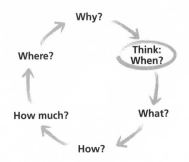

WHEN DO I WANT TO EAT?
PART 1: AM I HUNGRY?

When do you feel like eating—when you're physically hungry or when there's some other trigger? Learning to tell the difference and deciding how to respond is critical. The next three chapters are devoted to the "When" part of the Eating Cycle to help you respond mindfully whenever you feel like eating.

Let's start with the sensations of hunger and satiety because they are the simplest yet most powerful tools for reconnecting yourself with your instinctive ability to know what your body needs. Do you see hunger as your enemy and blame it for your weight problems? Have you ignored hunger for so long that you've forgotten how to recognize it? Do you ignore it until you're starving then eat anything you can get your hands on? Do you eat on a schedule so you never get hungry? Are you eating all day for all sorts of other reasons? Has it occurred to you that eating when you're not hungry causes you to gain weight?

Unfortunately, over time you may have learned to ignore your hunger and fullness signals and eat mindlessly. When you're disconnected from hunger and satiety, you lose the ability to naturally regulate your intake to meet your body's needs. When you reconnect with these signals, you can reach and maintain a healthy weight without restrictive dieting.

Hunger helps you eat what you love without gaining weight because you eat less food to satisfy physical hunger than when you eat to try to satisfy other needs. Think about it. If you aren't hungry when you start eating, how do you know when to stop?

MINDFUL MOMENT: When you wait until you're hungry, eating is more pleasurable and satisfying. Hunger is truly the best seasoning!

When you're mindful of your body's signals of satiety, you enjoy feeling comfortable at the end of a meal instead of feeling miserable. You find it easier to stop eating because you know you'll eat again when you get hungry.

Besides, food just tastes better when you're hungry. Close your eyes and think back to one of your most enjoyable meals. It is likely that you were hungry when you ate. The only way to feel fully satisfied with food is to eat because your body needs it. Once you've experienced the pleasure of eating to satisfy hunger, you'll begin to relish the prospect.

This time you'll relearn to trust your body wisdom and become your own internal authority for when, what, and how much to eat. My goal is to help you lose your obsessions with food, dieting, and your weight without giving you a long list of rules to follow. This should come as a relief.

It may feel scary, too. You may be asking yourself questions like these: "If I don't have strict rules about eating, won't I lose control? If an outside 'expert' doesn't tell me, how will I know what to do? How will I know when to stop? How will I reach my healthy weight and stay there?"

Remember, you don't need to be in control; you need to be in charge. This time you'll become your own expert. After all, it's your body, your mind, and your life. Aren't you the best person to make decisions about how you should eat? Of course, you'll need accurate information and new skills to make the best choices for yourself, but you already have the most important tool you'll need: hunger.

Hunger Is a Primitive Instinct

Hunger and the instinctual drive to satisfy hunger are essential for survival. Hunger is a primitive yet reliable way of signaling your body's need for food and regulating your nutritional intake. Hunger and satiety are caused by complex biological pathways, but simply put, hunger is your body's natural way of telling you that you need fuel.

Consider a newborn baby. Within hours, she lets her caregivers know she's hungry by crying. When she's fed and her tummy is satisfied, her cries are soothed until she gets hungry again and the cycle repeats itself. Obviously, a baby also cries for many other reasons, but if you try to feed her (instead of changing her, holding her, or warming her), she'll spit out the nipple and turn away from the food. Soon, her attentive caregiver learns the meanings of her different cries and tries to satisfy each of them appropriately.

As a baby grows and begins to eat solid food, she lets you know when she's full by turning away from the spoon—or spitting the food back at you if you force the food in anyway. As a toddler, she seems to be in perpetual motion exploring her new world. She barely stops long enough to eat a handful of crackers here and a few slices of banana there. She never stops to ask the question "Am I hungry?" yet somehow manages to eat enough to grow and maintain a healthy weight.

If food is readily available and she's able to eat when she's hungry, she trusts she'll get what she needs. At the same time, her body trusts that there's enough fuel around, resulting in an active metabolism that burns energy freely as needed for survival, growth, and activity. Besides, she's too busy exploring and playing to bother thinking about food and eating until hunger tells her to.

As she grows she is gradually given more control over *what* she eats, but she continues to use her instinctive signals to tell her *when* and *how much* to eat.

How You Lost Touch with Your Body Wisdom

Internal and external influences may have caused your natural system of regulating your food intake to go haywire. Whether or not you're aware of them, past experiences and associations affect how you eat now.

For example, parents want to meet the basic nutritional needs of their child, but their beliefs and customs may lead them to feed him in a way that doesn't respect his instinctive ability to know when and how much to eat. This can set the stage for food and weight problems in the future.

If well-intentioned parents insist on feeding their son every time he cries, he learns that eating can soothe any discomfort. Once he's old enough to sit at the table, they serve the amount of each food they think he needs because they want him to eat a balanced diet. Then they urge him to eat everything, telling him to "be a good boy and clean your plate." This teaches the child to ignore the physical discomfort of being too full in favor of winning his parents' approval. Sometimes pressuring children to eat certain types and amounts of food backfires, and the dinner table becomes a battleground of intense power struggles.

The child who doesn't get dessert unless she finishes all her dinner learns that sweets are an incentive to eat more than she was hungry for. "Eat all your dinner or you don't get dessert" translates to "You have to overeat so I'll reward you by giving you more to eat." Of course, bribes work because children have a natural liking for sweets. Using certain foods to reward good behavior or as a prize for finishing their meal causes children to believe these foods are special, so they want them even more.

Children and adults may also learn to eat in response to environmental and emotional triggers. The triggers are different for each person at different times, but if you struggle with your weight, it's likely you're sometimes eating for reasons other than hunger.

For example, have you ever suddenly felt like eating when you walked by doughnuts in the break room at work? It's common for people to confuse this sudden urge to eat with true hunger, but environmental situations often trigger "head hunger" whether your body needs food or not. These triggers develop when certain activities, people, or places are paired with eating so often that they become linked in your mind: one automatically goes with the other.

Examples of environmental triggers include mealtimes, holidays, advertisements, entertainment, social situations, friends and family members, restaurants, and even certain rooms in your house. The abundance of high-calorie appealing foods in increasingly larger portions has become a significant environmental trigger for people in many cultures.

You may have also learned to use food to express, hide, or cope with your emotions. For example, if you've had a stressful day, you might comfort or reward yourself by eating a large bowl of ice cream.

Everybody has emotional connections with food including celebrating special events, showing love, or finding comfort in Grandma's apple pie. As one person said to me, "Food is the background music for my life." Emotional eating becomes destructive, however, when it's the primary way a person deals with such feelings as loneliness, boredom, anger, stress, or depression.

To be clear, this *does not* imply that you are psychologically disturbed if you have food or weight struggles. It simply means you may have learned to cope with certain feelings by eating, and you sometimes use food for purposes other than energy and nourishment.

When you become frustrated with your weight, you may decide to diet. Most diets focus on what you should or shouldn't eat; they overlook the fact that you are eating for reasons other than hunger. If you are eating to satisfy a need other than fuel, focusing on the form of the fuel isn't going to be very effective in the long run. But that's exactly what most diets do. In addition, diets typically have very specific rules about food and exercise, but ironically, you may have to ignore your hunger signals in order to follow them. You may be forced to eat on a schedule that never allows you to get hungry. You may even feel proud for not letting yourself eat when you are hungry. As a result, dieting further disconnects you from trusting yourself and knowing what your body really needs.

The feelings of frustration, deprivation, guilt, and failure can be so powerful that even stepping on the scale and thinking about starting another diet become triggers for overeating.

RELEARN INSTINCTIVE EATING

Can people who are out of touch with their hunger signals begin to recognize and once again use hunger to learn to eat instinctively? Definitely! Hunger is a natural, innate tool, and the skills for using it effectively can be relearned. In fact, at times you may already eat according to your hunger signals. The more

MINDFUL MOMENT: If you aren't hungry when you start eating, how will you know when to stop?

consistently you use hunger and satiety to guide your eating, the easier it will become to reach and maintain a healthier weight without dieting.

A remarkably simple but powerful way to become more aware of your body's cues is to ask yourself, "Am I hungry?" whenever you want to eat. This important question will help you distinguish an urge to eat caused by the physical need for food from an urge to eat caused by other triggers. Matt described it this way.

> While I was filling up my car at a gas station, I realized that asking myself if I'm hungry before I eat is like checking the fuel gauge before stopping for gas. There's a station that I could stop at on nearly every corner, but until I need gas, it's a waste of time. If I overfilled my tank, the gas would just spill out onto the ground. I guess my extra fuel just spills out over my belt.

What Does Hunger Feel Like?

It's very common for people who have struggled with food and their weight to be disconnected from the physical sensations of hunger. They simply don't recognize, pay attention to, or respond to the signals.

Perhaps you feel like you're hungry all the time. *Wanting* to eat isn't the same thing as *needing* to eat, and it's unlikely that your body constantly needs food. Could you be misinterpreting other physical symptoms and sensations like thirst, fatigue, or nervousness for hunger? Do you confuse emotional or environmental triggers, cravings, and appetite with hunger?

Maybe you never feel hungry. Could you be missing the signals of hunger because you don't really remember how hunger feels or you're too busy or distracted to notice? Have you learned to ignore hunger in order to control your weight? Or maybe you truly aren't hungry because you're feeding yourself so frequently for other reasons that your body never needs to tell you it needs more fuel.

Before reading ahead, stop and think for a moment. How do you know when you're hungry? What does it feel like? What are all the signs your body gives you to let you know when you need to eat?

STRATEGIES: MIND-BODY SCAN

When you learn a new skill—or, in this case, relearn a skill you've forgotten—it helps to have a strategy. Throughout this book I'll give you specific strategies to help you build the skills you'll need to eat instinctively again. Don't read them and set them aside. Instead, practice them over and over, like riding a bike, until they become so natural that you don't even have to think about them anymore.

To identify hunger, you need to know what to look for and how to find it. Some of the sensations of hunger are subtle and can be easily missed if you're not used to noticing them. A Mind-Body Scan will help you become fully present and mindful so you can identify what your true needs are.

Focus your attention. Move away from the sight and smell of food because people who struggle with their weight are usually *food suggestible*. In other words, when you're sitting in front of a big plate of appetizing food, it's hard to tell the difference between wanting to eat and needing to eat. Just seeing or smelling food, or seeing other people eat, can confuse you.

To minimize mixed signals, try to move away from any place or situation you associate with eating. This might be the kitchen, dining room, break room, or even the living room, bedroom, or car if you're in the habit of eating in any of those places. One woman said a bathroom is the best place for her to go to figure out if she's really hungry because that's the only place where she doesn't think about food! If you're going to eat at a restaurant, do a Mind-Body Scan before you get out of the car. At a party, you can step outside and admire the backyard for a moment in order to tune into your signals.

Focus inward. Once you're away from food and any food associations, close your eyes for a moment if possible. If you can't get away from the food or situation, just try to tune out your surroundings for a few moments. One woman I worked with said she adds a few seconds to her mealtime prayer to tune out the rest of the world.

Take a few deep breaths and calm yourself. Be aware that being near food or thinking about eating might cause you to feel excited or anxious, making it more difficult to identify the signs of hunger. By first taking a few calming breaths, you'll reconnect your body and mind so that it will be easier to focus on important sensations and feelings.

Focus on your physical sensations. Since hunger is a physical sensation, connect with your body by placing your hand on your upper abdomen, just below your rib cage. Picture your stomach. It's about the size of your fist when it's empty and can stretch several times that size when it's full. Think of a balloon and try to imagine how full it is.

Ask yourself, "Am I hungry?" What physical sensations can you identify? Are there pangs or gnawing sensations? Is there any growling or rumbling? Does your stomach feel empty, full, or even stuffed? Perhaps you're neither hungry nor full; as a result, you don't feel your stomach at all.

Notice other physical sensations. Do you feel edgy, light-headed, or weak? Are these signals coming from hunger or from something else? Are you thirsty or tired? Are you aware of any tension, discomfort, or pain? This is a great opportunity to become mindful of your body's signals and reconnect with your inner self.

Focus on your thoughts. Quite often, your thoughts will give you clues about whether or not you're hungry. If you find yourself rationalizing or justifying, "It's been three hours since lunch so I should be hungry," you may be looking for an excuse to eat. If you have any doubts about whether you're hungry, you're probably not.

Focus on your feelings. What emotions are you experiencing at the moment? Let go of any negative thoughts or feelings you're having about eating. Keep in mind that hunger is a normal sensation, and eating is the best way to satisfy it. There's no need to feel guilty about this natural process.

A Mind-Body Scan helps you tap into the wisdom you have within you all of the time.

Do you recognize any of these common hunger symptoms?

- Hunger pangs
- Growling or grumbling in the stomach
- Empty or hollow feeling
- Gnawing
- Slight queasy feeling
- Weakness or loss of energy
- Trouble concentrating
- Difficulty making decisions
- Light-headedness
- Slight headache
- Shakiness
- Irritability or crankiness
- Feeling that you must eat as soon as possible

What Causes Hunger?

What do all the symptoms of hunger have in common?

They are physical. They're not thoughts, emotions, or cravings. To become more aware of these physical sensations, it helps to understand what causes them.

Hunger symptoms are caused by a combination of your stomach's emptiness or fullness, your body's need for energy, and various hormones and other substances in your body. We'll focus on your stomach and blood sugar, however, since they cause the most recognizable symptoms.

Your stomach is composed of muscle-like tissue that squeezes food to break it apart, mix it with digestive enzymes, and move it into your intestines. When your stomach is empty, its muscular walls begin to contract, which causes the growling or rumbling you may feel or hear when you're hungry. You may also experience an empty or hollow feeling. Since the stomach produces small amounts of digestive acids even when there's no food there, some people get sensations of gnawing or queasiness.

At the same time, you may notice symptoms of your blood sugar (or glucose) dropping. Your body and brain primarily use glucose from your bloodstream for energy. As your blood sugar falls, you may notice your energy level begin to dip and find it harder to concentrate and make decisions. When you're extremely hungry, you may develop a headache or feel light-headed and shaky.

Hunger can also trigger mood changes. Many people become irritable, impatient, cranky, or short-tempered when they're hungry.

Hunger symptoms are initially subtle then become stronger until you reach a point when you feel you absolutely must eat. If you wait any longer you simply won't care what you eat as long as you get something into your stomach. That's why waiting to eat until you're ravenous often leads to mindless food choices and overeating.

So it's really pretty simple (though not always easy). Whenever you feel like eating, ask yourself, "Am I hungry?" and do a Mind-Body Scan to focus on your physical sensations, thoughts, and feelings.

What Happens When You Eat?

When you eat, your digestive system breaks down and absorbs the food, causing your hunger symptoms to subside. Food and fluids fill your stomach, and as you eat or drink more, your stomach begins to stretch. You'll begin to feel a sense of fullness, discomfort, or even pain. You may be tempted to loosen your belt or unbutton your skirt to make room for your expanding stomach.

When you eat, energy is drawn to the digestive system. That's why your mother told you to wait for thirty minutes after you ate to go swimming. When you eat a small amount of food, you won't even be aware of the digestive process going on. However, if you eat a large amount or heavy foods, you may notice that you feel drowsy or sluggish, and it may be difficult to concentrate and be productive.

The type of food and how much you eat determines how long the digestive process takes. After the food is broken down, your body will use the energy for its activities and store any extra fuel in the form of body fat until it's needed. When your stomach is empty, your body is ready to process more fuel and the cycle of hunger continues.

How Hungry Am I?

The Hunger and Fullness Scale is a useful tool for assessing your hunger and fullness levels before, during, and after eating. It will help you identify hunger cues, observe how different types and amounts of food affect you, and recognize when the urge to eat has been triggered by something other than hunger. This scale is not intended to set strict guidelines about when you should eat; rather, it is to help you develop a greater awareness of your body's subtle signals.

The Hunger and Fullness Scale ranges from 1 to 10. A level 1 represents ravenous—you're so hungry you could eat this book. A level 10 means you're so full that you're in pain and feel sick. Remember, smaller numbers, smaller stomach; larger numbers, larger stomach.

In the middle of the scale is a level 5, which equates to being satisfied and comfortable. At a 5, you cannot feel your stomach at all. It's neither empty nor full; it isn't growling or feeling stretched. This may be how your stomach feels after you've eaten breakfast. Most people don't want to feel sluggish in the morning, so they tend to eat light, which results in a comfortable level of satiety.

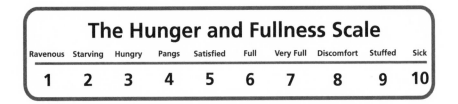

				The Hunger and Fullness Scale					
Ravenous	Starving	Hungry	Pangs	Satisfied	Full	Very Full	Discomfort	Stuffed	Sick
1	2	3	4	5	6	7	8	9	10

It may be challenging at first to label your hunger and fullness levels with numbers, but as you practice, it becomes second nature. Here are some descriptions to help you learn what the numbers mean.

1—Ravenous: Too hungry to care what you eat. This is a high-risk time for overeating.

2—Starving: You feel you must eat NOW!

3—Hungry: Eating would be pleasurable, but you can wait longer.

4—Hunger pangs: You're slightly hungry; you notice your first thoughts of food.

5—Satisfied: You're content and comfortable. You're neither hungry nor full; you can't feel your stomach at all.

6—Full: You can feel the food in your stomach.

7—Very full: Your stomach feels stretched, and you feel sleepy and sluggish.

8—Uncomfortable: Your stomach is too full, and you wish you hadn't eaten so much.

9—Stuffed: Your clothes feel very tight, and you're very uncomfortable.

10—Sick: You feel sick and/or you're in pain.

Hunger and Fullness

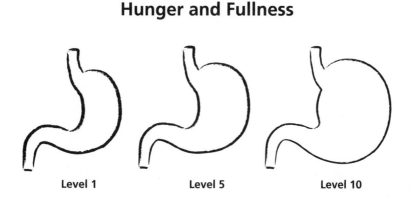

Level 1   Level 5   Level 10

It helps to develop a good mental picture of what's happening to your stomach at these different levels of hunger and fullness.

Make a fist with your right hand. When your stomach is completely empty, it's about that size. This is a level 1. One or two handfuls of food will take you from a level 1 to a level 5.

Another way to picture your stomach is to think of a balloon. When it's deflated you're at a 1. When you blow that first puff of air into the balloon, it fills out gently and takes its shape. That's a 5.

As you take a deep breath and force more air into a balloon, its elastic walls begin to stretch and expand. These are levels 6 through 10. Your stomach is able to stretch to a 10 in order to hold excess food; therefore, the numbers over 5 indicate how stretched or uncomfortable your stomach feels.

MINDFUL MOMENT: Your stomach is about the size of your fist so it only takes a handful or two of food to fill it.

If you blow too much air in, a balloon would continue to stretch and eventually pop. Fortunately, stomachs rarely rupture, but most of us have eaten so much at one time or another that we've said, "If I eat one more bite, I will explode!" When you feel this way, you're at a 10.

Of course, changes in blood sugar levels, energy levels, moods, and substances in the bloodstream resulting from the digestive process also signal hunger and fullness. These other clues also help tell you how hungry or full you are.

When Is the Best Time to Eat?

Once you're aware of your signals, you can use the Hunger and Fullness Scale to begin to fine-tune your eating patterns. Starting in the middle, let's work our way down the scale.

5 or higher—I'm not hungry:
If you're at a 5 or above and you want to eat or keep eating, you know something other than hunger triggered it. This is an opportunity to learn more about yourself and how you respond to your environment and your emotions. I'll deal with that in the next two chapters.

4—Wait or eat a small amount:
When your hunger level is at a 4, you're slightly hungry and starting to think about eating. You can begin to plan for it by making sure time and food will be available when you're ready to eat. There will be times when you'll want to eat even though you're only slightly hungry: for example, at a mealtime or when you won't have another opportunity to eat later. Just keep in mind that if you're only a little bit hungry, you need only a little bit of food.

2 or 3—Ideal time to eat:
At this point you're significantly hungry, so food will be pleasurable and satisfying.

1—Use caution:

If you put off eating or don't notice that you're hungry until you're famished, you may not think as clearly or make mindful decisions about what you want to eat. You're more likely to eat anything you can get your hands on and eat too quickly to notice when you've had enough. That's why you can easily go from starving to stuffed.

When you're aware of what can happen when you're at a level 1, you can slow down and think about your choices. Have a few bites of food then wait a few moments to take the edge off your hunger so you are less likely to overeat.

Hunger Rhythms

Now that you know the basics of hunger, you're ready to learn about other nuances that can help you understand your personal hunger rhythms.

Hunger doesn't follow a clock. If you tell yourself, "I should be hungry; it's dinnertime" or "I shouldn't be hungry yet," you're not listening to your body. You might feel hungry even when it's not a conventional mealtime.

Since it's not always convenient to eat when hunger tells you to, you may need to retrain yourself to be hungry around a particular time. For instance, if you're usually hungry at four in the afternoon but you want to be hungry for dinner with your family, plan a light afternoon snack so you won't be ravenous. Or maybe you aren't very hungry during your lunch hour. Try eating a little more protein at breakfast so you can skip your mid-morning snack or just eat less at lunch and be prepared to have a mid-afternoon snack.

On the other hand, you might not be hungry when you're supposed to be. For example, breakfast is an important meal to spark your internal thermostat and give you energy. If you don't usually feel hungry when you first wake up, however, check your hunger level an hour or two later. Maybe you ate a big dinner or a late meal the night before. Or maybe you drank several cups of coffee and rushed around all morning getting ready, so your hunger signals were suppressed.

Since studies have shown that people who eat breakfast are less likely to be overweight, it's worth retraining yourself to be hungry in the morning. You can retrain yourself by cutting down on late night eating, getting up a little earlier so you can slow down to eat, or waiting an hour or so then eating a light breakfast.

Hunger may seem erratic. Hunger comes and goes according to your body's needs. You may feel hungry frequently one day and rarely the next. For example, many women experience wide fluctuations in their hunger throughout their menstrual cycles due to changing hormone levels. Because of your activity levels and many other factors, you simply don't need the same type or amount of food at the same time each day.

This is contrary to the way most diets are structured and yet another reason why they usually fail. You were more likely to "cheat" when your hunger levels didn't match the rules of whatever diet you were following. This time, be your own expert by learning to understand and trust your body's signals.

Eating when you're hungry reassures your metabolism. Hunger is a natural biological signal that ensures that your body will get the fuel it needs, when it needs it. By eating according to your hunger signals, your body learns to trust that food will be available to meet its needs, so it allows your metabolism to run on high.

Eating small meals satisfies hunger best. When you don't overfill your stomach, you'll feel light and comfortable after eating. For a visual reminder, gently make a fist then open your hand. That's about how much food it takes for your stomach to go from a level 1 or 2 to a level 5. Surprising, isn't it, when you think about how large most serving sizes are. No wonder people struggle so much with their weight.

Of course, when you eat a small amount of food, you're likely to become hungry more often throughout the day. That is why so many people who eat instinctively seem to be eating all the time. This is also where the common diet rules "Eat six small meals a day" and "Eat every three hours" originated. However, instead of using an arbitrary schedule designed by someone else, listen to your body and eat an appropriate amount in response to your hunger signals.

This instinctive pattern of eating small, frequent meals will level out your blood sugar and supply a consistent fuel source. As a result, you'll experience fewer mood and energy swings.

Hunger is affected by what you eat, not just how much you eat. The types of nutrients and the number of calories the food contains all affect your hunger levels. Macronutrients (carbohydrates, proteins, and fats) are digested at different rates and cause the release of certain biochemicals. For example, protein-containing foods lead to the greatest level of satiety; foods high in fiber slow down digestion. That's why crackers with peanut butter literally stick with you longer than plain crackers, and why a palm full of broccoli affects you differently from a palm full of chocolate candy. When you're really listening to your body, you can adjust what you eat to regulate your hunger patterns.

Hunger may be specific for a certain type of food. Often when you're hungry, a specific food will come to mind. In future chapters we'll take a closer look at how you can use this information to make the most satisfying food choices.

It may take twenty to thirty minutes after eating to tell that you're full. You might feel satisfied immediately after eating but feel very full a short time later. If you tend to overshoot and eat too much, then slow down, chew your food thoroughly, and put down your fork between bites. Stop periodically in the middle of eating to ask yourself where you are on the Hunger and Fullness Scale. It's also helpful to stop eating before you think you're at a 5 or a 6. You can always eat more, later, if you need to.

Hunger can't be satisfied before it occurs. Eating to avoid feeling hungry later (when eating may be inconvenient) is called *preventive eating*. The food you eat when you aren't hungry will be stored for later. If you already have fat stores, there's no reason to add to them with more preventive eating.

Think of it like this. If you're comfortable in a room but you put on a heavy coat now because you might get cold in an hour, you'll probably get hot and uncomfortable in the meantime. Instead, if you wait until you feel cold, the coat will do what it's supposed to do—make you warm and keep you comfortable. Hunger works the same way. If you eat now because you might get hungry in an hour, you'll feel full and uncomfortable. If you wait until you're hungry to eat, you'll feel satisfied and comfortable.

Preventive eating is sometimes a response to a fear of hunger. Perhaps there was a time in your life when you were insecure about having enough food. Or perhaps you perceive your natural feelings of hunger as unpleasant and try to avoid them. To combat this fear, assure yourself that you'll usually be able to eat when you're hungry, and then be prepared by keeping food on hand. It's usually better to have healthy, satisfying choices rather than foods that call to you even when you're not hungry.

It's also helpful to remember that feeling hungry for a while won't hurt you. In fact, it'll help you become more aware of your hunger cues and allow your body to use some of its fat stores. In other words, it's better to be hungry for a little while than to eat when you're not truly hungry, forcing your body to store more.

Hunger can be postponed. If food isn't available or it's not convenient to eat when you get hungry, your hunger may disappear and return in an hour or two. That's because your body will turn to other fuel sources—an important survival mechanism. Keep in mind, though, that if you take advantage of this and ignore hunger too often, it may backfire and cause your metabolism to slow down in order to conserve energy. Also remember that when hunger comes back, it'll probably be even stronger.

Every urge to eat is an opportunity to become mindful of your hunger and fullness signals. Before long, using hunger to guide your eating will become instinctive and natural again.

CHAPTER 3

IT'S NOT ABOUT THE FOOD

I felt overwhelmed with everything I needed to get done and found myself wanting to eat something. I was tuned in enough to my body to know I wasn't hungry. Still, I could hear the ice cream calling my name from the freezer. "Michelle! Michelle! I'm in here!" As I got up from my computer and wandered into the kitchen, my little voice reminded me how hard I'd been working. I deserved this little reward. As I dipped the spoon in to take a bite, I realized I was still standing in front of the freezer. That was a clue. When I don't even bother to sit down, I know it's not about the food.

I put the lid back on, grabbed a glass of water, and went outside to sit on the patio. As I thought about it, I realized I was using eating as an excuse to take a break. As I pondered that, I found myself thinking that I didn't deserve to relax until I was done with everything I needed to do. I felt overwhelmed again and heard the ice cream calling me once more.

I took a deep breath and sipped my water. Since I'd never get through my To Do list, I'd never get to rest. I would continue to use food as an excuse unless I changed my mind about what it took to earn a break. Within a few minutes I felt a lot better and ready to attack my list again. This time I decided I'd stop in an hour and take my dog for a walk. As I passed through the kitchen on my way back to my office, I noticed the ice cream was quiet for a change.

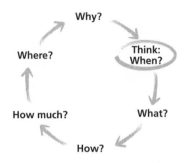

WHEN DO I WANT TO EAT?
PART 2: I'M NOT HUNGRY—WHAT NOW?

Now that you've relearned to tell when you're hungry, are you surprised when you want to eat without any physical indication that your body actually needs food?

You're in charge of what you do next. Notice how different that is from being in control. Being in control implies that you don't let yourself do the things you want and that you do other things even though you don't want to. Control is what you need to follow the rules of a diet.

Being in charge means you get to make choices. Marla figured this out pretty quickly.

> I am much more aware of whether I'm hungry or not when I feel like eating, and that has helped a lot. The problem is that there are still lots of times I want to eat even though there are no signs of physical hunger whatsoever. If I start thinking, "I'm not hungry—I shouldn't eat," it makes me want to eat more!

Remember, whenever you have an urge to eat, ask yourself, "Am I hungry?" I didn't say, "You may eat *only* when you're hungry" or "If you aren't hungry, you're not allowed to eat." If I had, this wouldn't be any different from all those diets that gave you rules to restrict your calorie intake. When you want to eat (or keep eating) even though you aren't hungry, you get to decide what you'll do next.

WEIGH YOUR OPTIONS

If you want to eat or continue to eat when you aren't hungry, you have three options to choose from: eat anyway, redirect your attention, or meet your true needs. Each choice is valid, and each has its advantages and disadvantages.

Option One: Eat Anyway

Your first option is to go ahead and eat anyway. Yes, that *is* one of your options. Even people who eat instinctively sometimes eat or overeat when they aren't particularly hungry—because of a special occasion, because the food looks or tastes wonderful, or simply because it's convenient. They just don't do it all the time.

When you've weighed the advantages and disadvantages and made a conscious choice, eating anyway is less likely to drive your Overeating Cycle or force you back into your Restrictive Eating Cycle.

I need to make an important point here. Because of past dieting, many people still eat when they aren't hungry but choose "allowed" or healthier foods. Although you might rationalize that it "does less damage," it's important that you acknowledge that you're still choosing to eat even though your body didn't ask for food.

What are the advantages of choosing to eat or continuing to eat even though you aren't hungry? There must be some; otherwise, you wouldn't have done it thousands of times before. Stop reading to think about it for a moment.

Advantages: Eating Anyway
- It's easy—Eating anyway requires no effort, thought, or energy because you've done it so many times before. You can eat on autopilot without having to think about what you're doing or why.
- It may give temporary pleasure—Food tastes good and can be used for short-term pleasure, reward, or celebration.
- It may distract you temporarily—Eating can be used to avoid certain thoughts or feelings or to postpone something.

MINDFUL MOMENT: You can eat when you aren't hungry; just be aware that you're doing it.

Disadvantages: Eating Anyway

- It may cause discomfort—Eating or continuing to eat can lead to feeling physically uncomfortable, bloated, and lethargic.

- You may eat more than if you were hungry—If hunger doesn't tell you to start eating, what's going to tell you to stop? You'll stop when the food is gone, when someone comes in, or when you feel uncomfortable or numb.

- You may feel regretful—Notice my intentional use of the word *regretful* instead of *guilty*. There's no need to feel guilty if you made a conscious choice to eat even when you're not hungry. Guilt leads to shame and negative self-talk, which adds fuel to your Overeating Cycle. (In chapter 5 I talk more about getting rid of guilt.) On the other hand, regret implies that you made a decision and now you wish you'd made a different choice. That leaves room for you to experience and learn from the consequences.

- It causes weight gain—When you eat food your body didn't tell you to, it has no choice but to store it. This survival mechanism has been in place for centuries, but in an abundant food environment, it may actually lead to decreased survival. Besides, carrying extra weight may cause you to have less energy and less motivation to engage in other activities, further compounding the problem.

- You don't meet your true needs—When you eat instead of addressing your triggers, you're not meeting your needs. When your true needs are unmet, your triggers will return again and again.

In short, eating even though you aren't hungry is easy and may give you temporary pleasure or distraction. The downside is that it has strings attached. You might feel better temporarily, but when you grab food out of habit or to meet a need other than to satisfy true hunger, you're more likely to overeat, leading to weight gain and the discomfort of feeling too full, sluggish, and regretful afterward. It reminds me of that old antacid commercial with the tagline "I can't believe I ate the whole thing!"

Ironically, even if you believe you overeat just because you love food, the true purpose of eating is to nourish your body. Eating or continuing to eat when you aren't hungry can't possibly give you the same level of enjoyment as eating to satisfy physical hunger.

Most important, eating anyway fuels your Overeating Cycle because it doesn't allow you to address your underlying needs. Marla shared one of her challenges.

> Almost every day after lunch, I put my toddler down for a nap and turn on the television for a little break. There's usually nothing good on, so I watch the shopping channel or one of those cooking shows. I always want a snack, so I poke around in the cupboard until I find some crackers or cookies. Sometimes I even eat chocolate chips right out of the bag! I don't know why, but I find myself rummaging around in the refrigerator, munching on some cheese or grapes or even the leftovers from dinner. This can go on for an hour or more until I am just stuffed or my toddler wakes up. I get so mad at myself because I know that if I keep it up, I'll never lose this weight. I always promise myself I won't do it again tomorrow, but I usually do.

No matter how much she ate, Marla didn't feel satisfied because she wasn't hungry. Her promises to herself weren't working because her eating wasn't about the food.

Option Two: Redirect Your Attention

When you choose to redirect your attention, you're making a conscious decision to focus on an activity other than eating (or thinking about eating) because you're not hungry yet. Sometimes the answer is as simple as moving a candy dish out of sight or knitting instead of munching while you watch television. Sometimes distracting yourself is more involved, like working on a scrapbook page for an hour or calling a friend to go for a walk.

Advantages: Redirecting Your Attention

- An urge to eat will likely pass—When you engage your mind in something else, the desire to eat usually goes away within a few minutes. Redirecting your attention works especially well for environmental triggers like a TV commercial or the sight of food.

- It's a more productive use of time than eating—How much time do you spend thinking about eating, looking for or preparing food, eating, then feeling regretful afterward?

- It disrupts your Overeating Cycle—Eating in response to your triggers is a habit; choosing to do something else breaks the cycle.

- Waiting until you're hungry makes eating more satisfying.

Disadvantages: Redirecting Your Attention

- It requires some thought and effort—Habits are like deep ruts in a road; you have to turn your steering wheel hard and give the car some gas to pull yourself out.

- It requires some preparation—You need to have ideas, and sometimes supplies, ready so it's as easy as possible to find something else to do besides eat.

- It works temporarily—Fortunately, that is often all you need since an urge caused by an environmental trigger will usually pass quickly.

- It may not meet your true needs—As with eating anyway, you may not meet your real needs when you distract yourself—but sometimes you do. For example, if you feel like eating when you're stressed but you take a walk instead, you'll be distracted from the food and reduce your stress, too.

Redirecting yourself is often an effective short-term strategy. Marla tried it.

The day after we talked about trying to distract myself instead of eating, there I was again, wanting to snack while I watched TV after lunch. I knew I wasn't hungry, so I decided to pay my bills instead of eating. It didn't help at all. I wasn't ready to give up yet, so I called my friend Jean and we talked for over half an hour. Before I knew it, my son was awake. I took him to the park to play and by the time we got back, we were both hungry so we had a snack together. I felt great! For the rest of the week, whenever I started watching TV and got an urge to eat, I called a different friend. It really worked—but I am running out of friends to call!

How to Redirect Your Attention Away from Food If you've ever been on a diet, distracting yourself from eating isn't a new technique for you. Here are some specific strategies, however, that will make that technique more effective.

1. **Make a list of activities that appeal to you before you need them.** Write down both simple and more complicated ideas; be sure to include a few that don't require any preparation or equipment. You may have different ideas for home, work, and other settings. Add new activities to your list as you think of them. Having a variety of ideas ensures that you'll come up with something that fits your mood or situation. Use your imagination. One of my workshop participants, for example, is an engineer who has lost more than fifty pounds. She keeps a few Lego sets on her desk to play with when she feels like eating.

2. **Choose activities that are enjoyable—or at least not unpleasant.** If you're going to make a choice not to eat, the alternative must be somewhat appealing. Now you know why it didn't help Marla to try to pay her bills.

3. **Choose an eating-incompatible activity if possible.** This is any activity that requires your hands or full attention. For example, it's difficult to eat while you are playing the piano, building something, or sewing.

4. **Be prepared with things to do.** Choose a few of the distractions from your list and have everything you'll need ready to go. For instance, if you plan to play a game of solitaire, keep the cards nearby. If you're going to try meditation, do a little reading about

it ahead of time so you know what to do. Keep a distraction kit or drawer in your home or office stocked with things to do—stationery, a favorite book, puzzles, tools, crafts, or anything else that appeals to you.

5. **Establish a "Food Free Zone" at home and at work.** Create a pleasant, comfortable space that you don't associate with eating. Promise yourself you'll never eat in that place, though drinking water, tea, or coffee is fine. Keep your distraction kit there so you can retreat to your Food Free Zone until the urge to eat passes.

6. **Promise yourself you'll try distraction for at least a little while.** Although it's easier to eat anyway, you stay trapped in your Overeating Cycle when you do. Try to redirect your attention away from eating even if it is for only a few minutes at first. For example, say to yourself, "I'll work on this puzzle for ten minutes, then see how I feel." You'll quickly learn that you can postpone eating with no adverse consequences, and that will encourage you to try distraction again next time.

Remember, you're redirecting your attention away from food because you don't need it yet, not because you're depriving yourself. Remind yourself that you'll eat when you're hungry.

Distracting yourself from eating works best when something in your environment triggered your urge to eat, like the sight of food. For Marla, watching cooking shows could have been triggering her afternoon binges. Like many people, she probably also associated relaxing and watching television with snacking. Getting away from the television was a good idea.

Deciding to engage in another activity is also very effective when you feel like eating because you're bored, you need a break, or you're trying to avoid some other activity. In these situations, eating is certainly something to do, but there are lots of other options that don't have strings attached.

Redirecting your attention is helpful when you don't have the time or energy to figure out why you want to eat or how to deal with that urge right at that moment. In that case, promise yourself you'll take time to address the trigger later. If you always choose to distract yourself and never address the

> **MINDFUL MOMENT:** Put a sign on your refrigerator that says, "If I'm not hungry, what I'm looking for is not in here."

underlying problem, it will continue to cause an urge to eat and trigger your Overeating Cycle. This brings us to your third option.

Option Three: Meet Your True Needs

Your third option is to focus, figure out what triggered your urge to eat, and decide what to do about it.

Advantages: Meeting Your True Needs

- It decreases your triggers—Discovering what's triggering the urge to eat and addressing the underlying need eventually causes that trigger to decrease.

- Weight management becomes easier—When you don't use food to meet your needs, you'll lose weight, or at least you'll have more success at weight maintenance.

- It improves your overall health—When you recognize and meet your true needs, you take better care of your whole self—body, mind, heart, and spirit.

- It builds new skills—This process also helps you learn how to cope better with other issues in your life.

- It leads to the best long-term results.

Disadvantages: Meeting Your True Needs

- It's the most challenging option, but it's also the most rewarding!
- It may require time, effort, and energy.
- It requires openness and honesty with yourself and others.
- It requires you to build new skills.
- It may require you to ask for help from others to work through issues, develop new skills, and provide support.

STRATEGIES: IDENTIFYING FEELINGS

At first when you try to focus on your feelings, you might notice that you're thinking only about food, your weight, or other superficial thoughts like "I feel fat." Keep in mind that a thought is usually a sentence or phrase like, "I probably shouldn't eat that or I'll gain weight," whereas a feeling can usually be described in two or three words like, "I feel sad," or "I'm mad." Realize that "I feel fat" is a physical sensation, not an emotion, so keep going even if your feelings aren't obvious at first. Instead, picture them like the layers of an onion or the petals of a rose that you gently peel away to get to the center.

Try the following strategies for identifying what you are feeling:

- Become aware of your breathing for clues about your emotions. Are you holding your breath? Is it rapid and shallow? Slow and rhythmic?

- Inhale and exhale deeply as you "sit" with your feelings for one minute. Observe and label the emotion—for example, "frustration." If you feel confused about your emotions, consider these common feelings: anger, sadness, fear, stress, guilt, love, or pleasure. Keep in mind that feelings fall on a continuum: anger, for instance, can range from annoyed to enraged; sadness can range from disappointed to grief stricken.

- Notice your emotions ebb and flow; even intense emotions will subside as you observe them. If they are too much to bear for more than a minute, you can then make a conscious decision to redirect your attention or eat if you wish.

- Write your feelings down using a journal, computer, or even a scrap of paper.

- Complete the sentence "I feel . . ." or "I am . . ." For example, "I feel lonely" or "I am angry with my boss" or "I am worried about my child."

- Picture a close friend or family member observing your thoughts and feelings nonjudgmentally. What would they describe?

- Invite the part of yourself who is a good friend to others, who gently parents your children, or who effectively manages a work team to help you sort out your feelings.
- Imagine that there's a pressure valve on your body that you can turn to release some of your feelings. You can turn the valve higher or lower to control the flow of emotions.
- Describe your feelings as a picture or a metaphor. Start with, "My feelings are like . . ." and compare them to a color, an animal, a familiar story, or whatever images surface.
- Draw images or scribble on a pad of paper to see what emerges.
- Notice whether cravings for a certain food give you clues about what you're feeling or needing. For example, a desire for a comfort food from your childhood could be a signal that you're feeling stressed.
- Talk about your thoughts and feelings out loud or into a tape recorder.
- Discuss your feelings with a trusted friend or family member.
- Seek the assistance of a counselor or therapist if you feel overwhelmed, scared, or unable to identify or work through your emotions.

FEAST

When you don't meet your true needs, those unmet needs drive your Overeating Cycle. Clearly, although this is the most challenging option, meeting your needs is the most satisfying choice.

I'll describe the steps for discovering and meeting your true needs using the acronym FEAST:

- **F**ocus
- **E**xplore
- **A**ccept
- **S**trategize
- **T**ake action

FEAST: Focus The first step is to focus on your body, your thoughts, and your feelings using the Mind-Body Scan you learned in the last chapter. At that stage, you were primarily focused on your physical sensations to identify hunger; now focus on your thoughts and feelings too.

Approach the Mind-Body Scan with curiosity, as in "I wonder what I will discover."

Focus your attention: Try to give yourself several minutes away from the sight and smell of food. It may feel challenging at first, but with practice it becomes easier.

Focus inward: Sit upright so you're open and not blocking any sensations or thoughts. Close your eyes if possible. Become aware of your breath; it is a bridge between your mind and body. Breathe deeply, all the way down to your lower abdomen. Bring your attention to the present moment as you become mindful of your sensations, thoughts, and feelings.

Focus on your physical sensations: Draw your attention to your body. Become aware as you scan from head to toe. What is your level of hunger or fullness? Are you thirsty? Are you energetic or fatigued? Are you experiencing any areas of tension, discomfort, or pain? Are you aware of any concerns about your health or well-being?

Focus on your thoughts: Observe the thoughts running through your mind. What is your little voice saying? Be aware that these are just thoughts, not reality. Don't try to change them even if you don't like them or they seem irrational. Just notice them as they are.

Focus on your feelings: What feelings and emotions are you aware of? Your emotions give you clues about what you really need and how to take care of yourself. Are they pleasant, unpleasant, or neutral? Don't judge yourself for your feelings even if they're uncomfortable. Just become aware of them as they are.

FEAST: Explore Your triggers can be just about anything physical, environmental, or emotional. Some triggers are not particularly dramatic or profound; they're just learned habits like eating popcorn at the movies. You'll be able to deal with many of these types of triggers simply by becoming aware of them. For example, if you realize the reason you feel like eating is that you

> **MINDFUL MOMENT:** When a craving doesn't come from hunger, eating will never satisfy it.

saw a burger on a billboard on your way into work, you might just smile at the thought and decide you aren't going to be manipulated by advertising.

Other times you'll need to dig a little deeper and explore the situation. Marla's story demonstrates this well. Because her cravings weren't coming from a need for food—after all, she had just finished lunch—no matter how much she ate, she didn't feel satisfied. Getting away from the TV and calling her friends was helpful. Not only did it distract her, it also gave her a connection with other people. Ultimately, however, the most effective long-term solution will be for her to further explore what's triggering her desire to eat.

Triggers like difficult emotions or challenging situations require you to develop deeper awareness. You might find it helpful to complete the sentence "I feel _____ because _____." Remember, you're peeling back layers, so keep asking yourself, "what else?" until you get to the core of the issue. If you find yourself stuck, you may want to seek out professional assistance from a doctor, counselor, therapist, coach, or some other trained and supportive person who can guide you through the process.

FEAST: Accept All too often people who struggle with eating have the mistaken belief that shaming themselves will somehow fix the problem, when in fact, it only makes it worse. Think for a moment about a parent and child. If the parent is always harsh and expects the child to be perfect, the child is likely to feel afraid, guilty, and even rebellious. If the parent is always permissive, the child is likely to feel entitled, uncertain, and even uncared for. On the other hand, when a parent sets firm but loving limits, the child always knows what the parent expects and is able to learn from her mistakes, but she also feels loved and accepted no matter what.

As an adult, you parent yourself. Are you harsh and judgmental? Are you permissive and lenient? Or do you set clear expectations and love and accept yourself no matter what?

As you focus and begin to explore your reasons for wanting to eat when you're not hungry, let go of any thoughts of right or wrong, bad or good, should or shouldn't have. Remember, eating may not have been the most effective way for you to cope in the past, but that doesn't mean you should feel guilty or ashamed. At least you've been coping in some way. Now you have the awareness and opportunity to choose a better way.

FEAST: Strategize At this point you're ready to come up with as many strategies as possible for dealing with the real reason you feel like eating. Be creative and try to come up with new ideas. As you'll see in the next chapter, these are things you *could* do, not what you've done in the past, nor even what you think you *should* do.

Your strategy might be as simple as screaming into a pillow when you're angry or reading for a while to reward yourself for working hard all day. Sometimes your underlying need is much greater. Even then, brainstorm several small steps that could get you closer to meeting that need. For example, if you feel overworked, exhausted, and in need of a vacation, you probably can't just get up and go. But you might come up with ideas like taking a hot bath while you take a mini-vacation in your mind, putting in a vacation request, taking a three-day weekend, picking up travel brochures on your way home, or searching the Internet to plan your next trip. Any of these options will get you closer to meeting your need for a vacation than eating will.

FEAST: Take action Consider all your options then come up with a plan. The goal here is to be *in charge* of what you do next. Unlike being in control, being in charge is not about having willpower or being willing to deprive yourself. It's about taking a step in the direction you want to go. Small changes you consistently practice gradually add up to new ways of thinking, feeling, and acting that feel better than eating.

Don't expect your plan to be perfect or to work every time. Your mistakes will help you learn and make adjustments until you figure out what works for you.

Here's what happened when Marla decided to Focus, Explore, Accept, Strategize, and Take action.

Turning off the TV and calling my friends really helped at first, but each afternoon it was the same thing; I still wanted to eat. After a week, I knew it was time to dig a little deeper. The next time it happened, I paid more attention to what I was feeling. It was obvious that I wasn't hungry, so I got up from the couch and went to my computer and just started typing my thoughts and feelings. I surprised myself by what I wrote.

> Here I am sitting in front of the computer because when I sit in front of the TV after Josh goes down, I could eat myself out of house and home. I know it's worse when I watch cooking shows—all that great food and stuff. But it even happens when I'm watching the shopping shows. One minute I'm thinking about some new gadget or piece of jewelry I want, and the next minute I want food. But it's not just stuff I want; I want something exciting to happen. I love being Josh's mommy, but I loved working, too. I kind of feel like my life is on hold and I'm losing part of who I am.

When I read what I wrote I felt guilty at first, but then I figured it was probably normal to feel this way. I thought about going back to work, but I'd really rather be home with Josh, at least until he's in preschool. I decided to start taking some online classes so I can finish up my degree. I feel reenergized! I don't even want to watch TV—much less eat all afternoon.

When you feel like eating even though you're not hungry, instead of automatically reaching for food, make a conscious choice to eat anyway, redirect your attention, or meet your true needs. Like my experience with the ice cream, when you give yourself the opportunity to discover what you're thinking and

MINDFUL MOMENT: When I'm hungry, I eat what I love. When I'm bored, I do something I love. When I'm lonely, I connect with someone I love. When I feel sad, I remember that I am loved.

feeling, you'll probably realize that most of the time it's not about the food. In Marla's case, she had been handling the transition of being a stay-at-home mother by watching television and eating. Once she realized that, she was able to create a new plan. Isn't it interesting that her overeating finally led her to discover what she really needed? Little by little, as you begin to meet your real needs, you'll find yourself not only eating less but also feeling better.

CHAPTER 4

WHAT AM I REALLY HUNGRY FOR?

Within weeks of becoming a "real doctor," I started my residency and spent most of my waking hours at the hospital. The long days and nights, challenging patients, and constant stress were expected but nonetheless difficult. One of the few highlights was the free food in the cafeteria. At any time of day or night, I could find company in the residents' lounge and comfort in the special of the day.

It didn't take me long to discover the double-dipped malted milk balls in the bulk bin. A wax paper sackfull slipped into my white coat pocket would last me all night. Each little sphere was a gift that gave me the consolation, the confidence, the energy, the reward, and the pleasure I desperately needed and often didn't know how to get. I gained a lot that first year—a whole new resilience and spirit—and at least ten pounds in malted milk balls.

Even now my husband will sometimes surprise me with a small sackfull and I still love them. They're just not my best friends anymore.

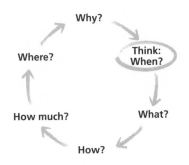

WHEN DO I WANT TO EAT?
PART 3: COPING WITH HEAD HUNGER

Head hunger is your little voice telling you to eat even when your body doesn't need food. It might say things like:

Maybe a little chocolate will pick me up.

I hate to waste perfectly good food.

Mmmm, that looks so good.

I already blew it; I may as well eat the rest.

I better have one now before they're all gone.

I'll just eat these last few bites; it's not enough to save anyway.

I better eat now since I don't know when I'll get another chance.

I'll get started right after I have a little snack.

I worked so hard. I deserve it.

I can hide the wrapper and no one will know.

Just a spoonful of ice cream won't hurt.

I'm not even going to ask myself if I'm hungry because I just want
to eat.

As you explore the sources of your head hunger, it's important to realize that what you believe and think causes you to feel a certain way, which causes you to do certain things, which ultimately leads to specific results. In other words, your thoughts become self-fulfilling prophecies. And since your results tend to reinforce your beliefs and thoughts, your results continue the loop.

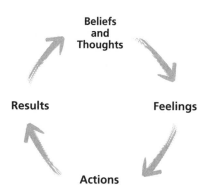

For example, if your little voice says, "I'll never get all this done!" you'll probably feel overwhelmed and hopeless. If your habit is to try to make yourself feel better by eating, you'll shift your attention to food instead of figuring out what to do next. You'll get further behind and think, "See. I knew I'd never get all of it done!"

It's common for people to try to change the *actions* and *results* they don't like without first recognizing and dealing with the *beliefs*, *thoughts*, and *feelings* that led to those unwanted actions and results in the first place. In the preceding example, going on a diet would address your eating (the action), not the thoughts and feelings that caused it. When the thought "I'll never get all this done" causes you to feel overwhelmed again, you'll struggle to stay on the diet.

Thinking thoughts that lead to undesirable results is a habit—a habit that can be changed through awareness. Granted, it's not always easy to recognize when a thought is driving unwanted results, especially if you've been thinking a particular way for a long time. That is where those first two steps in FEAST—Focus and Explore—can really help.

As you become aware of thoughts that are leading to results you don't want, it's important that you don't judge yourself for them. Remember, it's a loop, so feeling bad or blaming yourself only leads to negative actions and results. Instead, remember the importance of the Accept step in FEAST.

You have the power to change the thoughts that aren't working for you. When you change your thoughts, you change your results. This is where the Strategize and Take action steps come in. In this example, you could choose to think, "There's a lot to do. I can do only one thing at a time, so I must decide what's most important." In place of feeling overwhelmed, you'll feel in charge. You'll decide what to do first, then what to do after that. You may or may not get everything done, but you'll know you did what you could.

As you begin to explore your head hunger and create new, healthier habits, you'll probably find that at first you're still tempted to eat. Eating is easy, familiar, and comfortable, whereas change and growth can be challenging and uncomfortable initially. By trying new strategies and taking small steps, you'll eventually rewire what feels good to you. Your new habits will become more natural and your old habits will lose their appeal. Jerry shared a good example of this process.

> I used to always overeat at buffets. At first I found it hard to break that habit because I felt like I wasn't getting my money's worth if I didn't eat until I was stuffed. So I started telling myself, "I've gotten my money's worth when I've eaten what I need." Once I started eating a little less, I noticed that I felt a lot better when I got home. I eventually lost interest in all-you-can-eat buffets, and now I prefer restaurants where I can order exactly what I want and take home my leftovers.

In the following pages, we'll explore many examples of head hunger and strategies for coping with it. I've categorized the head hunger examples by three main types of triggers I introduced in chapter 1: physical, environmental, and emotional.

MINDFUL MOMENT: If you don't like your results, first ask yourself what you were thinking.

STRATEGIES: CREATING NEW HABITS

Here are some strategies for getting through the necessary discomfort of changing old patterns. Not surprisingly, these strategies have a lot to do with how you think.

- **Be a problem solver.** Consider all your options and choices and look for creative solutions.

- **Think direction, not perfection.** Don't get trapped into thinking you have to do it perfectly and nothing else will do. Instead, think in terms of making a step, any step, in the direction you want to go.

- **Take it slow.** Reasonably sized changes, even baby steps or micro-movements, will help you move forward little by little.

- **Be realistic.** Ask yourself, "What can I actually see myself doing?"

- **Weigh the pros and cons.** Consider the rewards and consequences of your options and think about the likely outcome of your decision. For example, if you're considering having another brownie, ask yourself questions like these: "How will I feel later if I eat it? How will I feel later if I don't? Is it worth it? Is this the choice I wish to make?"

- **Remember there are no right or wrong choices.** Choose what's most effective for you under the circumstances.

- **Be flexible.** Circumstances can change rapidly, so what works for you may be different at different times.

- **Learn from your mistakes.** Every mistake brings you one step closer to being an expert as you discover what's most effective for you. Just do the best you can.

- **Practice, practice, practice.** Consistency and repetition are the keys both to reducing the necessary discomfort of change and to energizing new behaviors.

PHYSICAL TRIGGERS: FEED MY NEED

Food can be calming, energizing, and pleasurable. Certain foods even activate the pleasure centers in the brain and reduce awareness of physical pain, illness, and fatigue. To effectively reduce overeating in response to physical triggers, you'll need to learn to substitute other activities that stimulate those same pleasure centers. Here are some of the most common physical triggers for overeating and some strategies to get you started in changing your habits.

Thirst

Many people feel like eating when, in actuality, they need water. Thirst is a physical sensation, but food is an inefficient way to meet your body's need for fluids.

Strategize Try drinking a glass of water before you eat. (Read chapter 11 for practical suggestions about how to deal with this common trigger.)

Fatigue

Your little voice might say, "I'm so tired; I need a little pick-me-up." Although hunger sometimes causes a feeling of low energy, eating when you actually need to rest makes you feel more tired because your body has to work to digest and store the unneeded food. In addition, studies have shown a link between poor sleep and weight gain.

Strategize Take a break and rest when you need it. Get enough sleep each night to reduce fatigue as a trigger and to feel your best each day.

MINDFUL MOMENT: Small changes will gradually rewire what feels good to you.

Salivation

Salivating is a normal physical response to the sight, smell, or the thought of appetizing food. Since salivation occurs with or without hunger, it's not a reliable sign that your body needs food.

Strategize Look for other physical signs of hunger besides salivation.

Urge to Chew, Crunch, or Suck

A desire to chew, crunch, or suck is a physical urge but that doesn't mean your body needs food. For example, some people feel like eating crunchy food when they're angry.

Strategize If the urge is strong, look for noncaloric ways to satisfy it such as chewing sugar-free gum or sucking on ice. Using tobacco is not a healthy way to satisfy this urge.

Pain

Pain and physical discomfort are powerful triggers for some people. Eating certain foods may cause the release of endorphins, which have pain-relieving properties. However, the effects are very short lived and overeating and weight gain often compound the problem, especially for conditions like arthritis and fibromyalgia.

Strategize Depending on the source of the pain, gentle physical activity, relaxation techniques, massage, alternative therapies, medications, and other pain management strategies can provide effective and sustainable relief. Talk to your health care professional for advice.

Hormonal Cycles

Cyclical hormonal changes in women may cause them to eat a disproportionate number of calories and prefer certain foods like chocolate and carbs right before their menses. Since this kind of eating is against most diet rules, it can lead to guilt and bingeing.

Strategize Don't use PMS as an excuse to binge; you'll feel far better when you continue to use balance, variety, and moderation to guide your eating. However, rather than trying to resist hormonal fluctuations, see what happens when you listen to your body and allow your hunger and cravings to ebb and flow naturally. You'll probably notice that you want to eat less the following week so everything evens out.

Medication Side Effects

Certain medications can cause increased appetite and/or weight gain.

Strategize Talk to your health care professional about your medications and ask if there are other kinds that won't cause increased appetite and weight gain. If you must be on a certain medicine for medical reasons, put a little extra effort into making healthier choices, using moderation, and being physically active to counteract any weight-gain side effects.

Medical Conditions

Low thyroid (hypothyroidism), menopause, and other conditions can cause weight gain or make it more difficult to lose weight. Some age-related changes are related to the metabolism issues discussed in chapters 7 and 9.

Strategize See your health care professional if you suspect there's an underlying medical cause for abrupt weight gain. A word of caution is needed here, though. Although many patients request hormone testing to explain their weight gain, it's uncommon to find abnormalities that will completely explain and resolve the problem. The tests may be well worth doing, but I also encourage you to continue to focus on making healthy lifestyle changes.

MINDFUL MOMENT: Begin to think of a "meal" as exactly the right amount and type of food for you at the time when you need it.

ENVIRONMENTAL TRIGGERS: WHAT ARE MY BELLS?

A famous scientist, Ivan Pavlov, measured the saliva that dogs produced when they ate. He then rang a bell every time he fed them. After a while, he found that the dogs would salivate whenever he rang the bell—even if he didn't feed them. Environmental triggers are like Pavlov's bell. If you pair eating with an activity often enough, eventually the activity itself triggers the urge to eat. You may have hundreds of bells—sights, smells, people, places, events, and situations that can trigger mindless eating. When you stop responding to your bells automatically, you'll begin to change the way you think, feel, and react to them.

Mealtimes

Society programs you to follow a schedule and conditions you to eat certain foods and certain amounts at certain meals. While it may be more convenient or necessary for you to eat meals at conventional times, those mealtimes don't always coincide with your internal clock or natural hunger rhythms. Perhaps you're also in the habit of eating traditional meals that include a main course, side dishes, and even dessert, or it doesn't "count" as eating.

Strategize Though it's challenging to change your mealtime routine, you can adapt it to fit your needs. Keep a healthy snack handy in case you get hungry. If you're consistently tempted to snack right before a meal, consider moving the mealtime up or eating differently the meal before. For example, I've found that if I know I'm going to be tied up in a meeting, I can add peanut butter to my breakfast so I can skip my usual mid-morning snack. This is another place where using a journal can really help you figure out what works for you. And remember, you don't need to eat a whole meal if you're only a little hungry. Sometimes just a few bites are all you need.

Eating on a Schedule

Many diets promote scheduled eating to prevent hunger or to fuel your metabolism. This rule comes from the observation that many thin people eat frequent small meals. But they do that by eating when they're hungry and stopping when they're satisfied—not by watching the clock.

Some experts presume that you'll lose control of your eating if you get hungry. But now you know that exactly the opposite occurs; you're more likely to eat in a satisfying way when you're hungry—as long as you're not *too* hungry.

Strategize Learn to pace yourself by observing your natural hunger rhythms then establishing a consistent meal pattern that matches them. Rather than automatically eating every three hours, do a Mind-Body Scan every few hours to see how you're feeling. You'll probably notice you get hungry every three to six hours depending on what and how much you ate at your last meal and how active you've been. Research suggests you'll function better on frequent small meals (grazing) rather than three large meals a day, so experiment with this to see how you feel.

High-Risk Times

Many people have times of the day that are high risk for overeating. For example, you may experience a late afternoon energy slump or a tendency to munch when you come home from work to help you transition into your evening.

Strategize Know when you're most at risk and develop an alternate strategy. For example, create a "recharge" or transition ritual to help you relax or unwind after work. Perhaps you could save a favorite magazine or book to read, call a friend, or walk your dog instead.

Holidays and Weather

Many people eat more in colder weather or crave different types of foods in different seasons (winter stews, summer salads). Holidays can be especially difficult because of all the social ties to traditional foods and certain people. In addition, many of the foods you eat during this time may seem "special" and therefore harder to eat in sensible quantities.

Strategize These occasions repeat themselves year after year, so anticipate what typically occurs and create a plan for dealing with your triggers. Make it a point to really listen to your body instead of the external cues. Keep in mind that special foods will be even more special when you eat them mindfully, focusing on the appearance and flavors of the food, the ambience, the other people, and the reason you're all together. Try tasting small amounts of some of the foods you're hungry for, asking for recipes, and taking foods home with you to eat when you *are* hungry. And don't forget, those holiday cookies will be back before you know it—and you *can* make turkey and mashed potatoes in July if you want.

Preventive Eating

Fear of being hungry when it isn't convenient to eat can drive you to want to eat before you need fuel.

Strategize You wouldn't put a coat on *before* you need it because it would make you feel uncomfortable. Eating is no different. As with a jacket, have food with you just in case, but remember, you can't satisfy hunger ahead of time. Besides, you probably have enough energy stored to last you until it's more convenient to eat.

Sight of Food

Many people are "food suggestible." This means you might begin to salivate and think you're hungry when you see appetizing food. Seeing displays of food like candy or nuts in dishes and tempting foods when you open your cabinet or refrigerator can trigger you to want them. Even if you weren't thinking of food before, your little voice might say, "Oh, I want some of that!"

Strategize If you see food and suddenly feel like eating, go somewhere away from the food for a quick Mind-Body Scan. If you're not hungry, it's still fine to appreciate the appearance and aroma of appetizing food without eating it. Just think of it as a "feast for the eyes." Admire it and say, "That looks wonderful!" and walk away.

It also helps to decrease your exposure to the sight and smell of food when you're not hungry. Out of sight, out of mind. Examples of strategies you could try: Don't meet your friend for coffee if the pastries always tempt you. Keep water at your desk instead of going to the break room if there are usually snacks there. Don't use food as decorations or leave appetizing foods in plain view. Try putting tempting foods behind other foods in your cabinets and refrigerator; you'll be surprised by how often you actually forget about them. If coworkers keep food out, politely ask them to put it in a drawer instead. At a party, socialize away from the food.

Trigger Foods

Trigger foods are foods that you associate with overeating: for example, the one bowl of ice cream that always turned into a whole carton. Often, these are foods that you have tried to resist in the past, and when you finally gave in and ate them, you felt out of control. In the next two chapters, I'll show you how to eat these foods in a more enjoyable way, but in the meantime, try these strategies for handling them.

Strategize   Remind yourself that you don't have to be in control because now you're in charge. There are different ways to deal with foods that have triggered you in the past; the most important thing is to discover which way works best for you.

One way is to keep trigger foods away until you feel more in charge of your eating. Keep other foods on hand that you really enjoy so you won't feel deprived. Then when you crave a particular food that you're concerned about overeating, go to a restaurant or a store and buy one serving. If there are other people who want to keep problem foods around, ask them to choose types you don't particularly like, keep them in a separate place, or keep them in small amounts that aren't overwhelming. It will also help to remind yourself that it's *their* food, not *yours*.

Another way to deal with trigger foods is to keep a small amount around at all times. Some people find they are less prone to bingeing on that food when they know it will always be there. I use a combination of both strategies: I generally don't keep potato chips in the house, but I almost always have a little bit of chocolate in my cabinet or purse. Whichever strategy you use, when you choose to eat a food you've struggled with in the past, make it a point to enjoy it thoroughly without guilt so you'll feel truly satisfied.

Advertising

Food is everywhere—on billboards, on television, and in magazines (ironically, often next to the articles about the latest wonder diet!). That's because marketers know how food suggestible most people are.

Strategize Get yourself a glass of water during commercials, avoid watching programs that focus on food, and skip quickly over the food ads and recipes. Break the habit of eating while watching television—usually a mindless, high-calorie activity. One man I worked with said that just sitting in a different chair to watch TV broke his association with eating. When you're exposed to food marketing, remind yourself that you're the one who decides when and what you'll eat.

Social Events

Many people have a tendency to ignore or become distracted from their hunger signals and eat mindlessly in social settings. Movies and popcorn, sports and hot dogs, dates and dinner—these are common social triggers for eating out of habit.

Strategize Instead of making food the main event, focus on the movie, the game, and other people. The key is to decide to make eating a conscious activity while enjoying the whole experience, not just the food. It really helps to time social meals to match your natural hunger rhythms or adjust your eating that day so you'll be hungry (but not too hungry!).

At a buffet or social event, survey all your options, focusing on quality instead of quantity. Be selective and take small samples of the most appealing foods. If you attempt to taste everything, you'll end up feeling too full. In some situations, you can provide your own food: a dish to share at a party or snacks for a ball game. This strategy often saves you money, too. If you'd feel deprived if you didn't have the popcorn, buy the smallest bag, decide whether it really needs extra butter, and savor every bite.

Grocery Shopping

There's a marketing science behind grocery store layout and the placement of food and sale items to trigger impulse purchases. Have you ever wondered why they have candy in the checkout lane at hardware and craft stores?

Strategize You've probably heard these strategies before, and for good reason—they work! Make a list to shop from and don't shop when you're hungry. Try shopping around the perimeter of the store where the produce, dairy, bakery, and deli are located so you'll stick to the basics, venturing down the aisles only for items on your list. When you're in a nonfood establishment such as a video rental store that has tempting snack displays, tell yourself, "I won't be a puppet for their profit!"

Preparing Food

Just a few extra bites while you are preparing food can add up to a lot of extra calories and spoil your appetite for the meal. My mom used to say, "I just want to make sure it's good enough for you!"

Strategize Avoid tasting food while you're cooking. If you need to taste to adjust seasonings, take only a small amount. Be sure to notice whether you're less hungry as a result, then eat accordingly during the meal. If you feel overly hungry while you're cooking, go ahead and eat a little bit of what you've planned to serve to take the edge off.

Food Associations

If you have a habit of eating while sitting in front of the TV, propped up in bed, or standing in the kitchen, you may get an urge to eat whenever you're in those places.

Strategize You can make it a family rule to limit eating to one or two rooms in the house and to eat only while sitting at a table. This will decrease triggers like watching TV and reading and help you focus on enjoying your food without distractions.

Eating in the Car

Eating while you're driving will distract you from the road and from enjoying your food. Additionally, your choices may be limited to fast-food restaurants and convenience stores.

Strategize Try not to eat in your car, and avoid eating while driving. If you have to be on the road for work or travel, pack a snack or lunch and park to eat.

Talking on the Phone

If you eat while you're on the phone, your body won't register satisfaction because your attention will be on the conversation. Besides, it's rude!

Strategize Don't eat while talking on the telephone. Period.

Obligatory Eating

Beware of eating something just because someone offered it to you or handed you a sample. Your little voice might say, "It's rude to refuse food" or "You can't pass up free food." This is particularly difficult when a friend or family member makes something especially for you.

Strategize Be polite but firm when turning down food other people want you to eat. You're in charge. If you're concerned about hurting someone's feelings, thank them then ask for the recipe or ask to take some home to eat later when you're hungry.

Eating What's Left

Eating those last few bites of food left in the bowl or on your children's plates, or finishing off the leftovers while you are cleaning up, can push you past the point of satisfaction.

Strategize You're not a human garbage disposal! Don't keep the serving dishes on the table during the meal; this will decrease your temptation to finish off what's left and will make you consciously decide whether to get up to get more. Give yourself some time to feel full by cleaning up the kitchen before taking a second helping. While you're at it, pack a serving for lunch the next day to remind yourself you can eat it again when you're hungry.

Serving Sizes

Research has shown that larger portion sizes and larger serving dishes trigger people to eat more. Restaurants often serve overly large portions to make their customers feel they're getting value. The extra food costs them very little once they have you in the door, but these large portions will keep you super-sized.

Strategize Use smaller plates and buy or divide your snacks into single serving bags to decrease the chance you'll eat more than you need. Remember that when you have food sitting in front of you, you're more likely to keep nibbling. Estimate how much food you think you'll need and put the rest away before you start eating, or be prepared to wrap up the extra as soon as you feel satisfied. Remind yourself you'll get to enjoy that food again when you're hungry.

When eating out, you can choose to skip the appetizer, order a half portion, or request a child's serving. On the occasion I eat fast food, a kid's meal is the perfect size; I just never know what to do with the toy!

Most important, adopt the motto "quality over quantity." Is it well prepared? Attractive? Fresh? Healthy? My husband and I are both "foodies," and we love to share meals. We call it co-ordering and co-eating because we get to enjoy great food in portions that don't leave us feeling stuffed. Caution: Don't let sharing be an excuse to order too much food. Also be aware that trying to share food you really want all for yourself can cause you to feel deprived.

Dining Out

You go out to eat to enjoy eating when you don't have to cook and wash dishes. However, if you have a "special occasion mentality," you'll be more likely to order less healthy food and eat too much. You may also try to get your money's worth, especially at a buffet, and that can lead to overeating.

Strategize Ask yourself what you're hungry for to narrow your choices before you go to the restaurant or look at the menu. Decide which course is most important to you at that particular meal or that particular place. For instance, if you really want dessert, you'd probably be too full if you ate both an appetizer and an entrée beforehand. Finally, remind yourself you can come back to the restaurant another time to try the foods you choose to skip this time.

Business Entertaining

"Doing business," networking, and business travel often include lunch meetings, conference meals, and invitations to socialize over food and/or drinks.

Strategize If you need to meet over a meal, try to have healthy choices available and be mindful of what and how much you're ordering and eating during the meeting. When possible, make plans to do business socializing around activities where eating isn't the primary focus, such as golf, tennis, sporting events, or spa days.

Eating at Work

At work, people sometimes snack to alleviate stress, break up monotony, or give themselves a break or a reward—often without regard to physical hunger. Eating while at your desk or work area creates an association with food that may trigger urges to overeat. Furthermore, the break room can become a minefield of trigger foods like doughnuts, cookies, and snack foods—particularly around any holiday.

Strategize Make eating and working two distinct activities, and avoid eating while you are engaged in a work-related task. You may decide you'll eat only what you bring so you'll be less tempted to eat whatever shows up at the office. And steer clear of that break room; tell yourself, "It's not my food." Take a real break when you need one by getting away from your desk and getting some fresh air!

EMOTIONAL TRIGGERS: WHAT'S EATING ME?

Emotional connections to food are woven into the fabric of our social experience. From birth you were held and fed; you went to birthday parties for cake and ice cream; you go out for dinner to celebrate a new job or a raise. Think about how common it is for people to use food as a way to bond, nurture, soothe, reward, love, celebrate, and create pleasure and excitement.

Emotions are also common triggers for overeating. Eating is a way to change or manage emotions quickly: for example, stuffing or calming down feelings in order to bring yourself back into balance. However, it's important to understand that most people who struggle with food and weight do not have major underlying psychological problems. Eating to deal with certain emotions is simply a habitual way of coping.

It may not always be obvious to you when you are using food to cope with your feelings. You may think you are overeating "just because it tastes good" or because you lack willpower. If you don't really know *why* you overeat, you may be using food to cope. The *why* becomes clear only when you begin to explore the feelings that underlie your actions.

High-sugar, high-fat, and highly processed carbohydrate foods can temporarily activate the pleasure centers in the brain by triggering a release of "feel good" chemicals like serotonin and beta-endorphins. Although you may feel better while you're eating and for a short time afterward, the pleasure or peacefulness is short-lived. Furthermore, eating doesn't address the issue that caused the emotional discomfort in the first place. As a result, the discomfort returns after you're done eating. In addition, you may have made yourself physically and/or emotionally uncomfortable by overeating. This usually turns on your little voice, as in, "I'm no good," or "I'm so out of control."

Ironically, what began as an attempt to feel better leaves you with both the original issue and the additional physical and emotional discomfort. The way to break out of this pattern is to try to figure out what's eating you, and to learn to tolerate and deal more effectively with your emotions. When you do, you'll feel better, for longer. What follows are common reasons why people turn to food to temporarily comfort or distract themselves and strategies for addressing these emotional triggers.

Pleasure

Food often looks good, tastes good, smells good, and feels good; it's a way to delight the senses any time, day or night. The downside is that the temporary pleasure is usually followed by discomfort and regret.

Strategize What, other than food, delights and pleases your senses? Friends? Flowers? Bath oil? Candles? Sports? Find ways to create pleasure for yourself that don't involve food.

Reward

You might eat to reward yourself for your accomplishments or to treat yourself for getting through a difficult day or situation.

Strategize If you feel you deserve a reward, you do. Perhaps you could start a reward fund. Each time you want to reward yourself, put a dollar or whatever amount you choose into the fund. At the end of the week, treat yourself to something special (besides food). If you feel you need a more immediate reward, turn on some music, treat yourself to a phone call with a friend, read your favorite magazine, or take a stretch break. Don't forget to tell yourself what a great job you did—even if no one else does.

Love

Food is often used to show love and affection. Mothers and grandmothers cook for their families, husbands bring chocolate to their wives, and couples gaze into each other's eyes over romantic dinners. Food and love have been intimately connected throughout history.

Strategize You can enjoy connecting with people you love over food while still using hunger and fullness to guide you. Also recognize whenever you're pushing food on others as a way to express love. Look for nonedible ways to give and receive affection: attention, words, touching, cards, and small gifts, among many others.

MINDFUL MOMENT: "I want a brownie" may really mean "I want love," "I want attention," "I want comfort," "I want rest," or "I want someone to listen to me."

Boredom

Eating can be a way to pass the time, occupy your attention, or put off starting a mundane or unpleasant task. Some people find themselves in front of the refrigerator when they're looking for something to do—or postponing something they need to do. Of course, as soon as you stop eating, you become bored again and so you eat again.

Strategize When you're bored and need something to do, remind yourself that eating is merely one of literally thousands of options. Review the section called "Redirecting Your Attention" in the previous chapter for great strategies. If you're eating as a way of procrastinating, break your task into small goals that don't seem as unpleasant or overwhelming.

Feeling Overwhelmed

Life places many demands on your energy and time; these demands are often exacerbated by unrealistic expectations and a sense of urgency. Eating can be a way of distracting or soothing yourself, but it often compounds the problem instead.

Strategize Respect your own personal strengths and limitations; learn to say no and do less. Make a list and prioritize what needs to be done. Increase the time you give yourself to do things and reduce the number of obligations and complications in your life. Make a conscious decision to slow down and become completely aware and focused on the moment and on one task at a time. You'll be more efficient, more effective, and more likely to notice life's little pleasures.

Stress

When you feel stressed out or don't have the skills you need to cope with stress, it takes a toll both physically and emotionally. This has a direct effect on your ability to manage your weight if you overeat in response to stress or use stress as an excuse for not exercising. The hormones produced during stress actually accelerate the storage of fat, another reason to learn to decrease and cope effectively with stress. Since you cannot get rid of stress completely, it's important to learn to manage it before it manages you.

Strategize Keep things in perspective by asking yourself two key questions: "What difference will this make one week or even one year from now?" and "Is this really important to me?" Create a buffer zone of self-care activities to make yourself more resilient and able to bounce back more easily from the stresses and demands of daily life. Don't waste time on "pseudo-relaxation" like watching TV; instead, use more-effective stress relievers like exercise, meditation, relaxation techniques, having fun, and connecting with friends and family. I'll share more self-care strategies in chapter 8.

Loneliness

Food is a loyal companion that doesn't ask much from you in return. However, food is a poor substitute for human interaction and relationships.

Strategize Combat loneliness by learning to enjoy your own company. Explore and expand your interests and work on your own personal development. Challenge yourself to deepen your existing relationships, and make new connections based on mutual interests. Spend time in places where you can meet and interact with other people who have similar interests. This might include work, community activities, religious organizations, hobbies, classes, clubs, sports, volunteering, and travel.

Worry and Tension

Feeling worried, nervous, or tense is common and can trigger overeating because of its temporary distracting or soothing effects. If you have anxiety that is frequent, persistent, or severe and out of proportion to the seriousness or likelihood of the feared event, you may have an underlying anxiety disorder. Please see your health care professional. For additional information about anxiety, see the Health Notes in the appendix.

Strategize Worrying about the past or the future robs you of the present. Ask yourself, "What can I realistically do to change this situation?" If there's a small step you *can* take, take it. If not, decide if you're willing to continue to focus on the thoughts even though they are causing discomfort. Worrying, like any habit, can be changed through awareness and making the choice to redirect your attention and energy.

Sadness

Feeling disappointed, unhappy, gloomy, depressed, hopeless, or grief-stricken may lead you to seek out food for comfort or distraction. Again, food cannot truly soothe your pain and will only distract you temporarily. If sadness is persistent or disruptive, you may have depression. Trying to manage your weight when you have untreated depression can be an uphill battle, so please see your health care professional.

For additional information about depression, see the Health Notes in the appendix.

Strategize When you're experiencing sadness, soothe and comfort yourself the way a loving parent might respond to a child. Be gentle, encouraging, and compassionate with yourself. Remember, even intense feelings will eventually dissipate as you allow yourself to experience them. If the feelings seem intolerable, try ways other than eating to comfort yourself. You may find it helpful to write in a journal, talk, pray, meditate, or just cry for a while.

Guilt and Shame

People sometimes overeat to punish themselves when they feel guilty or ashamed about their eating or about something else that happened—even something in the distant past.

Strategize Nobody's perfect, and acknowledging your mistakes makes it possible to learn valuable life lessons. If you're feeling guilty, ask yourself how your actions contributed to a particular situation. Pose the question this way: "If I knew then what I know now, and if I were operating at my best, what do I wish I would have done differently?" Rather than shaming yourself, this is an opportunity to accept appropriate responsibility, ask forgiveness, learn the lesson, and move on.

Anger

Anger is a normal emotion that ranges from annoyed, irritated, frustrated, and resentful to hostile, infuriated, and enraged. It often results from another emotion such as hurt, frustration, or fear of losing something or someone. Some people have been taught that anger is bad and they shouldn't feel it or show it, so they use food to stuff or express it instead. Eating can be a way to turn the anger against themselves or to punish someone else. However, when people stuff anger, it can erupt even more fiercely at a later time, often in response to an unrelated or minor event, affirming the belief that anger is bad.

Angela, a participant in our Facilitator Training, shared this insight.

> I've noticed that sometimes when I am feeling resentful about something, I reach for food as a sort of compensation. But if someone offered me food under those terms, I would never accept it. Just imagine someone saying, "Listen, I've decided to treat you unfairly, but I'm happy to buy off your bad feelings with this plate of goodies." Yet that's precisely what I'm doing each time I'm angry and I reach for food to soothe myself.

Strategize The next time you find yourself reaching for food to soothe anger from a hurt, an insult, or an injustice, ask yourself, "If this person offered me food to apologize for their action, would I take it?" Assure yourself that anger is a healthy feeling that should be expressed in a healthy way. That might include telling someone how you feel, writing an angry letter you don't intend to send, screaming into a pillow, or exerting yourself physically through exercise or a hobby like woodworking.

After dealing with difficult emotions like anger, it helps to shift gears by focusing on something that inspires the opposite feelings. For example, you could watch a funny movie or talk to a friend who always makes you happy. I remember feeling really angry when I was stuck in a traffic jam. I started digging around in my purse for a piece of candy when I suddenly realized that I was frustrated and worried about being late. I glanced around to make sure nobody was looking and then screamed a couple of times as loud as I could with the car windows rolled up. I immediately felt better and turned the radio from news to my favorite music station.

Avoidance

In avoidance eating, people eat to numb out emotional pain that they feel they can't resolve. Using food for sedation is similar to using drugs or alcohol to avoid experiencing feelings. Sometimes people eat to stay in denial about an important issue that's painful to address, such as whether to leave an unhappy marriage. People who avoid confrontation and conflict may also stuff feelings, thoughts, and opinions down with food rather than expressing themselves assertively. This can quickly take on an addictive quality and spiral into a pattern of abusing food.

Strategize FEAST is very helpful for identifying whatever you're trying to avoid. However, be quick to ask for help from your physician, counselor, therapist, or other trusted adviser if you're using food in an abusive manner. Take good care of yourself by seeking support and new skills when you need them.

Negative Self-Talk

Your beliefs and thoughts are the primary creator of your emotions, which then inspire your actions and lead to your results. Therefore, negative thinking leads to negative feelings and actions that create self-fulfilling results. For example, when your little voice says, "I can't do that," you'll feel inadequate, so you won't try, and therefore you prove that, indeed, you can't do it.

Your negative little voice may also serve up hypercritical messages to try to keep you in line. However, you're not motivated long term by criticism from yourself or others. As a result, you probably won't do your best, which only proves that your inner critic was right—and leads to more harsh criticism and feelings of inadequacy and hopelessness.

Strategize The first step in developing a more positive internal dialogue is to begin to notice, without judgment, what you're thinking and how it impacts your feelings and your resulting behaviors. You'll probably recognize that much of your self-talk is inaccurate, overly harsh, ineffective, or limiting. (For more examples of negative self-talk, see chapter 18.) Observing your thought patterns can help you see what is driving the feelings that lead you to overeat.

Once you recognize the internal conversations behind your feelings, actions, and results, you can choose to change your self-talk. Try using the nurturing voice you use when speaking to people you care about (especially children). It's gentle, reassuring, and understanding without being critical or judgmental. Practice using this kinder voice to generate the feelings, behaviors, and results you really want.

Perfectionistic Thinking

Expecting perfection from yourself or others guarantees that you'll never be satisfied. The frustration that results from missing the mark can lead to overeating. While it's important to do your best, perfection isn't possible or necessary. Constantly striving for it just chews up your time and energy.

Strategize Ask yourself: "Is there a more reasonable expectation I could have about this situation or myself? What would be a more realistic and empowering way of talking to myself about this?" Be flexible and willing to make mistakes since they are an opportunity for learning and growth.

Communicating with Body Size

Different cultures have different standards and associate different meanings with body size. For example, in some cultures, men are expected to be big because it's seen as a sign of strength or prosperity. In other cultures, large or "curvy" women are seen as sexy.

Sometimes people eat (or don't eat) to communicate information to others with their body size. For example, a large body may be a way of telling other people that you are powerful and strong, that you don't want to be ignored, or that you don't want to be noticed or approached.

Strategize Consider whether you eat to maintain a certain body size or shape because of cultural messages, even if it isn't what *you* want. Are there other ways you can honor your culture without disregarding your personal wishes and health?

Using your body to communicate other messages to those around you is a fairly complicated issue and one that you may wish to explore with a counselor or therapist. The goal is to learn to communicate your needs, wants, and boundaries in the most effective ways possible.

Diet Mentality

Diet thinking is a powerful trigger for overeating. You may feel virtuous for eating allowed foods and guilty for eating illegal foods. Your little voice will say you *should, shouldn't, must, ought, always,* or *never.* This usually backfires because when you don't do what you think you should, you'll feel guilty and rebellious. Moreover, restriction can cause you to become more sensitive to the sight and aroma of food. You may develop powerful cravings and say you're "hungry all the time." Ironically, diet thinking is often a way of avoiding or coping with emotions, just as overeating often is. When you're obsessing about food rules and weight, you can't focus on meeting your true needs.

Be sure you haven't turned this process into a diet, too. In other words, don't beat yourself up when you eat even though you aren't hungry; that will have the same effect as diet thinking. Eating is a legitimate option when you're in charge.

Strategize Develop a whole new relationship with food, one built on satisfaction and health, not guilt and shame. Instead of rules, practice using hunger and satisfaction to guide when and how much you eat. There are no good or bad foods; you make the best decisions for yourself when you consider the principles of balance, variety, and moderation. Try to use words that indicate a choice such as *could, can, may, prefer,* and *sometimes.* For example: "I can choose to eat (fill in the blank) if I want it" or "I'd prefer to eat a salad" or "I'll make healthy choices for myself, but I'll make them because I want to, not because I have to."

Eating Disorders

Eating disorders such as anorexia nervosa, bulimia, and binge eating are important and treatable medical problems. Symptoms may include starving yourself, bingeing, purging by forcing yourself to vomit, using laxatives, or exercising excessively. For additional information about eating disorders, see the Health Notes in the appendix.

Strategize If you experience symptoms of an eating disorder, seek help from a doctor or therapist immediately.

Negative Body Image

The obsession with thinness in our society often leads to distorted, irrational, and unrealistic beliefs about your weight and your body. Body bashing and wearing clothes that make you feel uncomfortable can also lead to a negative body image, which in turn can lead to overeating.

Weighing yourself too often can lead to negative feelings that lead to overeating. People sometimes eat when they've gained weight, but they also eat to celebrate weight loss. Weighing yourself too often may also cause you to focus on a number on the scale rather than your behaviors and how you feel.

Strategize When your little voice begins to say unkind things, ask, "Would I say these things to a friend?" If you wouldn't, don't say them to yourself either. What can you do or say instead that would help you feel good about yourself? Remind yourself that all bodies are okay, including yours. Wear clothes that make you feel comfortable and attractive, and always focus your attention on your best attributes—and not just the physical ones.

If you feel it's helpful to weigh yourself, limit it to just once a week or even once a month. Focus on your decisions and other personal measures to let you know whether you're developing new healthier habits. See Strategies: Don't Measure Your Self-Worth in chapter 9.

Spiritual Needs

When people have unmet spiritual needs, they may experience a vague longing for something. They may be searching for meaning or purpose in their life but reach for food to fill the void instead.

Strategize Prayer, meditation, worship, and reading inspirational works will help you connect spiritually. You may also wish to seek out a faith community or a guide to help you on your spiritual journey.

When a craving doesn't come from hunger, eating will never satisfy it—but your cravings can be a powerful source of information about your true needs and wants. Remind yourself to think first by putting a sign on your refrigerator that says "If you're not hungry, what you need isn't in here." Sometimes eating is a response to a deep-seated emotional issue, but most of the time it's a habit—a way of coping with the demands of daily life or an attempt to bring yourself back into balance. Once you've identified the cues and emotions that trigger your urges to eat, you can gradually find ways to distract, comfort, calm, and nurture yourself without turning to food.

CHAPTER 5

FEARLESS EATING

used to worry a lot about what I "should" eat. Depending on what year it was, I worried about calories, exchanges, fat grams, or points. I couldn't even enjoy a cookie without wondering how many minutes it would take to burn off the calories. My favorite part of relearning to eat instinctively is the freedom I have now to eat whatever I want. And the irony is that now that I can eat whatever I want, I make healthier choices more often than I used to.

Let me give you an example. I had an early flight for a speaking engagement, but I wasn't hungry when I left my house. By the time I checked in at the airport and made it through security, I was in the mood for my usual bowl of cereal with fruit and milk— or at least something crunchy, cold, and fresh. Apparently that sort of thing isn't a big seller at the airport because all I could find were hot egg-and-sausage sandwiches, bagels, Danishes, bruised apples, and giant chocolate chip cookies. I was wishing I had taken the time to pack something to eat for the four-hour flight. In my old eat-repent-repeat cycle, I would have used this as an excuse to have the giant cookie even though it wasn't what I really wanted. As I moved up to the counter, I saw a woman assembling chicken Caesar salads for the lunch rush. Crunchy, cold, and fresh. That would do!

I got some strange looks while I was eating my salad on the airplane at eight in the morning, but it was delicious, and I didn't care. The truth is, if I had really wanted a giant cookie, I would have eaten that without caring what anyone thought either.

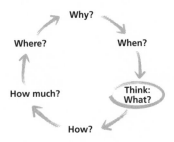

WHAT DO I EAT?

So you're hungry. Good. Now you get to decide what to eat.

At this point, I could give you a list of allowed foods and portion sizes to choose from, but then you'd be right back where you were on your last diet. Instead, think of Tom and Angie from chapter 1, two people who eat instinctively. What would they do?

They would eat what they want.

You might be thinking, "That's fine for them since they're thin, but I seem to want only 'bad' food." Life is different now. All foods can fit into a healthy diet; you get to choose what you'll eat. Let's take a look at what Angie ate in one day.

I ate my favorite breakfast, fiber cereal with fruit and low-fat yogurt and a cup of coffee. I put a Crock-Pot of beans on before I left the house and packed up the casserole I was taking to the office for our holiday potluck. As usual, I was hungry again by mid-morning, so I decided to eat half of one of the oranges that I keep at my desk. At lunch, I looked over everything on the buffet table, and just as I expected, my coworkers brought all kinds of delicious things to eat. There was a veggie platter with dip, chips and salsa, a colorful spinach salad, a Crock-Pot of chili, two casseroles—including the one I brought—and two of my favorite desserts. I chose chips and salsa, spinach salad, a small amount of the other casserole, and half of a serving of each of the desserts. I wasn't hungry for my usual afternoon snack that day, so I was glad the beans were ready when I got home. All I had to do was throw together a salad and dinner was ready.

Let's take a closer look at how and why Angie made her decisions.

Angie has a weekday breakfast routine that is nutrient rich and that she feels keeps her regular. She took a few minutes in the morning to start something for dinner so it would be ready when she got home. She always makes a point of having healthy food available at her desk to eat when she gets hungry, but that day she ate only half of her orange, wanting to be sure she was hungry for the potluck.

At the potluck, Angie didn't try to take a little of everything. Even though she loves vegetables and tries to eat plenty to keep her healthy, she didn't bother with the veggies and dip because she can get those anytime and she didn't want to be too full to try the desserts. She skipped the chili because she was already planning to have beans for dinner and too many make her feel bloated. The spinach salad was both healthy and delicious, so that was an easy decision for her. She passed on her own casserole, knowing there would probably be leftovers she could have for lunch the next day. She loves sweets, so she was careful to save room for dessert. She skipped her afternoon snack because she wasn't hungry after her larger-than-normal lunch, but she was hungry again by dinnertime.

The most effective way to make permanent healthy lifestyle changes is to learn to eat according to your body's signals and to eat as healthfully as possible without feeling deprived. This balance can be achieved when you use reliable nutrition information in making your food choices while still having the freedom to eat what you love without judging yourself or feeling guilty. Choosing food this way meets your natural need for nourishment and enjoyment.

Although Angie didn't need to analyze each of her decisions, they can be summarized by three questions:

- What do I want?
- What do I need?
- What do I have?

You can use these questions to help you make food choices that are healthful and satisfying.

WHAT DO I WANT?

Most of the time when you're hungry, a specific food, flavor, or texture will come to mind. As you get used to listening to your body's signals, you'll begin to recognize what type of food or taste will match your particular hunger at that time. Kim gave us a good example of why this is important.

> I was hungry and I really wanted a few of the chocolate chip cookies I bought for my kids' lunches. I've been trying to lose weight, so I decided to eat rice cakes instead. At first I felt good about it, but I just didn't feel completely satisfied. I decided to eat some yogurt, then I ate some baby carrots, and then some cheese. I took a few bites out of the ice cream carton, then a few more—for some reason, I always feel like I have to level off the top. I finally gave in and had the chocolate chip cookies after all. I felt so guilty that I ended up eating almost half the package before my kids came home. Afterward, I felt sick and thought, "What did I accomplish here?" It would have been better to eat a few chocolate chips cookies in the first place and really enjoy them while I was actually hungry.

Satisfaction is not just physical fullness. Satisfaction comes from enjoying the food you eat. When you don't eat the food you really want, you may overeat other foods then eventually get around to eating what you wanted anyway. But when you match the food you choose to what you're hungry for, you'll experience greater satisfaction and more enjoyment—with less food.

If a specific food doesn't come to mind, try to identify what you're hungry for by asking yourself these questions:

- What taste do I want—sweet, salty, sour, spicy, or bitter?
- What texture do I want—crunchy, creamy, smooth, or juicy?
- What temperature do I want—hot, moderate, cold, or frozen?
- What type of food do I want—light, heavy, or in-between?
- Do I want a certain category of food—protein, vegetables, or bread?
- Is there a specific food I have been craving?

> **MINDFUL MOMENT:** Get rid of guilt and make eating for enjoyment an intentional decision.

As you learn to ask yourself what you want, you'll discover that your body has wisdom. Listen to what Gary had to say.

> When you said, "Ask yourself what you want," I was sure all I would eat was steak and potatoes—and I did, for a couple of days. Then I noticed I actually wanted a salad sometimes. By the end of the week, I was eating chicken, trout, fruit, soup, and even quiche. It was exciting to see what my taste buds would come up with next.

I've found that, like Gary, most people eventually gravitate toward balance, variety, and moderation when they begin to ask themselves what they really want.

Eat What You Love

Let's face it. Food is wonderful. It's truly one of life's many pleasures. Enjoying food is only a problem if it's your *primary* source of pleasure.

The purpose of letting go of restrictive eating is to remove the false sense of value you place on certain foods. In essence, by letting go of the guilt, you eliminate the power that certain foods have over you. Amazingly, your desire to overeat them usually diminishes.

The key to eliminating guilt is to give yourself unconditional permission to eat any food. This means you place all foods on an even playing field where the choice to eat cake evokes no more guilt than the choice to eat an apple. In order to eat without guilt, strive to:

- Stop thinking of certain foods as "good" and others as "bad."
- Eat what you really want, paying attention to your body's natural signals.
- Eat without having to pay penance (as in, "I'll eat this today, but I'll diet the rest of the week," or "I'll eat this now, but I'll have to spend more time exercising tonight.").

Change Your Little Voice

Even when you know that deprivation has led to overeating in the past, you may still be afraid to ask yourself what you're hungry for. If you've been stuck in an eat-repent-repeat cycle, you may doubt that you can freely choose to eat what you want without losing control. But remember: as you learn to eat instinctively again, you no longer have to be in control, just in charge.

What does your little voice say that can get in the way? Your beliefs and thoughts ultimately cause you to make certain decisions. By recognizing when your little voice is derailing your intention with fear-based thinking, you can begin to think more fearless, empowering thoughts. Let's look at some examples.

Fear-Based Thoughts vs. Fearless Thoughts

Fear-based: I won't make healthy choices. You may be worried that if you ask yourself what you want, you'll always want sweets, fried food, or other foods you've tried to avoid. Initially, that may be true, especially if you've felt deprived.

Fearless: I enjoy a variety of healthy, satisfying foods. Once you let go of the guilt about eating certain things, you'll gradually discover that you want a variety of foods to help you feel healthy and satisfied. Once you stop labeling foods as good or bad, you can develop a greater appreciation for the taste of fresh healthful ingredients instead of seeing them as diet foods. In addition, you'll notice you feel better physically and emotionally with a balance of nutritious foods, and your body will actually begin to crave them.

Fear-based: I should feel guilty when I eat what I love. Many popular food and diet ads feed into the fear that eating for pleasure is sinful and that you should eat only foods that are "guilt free."

Fearless: I eat what I love, and I love what I eat. In the long run, you'll be more satisfied if you choose a variety of foods you like and allow yourself to enjoy them without guilt.

Fear-based: I really shouldn't be eating this. You are just giving yourself "pseudo-permission" if you don't really believe you can eat certain foods. When you choose a food you think you shouldn't, instead of fully enjoying it, you'll be planning to pay penance by exercising more, skipping a snack or a meal, or eating "light" to make up for it. Since you never really gave yourself permission to eat what you wanted, you'll continue to feel out of control, you'll overeat, and you'll punish yourself for it—the eat-repent-repeat cycle.

Fearless: I choose balance, variety, and moderation in my eating. Give yourself unconditional permission to allow all foods in your diet. If you repeatedly overeat a particular food, notice what you are thinking and feeling. You may be in a subconscious Restrictive Eating cycle and setting yourself up for overeating. All foods can fit into a balanced diet, so allow your common sense to guide your food choices by using the simple principles of balance, variety, and moderation.

Fear-based: I'll use the Hunger and Fullness Scale to control my eating. Feeling guilty if you eat when you're not hungry or judging yourself for eating past a 5 or a 6 is no different from dieting. This form of restrictive eating will lead to the same eat-repent-repeat cycle.

Fearless: I am in charge of all my decisions, including when I eat. When you want to eat, ask yourself, "Am I hungry?" knowing that you can choose to eat whether you are or not. Since being in charge means taking responsibility, you're free to choose to eat or overeat if you want, as long as you acknowledge the possible consequences and decide that for a given situation, the consequences are worth it.

Fear-based: I can't trust myself. You may believe you're addicted to certain foods and feel afraid that you won't be able to stop eating them if you start. This is a self-fulfilling prophecy because once you have even a bite, your mind

MINDFUL MOMENT: When you are free to eat whatever you want, food quickly loses its power over you. You are able to eat *anything*, without eating *everything*.

automatically prepares for a binge. Depriving yourself of certain foods gives them power over you; in fact, it causes the strong cravings in the first place. This lack of self-trust comes from a history of cycling between overeating and restrictive eating.

Fearless: I trust myself to eat in a way that nourishes my body, mind, and spirit.   When you know those previously forbidden foods will always be allowed, the urgency to eat them in large quantities eventually diminishes. Research has shown that people get tired of eating the same kind of food over time, even foods they love. Follow the steps outlined in "Strategies: Fearless Eating." Experiment with different foods and decide what foods you'll choose to eat based on how you respond.

STRATEGIES: FEARLESS EATING

Are there foods that you'd love to be able to eat without guilt or without binge-ing? If so, the following strategies for fearless eating will help you rebuild trust in your ability to listen to your body wisdom. These steps will help you try out one previously forbidden food at a time and eat it regularly until it loses its magic and goes back to just being delicious. Move through the steps at a pace that's comfortable for you.

- Make a list of your "forbidden foods," foods you enjoy but generally restrict yourself from eating.
- Choose one of the foods from your list and give yourself full permission to eat it when you're hungry and you *really, really, really, really* want it. This is the "four really" test.

- When you're hungry and decide you want that food (it passes the four really test), buy, prepare, or order one serving.

- Eat the food mindfully, without distractions, and focus on the aroma, appearance, flavor, and texture as you eat. You'll learn more strategies for mindful eating in the next chapter.

- Does the food taste as good as you imagined it would? Sometimes you'll discover it isn't as good as you thought it would be; you may even decide not to finish it or that you won't bother with it in the future. If you love it, continue to give yourself permission to buy or order it whenever you want.

- You may decide to keep enough of that food in your house so you know it'll be there if you want it. For some people, however, keeping certain foods in the house can feel too scary. In that case, promise yourself you'll purchase and prepare only as much as you'll need for one sitting or you'll go to a restaurant and order it when you want it.

- Don't be surprised if you want that food frequently at first; that's normal. Relax; the cravings will decrease when you realize the food is no longer forbidden.

- This strategy is also helpful if you find yourself obsessing about a particular food.

- When you're ready, choose another food from your list and practice the process again.

- If you find yourself overeating certain foods, ask yourself, "What was I thinking when I was eating it?" Thoughts like, "I shouldn't eat this," or "I'm going to eat it all in case I don't get another chance," can continue to drive overeating. Remember, you're in charge now, so replace those thoughts with more powerful, fearless thoughts.

- Repeat these steps regularly to banish the fear that you're not in charge of your eating.

When you give yourself unconditional permission to eat what you want, you'll notice that food quickly loses the power and strong attraction it once had. You'll begin to trust that you can choose from among all the wonderful food choices available when you're hungry. You won't have to stock up in anticipation of your next round of self-denial. Amazingly, you'll also find that you make healthier choices and feel more satisfied with less food.

WHAT DO I NEED?

Food decisions are neither good nor bad, but clearly, some foods offer more nutritional benefits than others. As you consider what food to choose, ask yourself, "What does my body need?"

Food fuels your body. It's wonderful to enjoy the food you choose, but keep in mind that the main purpose for eating is to provide your body with the energy and nutrients it needs to function at its best. Since your body is the finest, most complex machine ever created, it performs best and lasts longest with top-of-the-line fuel.

So, how do you implement this in your daily life? Paul explains how he did it.

It was great knowing that I'd never have to diet again. But that didn't mean I wasn't interested in eating more healthfully. As I learned more about carbohydrates, I wondered if I was eating enough fiber. I wrote down everything I ate and was surprised I was getting only about 10 grams of fiber a day—not even close to the recommended 30 grams a day. My "healthy" low-fat puffed rice cereal had only 1 gram of fiber per serving! The next time we went shopping, I looked for higher-fiber cereal and bought whole wheat pasta, wild rice, and whole-grain bread. I was already eating a lot of vegetables, but I switched to eating fruit instead of drinking juice. Within a month, I had gradually increased my fiber intake by almost 20 grams without adding any more food—in fact, I felt fuller with less food. The other bonus was, and don't laugh, I noticed I was going to the bathroom more regularly. I just feel better eating this way.

Nourish Yourself

Food can be used to your advantage when you learn to balance eating for nourishment with eating for enjoyment. Use the following strategies to help you with that process:

Make small, gradual changes. Forget "all or nothing." Healthy eating is simply the result of all the little positive decisions you make.

Choose food based on balance, variety, and moderation. Ask yourself what else you have been eating and what you are likely to eat later. Examples of helpful questions include: "Have I eaten a variety of fruits and vegetables today? Have I been eating a lot of junk food or fast food lately? Do I eat too much protein or not enough? Do I feel tired when I eat too many carbohydrates in one meal? Have I been practicing balance, variety, and moderation over the last few days?" Your answers to questions like these will help you decide which foods you could choose to meet your nutritional needs. (We'll discuss balance, variety, and moderation further in chapter 10.)

Eat for overall health, not just weight management. Health and weight management are not the same thing. In fact, as long as you eat fewer calories than your body burns, you'll lose weight no matter which foods you choose. However, your physical health and vitality would suffer if you chose to eat only potato chips and candy bars—or for that matter, just lettuce and apples. Eating like that would violate the principles of balance, variety, and moderation. More important, it's unlikely that your body's innate wisdom would tell you to eat that way for very long.

Learn about nutrition. Use nutrition information to make informed decisions, not to deprive and punish yourself or to make you feel guilty. Surprisingly, once you know how one appealing food compares to another, you'll often find yourself preferring the more nutritious food.

MINDFUL MOMENT: Nutrition information is a tool, not a weapon.

The chapters in part 2, "Nourish," provide information to help you understand the nutritional aspect of food. Without a doubt, science will continue to discover new and important information about nutrition and health. In fact, things are changing so rapidly in this field that even credible information from reliable sources may evolve and change over time. Find accurate and authoritative sources for nutrition information to keep up-to-date.

Be sure to examine how the information you learn applies to your life. Just because you hear or read something doesn't automatically mean you need to make a change. If you are unsure, your health care professional or a dietitian can help guide you through the maze of all the nutrition information that's available.

Consider your personal health needs. Take an honest inventory of your health. What specific issues do you need to consider when deciding what to eat? Think about the following issues and talk to your health care professional or a dietitian for specific recommendations if needed:

- Medical history (especially diabetes, high cholesterol, high blood pressure, risk of cancer)
- Family history (especially diabetes, high cholesterol, high blood pressure, cancer, heart disease)
- Allergies and reactions to certain foods (for instance, rashes, fatigue, digestive problems)
- Your health goals (for instance, fitness or weight loss)

Be willing to try new foods. You just might surprise yourself! It can take several tries of a new food to acquire a taste for it, but some of my favorite foods now are things I thought I wouldn't like. Don't persist in forcing yourself to eat foods you don't like, however, since that can backfire.

Make it taste great. Enjoy healthy choices by focusing on fresh foods, appealing combinations, new flavors, and interesting recipes. For example, learn to prepare healthy foods in exciting, delicious ways and learn to prepare your favorites in healthier ways by adjusting the ingredients or cooking method. (My family and I have shared some of our favorite recipes with you in part 4, "Eat.")

Look for healthful alternatives. Always ask yourself, "Is there a healthy choice that will meet my needs without leaving me feeling deprived?" For instance, could you be happy with frozen yogurt instead of ice cream this time? While eating out, could you decide to skip the fried appetizers and just enjoy the main course, order a great salad instead of a burger, or ask for a substitute for a less-healthy side dish with your favorite meal? Make it a habit to choose more healthful foods unless you feel you really need to eat a particular food to feel satisfied.

Keep an awareness journal. You may find it helpful to keep a journal for a while to help you recognize patterns and identify areas that you want to improve. Many of the people I work with initially say they hate the thought of journaling because it reminds them of a diet. The difference, however, is that an awareness journal is used to make connections between what you eat and how you feel (and for that matter, how you feel and what you eat) rather than tracking and accountability. Perfection is not necessary; you'll learn something about yourself even if you journal intermittently.

Become aware of how you feel after you eat. Notice how long certain foods stay with you, whether you feel more energetic or sluggish after eating certain foods, and whether any foods cause uncomfortable symptoms. To put this into practical terms, here's what Beverly noticed.

> I woke up late on Monday. I grabbed a cup of coffee with cream and sugar and headed out the door. On my way to work I noticed I was hungry, but I realized I'd been in such a hurry that I left my breakfast on the counter at home. I ate a glazed doughnut when I got to work. An hour later my hunger pangs came back so I had a small carton of orange juice. It seemed like I was hungry the rest of the morning. I had trouble concentrating and felt irritable.

What was going on? Throughout the morning Beverly had eaten low-fiber sugary foods, some fat, and an insignificant amount of protein. As a result, her blood sugars were spiking and dropping. If Beverly continued this pattern of eating, it would go on all day.

> On Tuesday, I woke up in time to have a cup of coffee and half a whole wheat bagel with peanut butter. I didn't get hungry again for over three hours. I ate a turkey sandwich and a cup of vegetable soup for lunch and almonds and grapes in the middle of the afternoon. I felt great all day.

What could account for the difference? The bagel, containing more fiber than the simple carbohydrates in the doughnut, along with the fat and protein from the peanut butter, helped slow down the rise in her blood sugar and her subsequent insulin response. This resulted in a more stable blood sugar, which contributed to her improved mood, attention, performance, and decreased hunger. It's just one example of how paying attention to the way your body responds to certain types and amounts of food will help you feel your best and meet your nutritional needs.

Resist restrictive diets. Without a doubt, you'll continue to hear about many wonder diets that promise amazing results. You may even be tempted to try one. Before you do, carefully examine the premise and science behind it. A good rule of thumb is this: If it sounds too good to be true, it is! Linda learned this lesson and shared it with the group.

> I loved being in charge of my eating, and I was seeing slow but steady progress in the way I looked and felt. However, when my daughter announced she was getting married in two months, I decided to do something more drastic to lose weight for the wedding. Someone at work was selling diet shakes and supplements, so I spent about $80 on a two-week supply. I lost four pounds in ten days, but I gained back five before the wedding! It took me a couple of months to get back on track again. The next time I want to speed up my weight loss, I'll bump up my exercise, work a little harder on eating fewer sweets and more vegetables, and be sure that I'm using hunger and fullness to guide me.

Be open to dietary guidance and more structure if needed. There's nothing wrong with making a decision to follow a specific dietary plan—after all, you're in charge. It's sensible to explore new ways of eating that are sound and make sense.

You may have a medical reason for following a specific dietary plan or find you need more structure and predetermined limits in order to lose weight. Just be sure to let hunger, satisfaction, and common sense guide you. A good rule of thumb here is this: If you can't imagine eating a certain way for the rest of your life, don't bother doing it for even a day.

Robert used the structure of a diet plan to help him.

> I understood instinctive eating, but I was still having difficulty staying on track, so I wasn't losing weight. Although I could never stick with a diet for very long before, I decided to try one again, this time using my hunger and fullness signals to guide me. What a difference! I used the diet to help me choose what foods to eat, but I didn't starve or deprive myself. I really feel I'm learning what it takes to manage my weight for life.

When it comes to eating for health, being in charge means taking personal responsibility for your food choices. Combine your knowledge of nutrition with your personal lifestyle and preferences to choose food that works best for you and your overall health.

WHAT DO I HAVE?

This step can be summarized with one word: planning. Having a variety of foods available is critical if you're going to learn to use hunger to guide your eating. If you feel hungry and the only food available is from a vending machine, you're likely to choose a snack that may not be very healthy, may not taste very good, and may not really be what you were hungry for anyway.

Recall that Angie had the ingredients for the breakfast she enjoys, started dinner before she left for work, and kept fruit at her desk to eat when she was hungry.

MINDFUL MOMENT: You are responsible for having food available for you to eat when you're hungry.

Be Prepared

The key is to keep a variety of foods available.

- Stock your home, workplace, and even your car, purse, or briefcase with different types of foods that meet the types of cravings you get.

- Ideas include fresh fruit and precut vegetables, dried fruit, whole grain crackers, pretzels, popcorn, packages of oatmeal, yogurt, string cheese, nuts, hard-boiled eggs, and cans of tuna or slices of turkey or lean roast beef. This way, you'll always have something satisfying available.

- Buy or separate the food into appropriate, convenient portions. Small snack bags work great for this.

- Focus on healthful options that you enjoy when you're hungry but that won't be calling out to you from their storage place saying, "I'm in here! Come eat me!"

- You may also decide to keep small amounts of chocolate or other favorite treats around when you're ready. Practice the "Strategies: Fearless Eating" outlined previously. If certain foods are too challenging for you to stop eating even when you're comfortably satisfied, introduce them more slowly.

- You're not always in charge of what is available, but you're still in charge of what and how much you choose. When you're eating from a menu or buffet, decide what you want and need first and then survey your options to see what will fit best.

Margo had a great way to be prepared at work.

> I used to eat out for lunch nearly every day, mostly because it was convenient. I knew I was spending a lot of money and I wasn't making the best choices for my health, so I decided to start taking my lunch to work. At the beginning of the week I bring a small grocery bag full of lunch items like soup, lunchmeat and whole wheat bread, frozen dinners, crackers, yogurt, fruit, precut veggies, and even a few snack-size candy bars. Now, no matter what I'm in the mood for, I can find something satisfying and I'm not as tempted to run out for a burger and fries.

If you're not used to choosing food mindfully and fearlessly, you may find it challenging at first. With practice, these strategies allow you to make choices that satisfy your body and your mind. Eating food you love while taking good care of your health is the best way to feel fully nourished.

CHAPTER 6

MINDFUL EATING

My husband and I visited wine country in Napa Valley with our friends. For us, it was heaven on earth. The scenery was breathtaking: rolling green hills, stands of huge trees, and perfectly symmetrical rows of grapes in carefully chosen valleys and on sunny hillsides. Through an old vine-covered building we entered hand-dug wine caves extending far into the rock. Our tour guide led us into the long, cool cave where subtle candlelight illuminated the wine barrels stacked as far as we could see.

Our guide handed us each a large wineglass that rang when we clinked them together. He approached one of his favorite barrels, uncorked it, and used a long glass "wine thief" to siphon samples and release them into our glasses. We swirled and sniffed and sipped the wine as he told us about where the grapes were grown and about the winemaker's passion for his craft. Later we tasted thin slices of fresh Parmesan cheese, small bits of dark chocolate, and sweet rich port as we admired the unusual art collection in the lobby.

Though not for everybody, this was mindfulness at its absolute best. We were thoroughly engrossed and swept away by this multisensory experience. Though food was just a small part of it, I can strive to make every meal I eat as satisfying as that was.

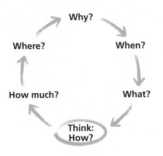

HOW DO I EAT?

You're now more aware about the decisions you need to make about *why*, *when*, and *what* you eat. Now decide *how* you'll eat.

Ironically, many people who struggle with their weight say they love food, but they don't eat in a way that shows they love food. Do you eat quickly, barely tasting what you're eating? Do you eat too fast to notice how full you're getting? Do you eat while you are watching TV, reading the newspaper, driving, or working? How often do you feel stuffed when you're finished eating? Do you ever finish something and wish you could have just one more bite? Have you ever eaten something and not even remembered it?

These are all clear signs of mindless or unconscious eating. Your brain and body cannot process information fully when you eat too quickly or when you're distracted by something else.

On the other hand, think about one of your most memorable eating experiences. How would you describe where you were, who you were with, what you talked about, what the ambience was like, what the food looked and smelled like, how it tasted, and how you felt while you were eating and afterward?

How often do you have eating experiences like that? How often would you like to have experiences like that? Mindfulness changes eating into a memorable, multisensory experience.

Love What You Eat

Eating is a natural, healthy, and pleasurable activity when you're eating to satisfy hunger. Choosing to eat mindfully—that is, eating with *intention* and *attention*—will give you optimal enjoyment and satisfaction from eating.

MINDFUL MOMENT: If you love what you eat, act like it.

Eat with *intention*. Be purposeful when you eat.

- Eat when you're truly hungry.
- Eat to meet your body's needs.
- Eat with the goal of feeling *better* when you're finished.

Eat with *attention*. Devote your full attention to eating.

- Eliminate or minimize distractions.
- Tune into the ambience, flavors, smells, temperature, and texture of the food.
- Listen to your body's cues of hunger and fullness.

When you eat with the intention of caring for yourself, you'll feel content, not deprived. When you pay attention, you'll enjoy the eating experience more while eating less.

Mindful eating helps you recognize the difference between physical satisfaction and fullness. When you eat on autopilot, you may only become aware when you're overly full. But at comfortable satiety, a 5 or 6 on the Hunger and Fullness Scale, your stomach may be just slightly distended. At that point, you could eat more, but your body isn't asking for it. Because it's a very subtle feeling of stomach fullness (less obvious than the signal to start eating) you must listen to your body carefully or you'll miss it. This is one place where mindfulness comes in.

Another benefit of mindful eating is that you'll notice how you feel, both physically and emotionally, when you eat certain foods, eat in certain environments, or eat in certain ways. This may affect your future choices about eating. However, it's important to observe how you eat from a neutral perspective. In other words, don't judge or punish yourself for the way you eat. Instead, use your heightened awareness to increase your satisfaction from eating. Here's how Donna explained it.

I always said I couldn't lose weight because I love food and eating too much. But as I look back on my eating, I can't see how I could have, really. I can remember so many times I ate dinner while I watched television, and the next day I could barely remember what I ate, much less how it tasted. I'd finish off a large bucket of popcorn at the movies, but I'd want just one more bite when it was gone because I'd eaten it without even noticing. Sometimes I'd eat something that tasted so fantastic that I just kept eating it. I don't think I really even tasted it after the first few bites. I think my mission was to finish it, not enjoy it. When I ate a really great meal, I'd usually ruin it by being so full when I was done that I felt miserable and guilty.

When I decided to start paying more attention to how I ate, I discovered a whole new world. I realized some of the foods I used to eat all the time don't really taste that great. Now I love to try new foods, new flavors, and new combinations. We go to new restaurants as much to experience the ambience as to eat the food. Eating has become a sensual experience for me. And surprisingly, I don't eat nearly as much as I did before—I just don't need to.

During our workshops we practice mindful eating by going out to dinner together or having a mindful eating potluck. Nearly everyone says that the experience has a huge impact on the way they eat. You too can experience eating with intention and attention by practicing these steps for mindful eating, either by yourself or with a friend over dinner.

Once again we're using the Eating Cycle as your guide for eating mindfully. If you have not learned the steps in the cycle already, this would be a good time to commit them to memory. That way you can easily recall them as you practice instinctive eating.

MINDFUL MOMENT: Set your intention to feel better when you've finished eating than when you started.

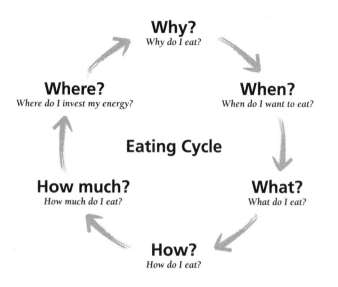

Why? *Acknowledge why you're eating.* Are you eating for fuel, nutrition, pleasure, convenience, or because of a physical, environmental, or emotional trigger? Why you're eating will affect every other decision in your Eating Cycle. Even when you're eating instinctively, certain situations, social occasions, and emotions will affect what, how, and how much you eat. When you're aware of why you're eating, you're more in charge of the rest of the decisions you make.

When? *Focus.* Get in the habit of checking in with yourself several times a day to see where you are on the Hunger and Fullness Scale. Begin eating when you feel significantly hungry (a 2 or a 3), but try not to wait until you're famished (a 1). One of the keys to conscious eating is to keep your body adequately fed to decrease the risk of overeating.

Set your intention. Decide how full you want to be at the end of eating. For example, if you're really working on losing weight, you might decide you'll stop at a 5. On the other hand, if it's a special occasion or special food, you might decide it's worth being a little uncomfortable afterward, so you plan to stop at a 7. Remember, you're in charge of how much you'll eat, but if you don't have a plan, you're more likely to eat more than you want or need.

What? *Choose food that will satisfy both your body and your mind.* To get the optimum level of satisfaction from your food and therefore eat less, remember to ask yourself these three questions: "What do I want?" "What do I need?" and "What do I have?" Because this is contrary to most of the usual diet rules it takes some practice. Review chapter 5 if necessary.

How? *Create a pleasant environment.* A pleasant ambience adds to your enjoyment and satisfaction from eating. Even when you're preparing food for yourself, make it attractive, as if you were serving it to someone special (you are!). Set the table, turn on music, and light candles, perhaps. Even a frozen dinner looks more appealing on a nice plate.

Minimize distractions. If you eat while you're distracted by watching television, reading, driving, working, or talking on the telephone, you won't be able to give your food or your body's signals your full attention. Some people have told me they get bored when they "just eat." That's particularly true as your hunger begins to fade, so use boredom as a signal that it's time to stop.

Sit down. Don't eat while standing over the sink, peering into the refrigerator, or propped up in bed. Instead, choose one or two places at home and at work for eating. This breaks or prevents the formation of triggers associated with other locations and minimizes distractions.

Purchase, prepare, or serve only the amount of food you think you'll need. With practice, you'll be able to predict how much food it will take to fill you up at different levels of hunger. If someone else fills your plate, visually determine how much you think you'll need and move or remove the excess. If you're at a restaurant, you may want to ask for a to-go container before you start eating.

Create a speed bump. Once you have the amount of food you think you'll need, physically divide it in half on your plate to remind yourself to stop halfway and check in again. This little "speed bump" will slow you down and serve as a reminder to become mindful again if you've lost your focus. When you reach that point, you'll stop eating for a couple of minutes to reconnect with your hunger and fullness level.

MINDFUL MOMENT: If you are distracetd when you eat, you may feel full but not satisfied.

Center yourself. Take a few deep breaths to calm and center yourself before you begin eating. This will help you slow down and give eating your full attention. If you're upset, anxious, or excited, take some time to calm down before you eat. Likewise, avoid having stressful conversations at the dinner table.

Express gratitude. In your way, take a moment to reflect on and give thanks for your food and the nourishment it provides, as well as the other blessings in your life.

Look at your food. Appreciate the appearance and aroma. Notice the colors, textures, arrangement, and smells. Imagine what it will taste like.

Taste your favorite first. Decide which food looks the most appetizing and start by eating one or two bites of it while your taste buds are the most sensitive. If you save the best until last, you may want to eat it even if you're full and you won't enjoy it as much.

Put your fork down. When you're loading your next forkful, you can't pay attention to the one in your mouth. Besides, when you're always paying attention to the next bite, you'll keep eating until there are no more bites because that's where your focus is.

Stay connected. Savor the aromas and tastes of your food as you eat. Mentally describe the temperatures, flavors, ingredients, seasonings, and textures. Stay conscious of all the different sensations you're experiencing.

Take small bites. Large bites are wasted on the roof of your mouth, teeth, and cheeks where you have very few taste buds. In addition, much of the flavor of food comes from the aromas. When you slowly chew a small bite of food, the aromas are carried from the back of your throat to your nose, enhancing the taste.

Appreciate the occasion. Appreciate the atmosphere, the company, or simply the fact that you're allowing yourself to sit down and enjoy your meal.

Enjoy your food. If you notice you're not enjoying what you chose, choose something else if possible. Eating food that doesn't taste good will leave you feeling dissatisfied.

How much? *Pause in the middle of eating.* When you get to your speed bump, stop eating for a couple of minutes. Ask yourself where you are on the Hunger and Fullness Scale now. Estimate how much more food it will take to fill

STRATEGIES: EATING MINDFULLY IN THE REAL WORLD

It's easier to become distracted from signals of physical hunger and satiety at restaurants and social gatherings, especially when food is the main event. Eating mindfully in the workplace also poses some common challenges. In these settings, you'll need to pay extra attention to your body's signals.

- Remember to ask, "Am I hungry?" It's common to have dishes of candy or snacks set out at parties and in many places of business, but don't eat food just because it's there. Before having a doughnut, bagel, or brownie from the break room at work or a sample at the grocery store, notice where you are on the Hunger and Fullness Scale.

- If you're hungry and really want that particular food, remember to sit down and eat it mindfully. If you're not hungry, save some of it for later or skip it altogether. It's likely it will reappear another day.

- Be careful of eating at your desk. Make enough time to enjoy a meal without work interruptions if possible.

- When eating while socializing or conducting business, make it a point to alternately shift your focus from eating to the conversation.

- Be aware of the effects of alcohol on your ability to eat mindfully.

- Don't allow the serving size or how much other people are eating determine how much you'll eat. Most of the time you'll get more food than you really need, so check in with your own hunger and fullness levels to tell you when to stop.

- Since meals tend to be longer at social events, you may need to have your plate taken away or put your napkin on it when you're satisfied to avoid nibbling unconsciously.

you to comfortable satiety, keeping in mind that there's a delay in the fullness signal reaching your brain. Don't be surprised if you realize you're already full or getting close.

Notice when your taste buds become less sensitive to the taste of food. When the food doesn't taste quite good as it did at first, it's a sign that your body has had enough.

Push your plate forward or get up from the table as soon as you feel satisfied. The desire to keep eating will pass quickly, so direct your attention away from food for a few minutes. Remind yourself that you'll eat again when you're hungry again.

Ask yourself where you are on the Hunger and Fullness Scale when you're finished eating. How close did you get to your original intention?

Where? *Notice how you feel after eating.* How do you feel? Where will you invest the energy you consumed? If you overate, don't judge or punish yourself. Just notice the physical and/or emotional discomfort that often accompanies being overly full, and create a plan to decrease the likelihood that you'll overeat next time. (We'll address this in more detail in the next chapter.)

If you're used to eating on autopilot, mindful eating may feel a little contrived and awkward at first. Like other strategies you've learned in this book, it becomes more natural with practice. By choosing to eat every bite with intention and attention, you'll find yourself eating less while experiencing more enjoyment than you ever did while overeating or dieting. Look at what happened when Marcia tried it.

> I love to munch on sweets or salty, crunchy snacks like chips or pretzels while I read. At first they taste really good, but then I get involved in the story and the next thing I know, I've eaten the whole bag. I feel so full, but I swear, I can't remember eating them all! I think I get into autopilot and I don't stop eating until the book ends, the food is gone, or I realize I'm totally stuffed.
>
> Well, chocolate is absolutely my favorite food. A good friend of mine brought a small box of truffles home for me from her trip to Europe. I was about to pop one into my mouth while I was reading when I thought, if I

love them that much, don't they deserve my undivided attention? I waited until I was hungry and really wanted one of those truffles. You'll probably think I'm silly, but I put the truffle on a china plate, cut it into eight little pieces, and sat in my dining room, savoring every little morsel. It was rich and creamy and absolutely wonderful. I think the only thing that could have made it any better would have been eating it in Belgium!

TASTING WINE AS A MINDFUL EXPERIENCE

Just as with learning to eat mindfully, you can learn to taste wine with *intention* and *attention:* with the *intention* of enjoyment without having to pay the price of excess and with *attention* to every detail of the experience.

Serve: Pour your wine into a clear, stemmed glass, filling it less than halfway so there's room to swirl the wine.

See: Hold the glass in front of a white surface and tip it slightly. Look through the wine and notice the color and viscosity (legs) of the wine.

Swirl: Set your glass down on the table and twist your wrist to make small circles with the glass to gently swirl the wine. This aerates the wine and brings the aromas up into the glass.

Sniff: Put your nose in the glass and inhale deeply to appreciate the aromas that hint of the terroir (the climate, soil type, drainage, humidity, and other factors in a particular vineyard) and the winemaking process used.

Sense: Sip a small mouthful of wine. Swish the wine over your tongue and open your mouth slightly as you inhale, bringing the aromas into the back of your nose.

Savor: Describe the flavors, identifying subtleties and similarities to other familiar flavors, and noting how the wine complements or detracts from any food you're eating.

Staying focused and fully present in the moment makes you aware of what you're thinking, feeling, and experiencing. This is what it means to truly love what you eat. Once you've experienced the pleasure of eating mindfully, become more mindful during other activities, too. Use intention and attention in your conversations, work, walks—no matter what you're doing. Living fully in the moment allows you to listen and trust your innate wisdom, increasing your effectiveness and contentment in everything you do.

CHAPTER 7

JUST RIGHT

love the holidays. Weeks before, our family begins planning for the significant meals we'll share. We're each assigned to bring the traditional dishes we've become known for—and with our large family, there's always plenty. During the blessing my uncle always gives thanks for the food that nourishes our bodies. Then the nourishment begins!

I know these types of gatherings take place all over the world, year after year. The comments are as traditional as the food. "Honey, this is the best turkey you've ever made. "Please pass the potatoes and gravy again." "I can't eat another bite or I swear I'll explode." "All right, just a little sliver of pie then." After dinner, people are sprawled out in front of the television, occasionally groaning or dozing off.

As much as I love these special occasions, I now know that there's an invisible line that I can cross if I'm not mindful. That line separates a great celebration with wonderful food from an evening of discomfort and regret. I constantly remind myself that I live in a land of abundance where turkey and potatoes are available year-round, and food will always taste good. So why eat until I'm miserable? Why not enjoy the event and still feel good when it's over?

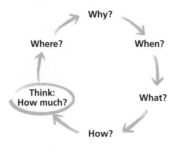

HOW MUCH DO I NEED?

When you live in a land of abundance, deciding how much food you *need* to eat is critical for lifelong weight management and health. Just as important, when you eat the perfect amount of food, you'll feel satisfied—just right.

Think for a moment about how that feels.

When you're satisfied, you simply don't need anything else. You feel content, fulfilled, pleased, and even happy. How wonderful it is to feel good when you're finished eating.

Stopping at "just right" can be challenging. You may eat past the point of satisfaction for many reasons: habits and learned behaviors, past dieting, and often, not paying attention while you're eating. When you eat more than you need, you'll feel unnecessarily uncomfortable, and your body will have no choice but to store the excess as fat. Eating too much may cause you to have less energy and be less active. In the past, it also led to feelings of guilt, which usually led to even more overeating.

As you practice eating mindfully, with intention and attention, your awareness will change your perception of overeating. For example, when you're disconnected from hunger and fullness and you overeat for emotional reasons, it may actually feel good, at least temporarily. However, when you're aware and more connected, you'll feel physically uncomfortable and recognize that eating did not meet your emotional needs very well.

To change old patterns, you'll need to rediscover how great it feels when you don't overeat—and learn what to do on those occasions when you do. It's critical for you to tune into your thoughts, feelings, and behaviors *without* judgment. You're not going through this process to punish yourself but to see what you can learn from the experience.

Compare teaching yourself to eat just the right amount of food to teaching a child to ride a bike. Do children learn easily when you get angry or criticize them for making mistakes? Will children feel like giving up if they are expected to do it perfectly right away? Will they want to try again if they're ashamed about falling off? Or do they learn best when you observe what they do, encourage each positive step they take, and offer gentle suggestions on how they can improve? Do they want to keep trying because you focus on how much they are progressing, not on what they do wrong? Will they feel encouraged when they notice it gets a little easier each time? Learning to stop eating when you're satisfied is exactly the same. You're most likely to learn when you're gentle, patient, encouraging, and optimistic with yourself throughout the process.

And, as with riding a bike, this process eventually becomes natural. Occasionally, something will throw you off balance, but because you've practiced and learned to make necessary adjustments and corrections, you'll keep cruising right along.

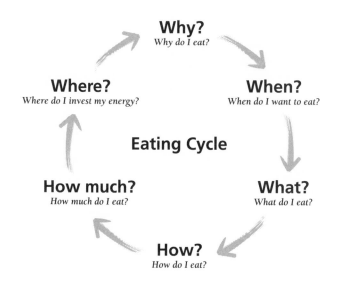

ENOUGH *IS* ENOUGH

As we've worked our way around the Eating Cycle, you've learned numerous strategies to help you eat the amount of food your body needs. You learned that mindful eating requires intention and attention. Your intention is to meet

> **MINDFUL MOMENT:** Notice how great it feels when you eat exactly how much you need.

your body's needs and to feel better when you're finished than you did when you started—in other words, satisfied. You pay attention to make it possible to eat less while enjoying it more. Let's pick up where we left off and build on those strategies. We'll also use the Eating Cycle to figure out why you overeat sometimes, and how to quickly move back into instinctive eating.

How Full Am I?

Your awareness and the Hunger and Fullness Scale are your most useful tools for helping you determine when enough is enough. Just as you use your hunger level to let you know when to eat, you'll use your fullness level to let you know when you've had enough.

Before you start eating, give yourself a hunger and fullness number and decide where you want to be when you're finished. Estimate how much food you'll need to eat to reach that level of fullness. Prepare, serve, or order only as much as you think you'll need; if you were served too much, move the extra food aside. Before you start eating, visually or physically divide the food in half to create a "speed bump." Eat mindfully and check your fullness level when you hit that speed bump, at the end of your meal, and again twenty to thirty minutes later.

Here are some questions you might want to ask yourself to help you determine how full you are:

- How does my stomach feel? Can I feel the food? Is there any discomfort or pain? Does my stomach feel stretched, full, or bloated?
- How does my body feel? Do I feel comfortable and content? Do my clothes feel tight? Is there any nausea or heartburn? Do I feel short of breath?
- How is my energy level? Do I feel energetic and ready for the next activity? Or am I sleepy, sluggish, tired, or lethargic?
- What do I feel like doing now?

The Hunger and Fullness Scale

Ravenous	Starving	Hungry	Pangs	Satisfied	Full	Very Full	Discomfort	Stuffed	Sick
1	2	3	4	5	6	7	8	9	10

Based on your answers to these questions, determine your number on the Hunger and Fullness Scale.

4 or lower: You're still a little hungry. You have several options:

- You could eat a little more; just a few bites may be all you need.
- You could wait a while to see whether you feel fuller; if not, you could eat a little more.
- You could stop eating for now. This is a great strategy if you're planning to have dessert, if you'll be eating again soon, or if you don't want to feel food in your stomach— for example, before you exercise.

5—You're satisfied and comfortable: You aren't hungry anymore, yet you don't feel the food in your body. You could eat more, but you don't need (or want) to. You may also notice that while you were eating, the flavor of the food went from fabulous to just okay as you became less hungry. It may have been harder to give food and eating your full attention. You feel light and energetic and ready for your next activity. Where will you invest that energy? There's a lot more on that coming up in chapter 8; in the meantime, just remember that the real purpose of eating is to fuel living.

6—You're slightly full: You can feel the food in your stomach, but it's not unpleasant. When you are a 5 or 6, you may want to move away from the table or move the food away from you to signal that you're finished. Pay close attention to this comfortable, contented feeling and try to remember it for next time.

7 or higher: You feel somewhere between very full to sick. Picture your stomach as a balloon, as we talked about in chapter 2. It can stretch far beyond its ideal capacity, but when it does, what is it pressing on or pushing out of the way? At a 7 or above, you think, "I ate too much!" You feel uncomfortable, regretful, and possibly sleepy and sluggish.

> **MINDFUL MOMENT:** Before you start eating, decide how full you want to be when you're done.

Notice that I intentionally used the word *regretful* instead of *guilty*. What happens when you feel guilty about eating? If you're anything like me, guilt is a powerful driver of your Overeating Cycle. Since you're in charge of the decisions you make, you don't need to feel guilty if you consciously decided to eat more than you needed.

Regret means you don't like how you feel and you wish you hadn't eaten so much. It leaves the door open for you to learn from the experience so you can do a little better next time. Even people who eat instinctively occasionally overeat for convenience or pleasure. They sometimes regret it later, but since they don't feel guilty about it, it doesn't lead to more overeating and compensatory restriction.

DON'T MISS THE LESSON

When you realize you've eaten too much, ask yourself, "Why did it happen?" Here are some other questions to ask to help you determine why you overate.

- Why was I eating in the first place? Was I in an Instinctive, a Restrictive, or an Overeating Cycle?
- When did I get the urge to eat? What was I thinking? What was I feeling? What else was going on?
- Am I able to identify hunger? Was I hungry? How hungry was I?
- If I wasn't hungry, what was the physical, environmental, or emotional trigger?
- What did I choose to eat and why? Did that affect how much I ate?
- How did I eat? Was I mindful or was I distracted?
- Did I set an intention for how full I wanted be when I was done eating?
- How much food did I have in front of me?

- What was I thinking about when I decided to continue to ea~~~~
  the point of satisfaction?

Most important, ask yourself, "What could I do differently next time?" By developing a strategy for what you'll do differently, you turn your mistake into a learning experience.

To help you sort it out, let's go back through the Eating Cycle to explore possible triggers for overeating and strategies for dealing with them more effectively. This will be a great review and application of some of the concepts you learned in previous chapters. Go back and reread any sections you're struggling with.

Why? *It just happened.* When you don't decide ahead of time how you want to feel at the end of the meal, you're more likely to overeat. In other words, start eating with an intention such as, "I'll eat only as much as I need to feel comfortable at a 5." You can always change your mind, but don't let it just happen; decide with full awareness of the consequences.

I've been feeling deprived. If you've been in a Restrictive Eating Cycle, you're more likely to overeat when you finally give in to your cravings. Remind yourself that there are no good or bad foods. You're less likely to feel out of control around food when you know you can have it again whenever you want it.

I was rebelling. If someone said you can't or shouldn't eat something, you may eat more to spite them. But ultimately, who have you punished? Since you're the one in charge of your eating, you get to choose when, what, and how much you'll eat.

I always overeat in that situation. Many people learn to associate certain events with overeating—Thanksgiving dinner, sporting events, dinner at Grandmother's house. Be aware of these triggers so you can think them through ahead of time and create new strategies that suit you better.

It was a special occasion. You're more likely to overeat if you give yourself permission to eat enjoyable foods only on special occasions. You don't need an

---

MINDFUL MOMENT: When you make a mistake, don't miss the lesson.

excuse to have a wonderful meal. Why use a special occasion as a reason to overeat? Just ask yourself, "If this occasion is so special, why would I want to ruin it by eating until I feel uncomfortable?"

I felt obligated. You may sometimes feel you're expected to eat, such as when someone else made or bought the food. Food pushers may urge you to eat for many reasons: for example, to make themselves feel good, to show you they care about you, or to avoid eating alone. Feeling obligated can cause you to ignore your body's signals of satisfaction in order to please someone else—or you may use it as an excuse to overeat. Remember, you eat to meet your body's needs, so come up with some polite but firm responses ahead of time.

When? *I wasn't hungry when I started eating.* When you eat before you're hungry, just about any amount of food will make you feel full. See how Ramona is working on freeing herself from eating on a schedule.

> My husband has always been an instinctive eater. Sometimes I'd get so mad at him because I'd work all afternoon preparing lasagna or something else special for dinner, but some days he'd just pick at it. He'd say he just wasn't very hungry because they'd gone out for lunch. I used to try to get him to eat anyway because I was thinking, "Hey, it's lasagna, and I made it and you should want to eat it no matter what else you ate today!" But now I understand, and I've stopped pushing food on him.
>
> In fact, I realized that a lot of the time I wasn't really all that hungry at dinnertime either. It dawned on me that I taste a lot while I cook. I'm trying to break that habit, but now, if one of us isn't hungry, we just wrap it up so we can have it for lunch or dinner the next day when we'll actually enjoy it.

I was too hungry when I started eating. When you wait too long to eat, you're more likely to eat too much, too quickly, and therefore overshoot your stomach's comfortable capacity. Pay more attention to your hunger cues and be prepared to eat when you get to a 2 or a 3. If you're at a 1, realize that it's a potentially high-risk situation. Slow down and just eat a little bit first to allow your blood sugar to come up; then be extra mindful of your choices.

I might be overeating to stuff other feelings. This is the most challenging reason for eating beyond satisfaction. It may also be the most important. If you're eating instead of feeling your feelings or coping with your emotions, you aren't able to meet your true needs. The first step is to become aware of what is happening; thereafter, make a decision to work on it, one step at a time. Remember FEAST—Focus, Explore, Accept, Strategize, Take action—from chapter 3? Those steps will help you with overeating, too.

What? *It tasted good, so I just kept eating.* Your taste buds are the most sensitive when you're hungry and when you first start to eat, so that's when food tastes the best. You might keep eating because you want to experience those first wonderful bites again, but at that point, you are really just eating a memory. It won't taste that wonderful until you're hungry again. In fact, you may even stop being aware that you're eating long before you actually stop eating. When you're eating a delicious food, don't get so caught up in the experience that you don't notice how you actually feel or you forget how you'll feel if you overeat. Check in and remind yourself that if you keep eating, the discomfort will eventually outweigh the enjoyment.

I wanted to taste everything. Studies have shown that having a lot of food to choose from causes people to eat more. If you know it's difficult for you when you have a lot of choices, you may wish to avoid buffets and similar settings for now. Better yet, turn it around. Decide that with so many choices, you'll get to eat exactly what you want. You can be extremely picky; decide that you will only eat what you love and that you won't bother with anything that's just so-so.

I was afraid I wouldn't get that food again. You may convince yourself this is the only time you'll get to have a particular food, so you should eat all you can. However, it's rare that a food will never be available again. You can ask for the recipe, take some home, ask if they'll make it for you again sometime, plan to return to the same restaurant, or enjoy experimenting with similar foods in the future.

I saved the best for last. If you save your favorite food for the end of your meal, you might eat it even if you're already full (this applies to dessert, too). Instead, have a bite or two when it will taste the best. Then, if you're too full to finish it, it will be easier to save the rest for later.

STRATEGIES: I ATE TOO MUCH! NOW WHAT?

After eating, sit quietly for a few moments and become completely aware of how you feel and where your energy is going. When you've eaten too much, your stomach is distended and you may feel sluggish as your body processes and stores the excess fuel you consumed. Again, don't beat yourself up; just focus on the sensations so you can remember them in detail. That way, the next time you're tempted to overeat, you can recall how you felt when you were too full, and you'll be less likely to repeat that mistake.

When you overeat, it's important to reenter your Instinctive Eating Cycle at your next decision point. By listening to your body wisdom, you can compensate for occasional overeating.

Why? People who eat instinctively sometimes overeat. However, although they probably feel regretful and uncomfortable, they don't typically feel guilty. Therefore, they don't think, "Well, I've already blown it; I might as well keep eating then start my diet tomorrow." Those thoughts would only trap them in an eat-repent-repeat cycle. Instead, they just listen to their body and return to eating instinctively by allowing hunger to drive their next cycle.

When? When you've overeaten, wait and see when you get hungry again. Rather than continue to eat out of guilt or because it's time, listen to your body. It probably won't need food again as soon; therefore, you may not be hungry for your usual snack or even your next meal.

What? Don't penalize yourself or try to compensate for overeating by restricting yourself. If you try to make yourself eat foods you don't really want, you'll feel deprived and punished—and you'll fuel your eat-repent-repeat cycle. When you get hungry again, ask yourself: "What do I want?" and "What do I need?" Trust and respect your body wisdom because it's likely that it will naturally seek balance, variety, and moderation. You might notice you are hungry for something small or something light: maybe a bowl of soup or cereal, a piece of fruit, or a salad.

How? Eat mindfully with intention and attention and you'll be less likely to repeat your recent mistake.

How much? You may not be as hungry, so pay close attention to how much you serve, order, prepare, and eat.

Where? Don't use exercise to punish yourself for overeating; instead, be active and use your fuel to live a full and satisfying life!

I ate food I didn't enjoy. If you choose food that isn't really what you want, you're less likely to feel satisfied. You may continue to eat, trying to reach satisfaction without realizing that the food choice, not the amount, is the problem. If you realize you're eating a food you're not really enjoying, stop and choose something else. If there are no other options, eat cautiously and promise yourself you'll eat something you like at the next meal.

How? *I wasn't paying attention as I ate.* You can't pay full attention to two things at once, so when you eat while you're doing something else, you're less likely to enjoy your food or notice when you've had enough. Instead, choose to savor each bite without other distractions.

 I ate too fast. When you eat quickly, your brain may not realize your stomach is full until it's too late. Slow down and pause for a couple of minutes in the middle of eating to reconnect and ask yourself where you are on the Hunger and Fullness Scale.

 I mindlessly picked at the leftovers. When you reach the level of fullness you intended, get up from the table, clear the food or have someone remove your plate, and package up leftovers for another meal. If you stay at the table, push your plate away or cover it with a napkin so you don't pick at the remaining food unconsciously.

How much? *I had too much on my plate.* Studies have shown that the larger the serving size, the more food people will eat. Make it a point to serve yourself only as much as you think you'll need. When you've been given a larger portion than you need, divide it into a more appropriate portion—or better yet, have the excess wrapped to go.

I was keeping up with someone else. You may overeat when someone else is eating a lot or eating very fast. You might be afraid you won't get your share or think you're not eating that much compared to the other person. Remember: you are eating for you, no one else.

I'm used to feeling full after a meal. Over time, you may have grown used to that full feeling you get from overeating. In the past, it may have even been your only signal to stop. If you're having difficulty letting that go, try drinking water when you eat, eating soup before your meal, and enjoying plenty of high-fiber fruits and vegetables and salads to fill you up without adding a lot more calories than your body needs. Also begin to practice noticing all the negative consequences that come from being too full. Eventually, most people begin to view fullness as an unpleasant state they want to avoid.

I wanted to get my money's worth. When you've paid for something, you may be tempted to eat more than you need so you won't feel you've wasted your money. You might also be tempted to buy (and then eat) more than you need because it's a better value. However, whenever you eat more than your body needs, your money has been wasted anyway.

I hate to let food go to waste. This may come from your childhood: "Eat all your dinner; there are starving children in (fill in the blank)." Eating all your food doesn't help children anywhere. If you're concerned about wasting food, take smaller portions, share meals, and save leftovers to eat later. Would you rather the food go to waste or to your waist?

I wanted to earn my dessert. You are an adult now; you don't have to clean your plate if you want dessert. Instead, remember that other familiar phrase: "Save room for dessert!"

Where? *I kept eating to avoid or postpone doing something else.* Sometimes eating is a lot easier or more fun than whatever else you think you should be doing. To combat this problem, make sure you have something to look forward to (or at least that you don't dread doing) when you've finished eating.

I'd rather eat than do just about anything else. If you don't have other things you enjoy doing and that make you feel good, you may eat for pleasure and to "fill yourself up." See chapter 8 for other ways to nourish your body, mind, heart, and spirit.

If your underlying reasons for overeating still aren't apparent, they may be buried under denial or other coping mechanisms. If your overeating continues without any progress toward identifying and addressing your triggers, professional guidance is likely to be useful.

Paula shared how she addressed one of her triggers for overeating.

> I had really cut down on my overeating. It didn't even feel good to be really full anymore. But I was still struggling with Sunday dinners at my grandma's house. The whole family had always joked about going off our diets once a week because she is such a wonderful cook. As soon as we get there, we start talking and nibbling on the cheese and crackers or other snacks she puts out. Then she serves this amazing dinner, but there's always way more food than one family should eat. Somehow she manages to goad us into finishing it all off so it won't go to waste.
>
> I noticed I always felt miserable by the time we left. When I observed her bribing my kids with dessert for finishing the huge plate of food she gave them, I thought, "I'm an adult now, and I'm in charge of what and how much I'll eat." I decided to be more aware of what I was eating instead of falling into old habits. I also decided to talk to my grandmother, but I was worried about hurting her feelings, so I practiced what I was going to say ahead of time—and made sure it was sincere.
>
> Finally, last week, when she was pushing another helping, I got up the nerve to say, "Grandma, this was another of your great meals! I couldn't be more satisfied. I hope you'll teach me how to make this sometime." She packed me up a to-go container to take to work the next day. Next time I'm going to gently ask her to let my kids fill their own plates, and I'll remind them to save room for her wonderful desserts.

Soon you'll prefer to feel content and comfortable after you eat. When you feel too full after eating, try to figure out why, and develop a plan for what you'll do differently next time. Perfection isn't possible, or even necessary, so just get right back into your Instinctive Eating Cycle by waiting to see when you get hungry again and what you're hungry for. With practice, it becomes easier and more natural to stop eating when you feel just right.

CHAPTER 8

SELF-CARE BUFFER ZONE

Our power went out unexpectedly one evening while I was trying to finish writing an article on life balance. It was summertime in Phoenix, so our house warmed up quickly. The kids were hungry, my husband was on the phone with the power company, and I was feeling a little stressed about the whole thing. Ironically, I was faced with the challenge of following my own advice.

As frustrated as I felt, I knew the situation was beyond my control. I took a few deep breaths, decided what was most important in that moment, and set about the task of lighting every candle in the house. I began to feel calmer, almost happy about the unforeseen change of plans. By the time it was dark, the house was aglow and our impromptu dinner of chips and salsa was laid out on the patio. The darkness and silenced video games kept the children closer than usual as we hung out together and talked. Without a computer, or even lights, we all got a much-needed respite from our full lives.

By the time the electricity came back on at our house, my own energy level and sense of peace had been fully restored. I promised myself I wouldn't wait for a "power failure" to occur to enjoy more balance in my life.

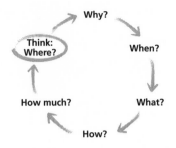

WHERE DO I INVEST MY ENERGY?

As you free yourself from thinking about food as good or bad, you can also free yourself from thinking about *where* you use your energy as just exercise and burning calories.

Where you invest your energy is more important than how many calories you burn. In this diet-crazed culture, what should be the natural process of consuming fuel to supply the necessary energy to survive and thrive has instead become a national pastime—or, more accurately, an obsession. Remember that the real reason you eat is to fuel your life and provide you with the energy to do whatever you need and want to do. So, what do you want to do? Where do you want to invest your energy?

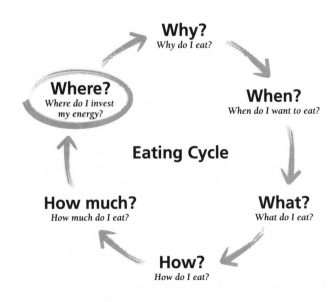

The Best Return on Your Investment

You've learned strategies for letting hunger and fullness guide your eating again so you can develop a healthier lifestyle without following a rigid diet or exercise regimen. But the most powerful result of freeing yourself from your Overeating and Restrictive Eating Cycles is that you'll have more energy to focus on what it really takes to make you a healthy person.

By *healthy* I mean a complete state of physical, intellectual, emotional, and spiritual wellness; in other words, health of your body, mind, heart, and spirit.

I don't mean perfect health; I mean *optimal* health—the best health you can have at a certain point in your life given your individual situation. For example, a person with cancer doesn't have perfect health, but it's possible for him to have optimal health through appropriate medical treatment and self-care, excellent emotional support and coping skills, feeling there's meaning and purpose for his life, and having a positive outlook.

Let's take a closer look at these four aspects of your health and where you invest your energy.

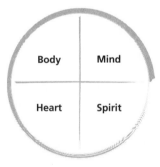

Body When most people think of health, they think of physical health first. Before anything else, your primary needs for shelter, safety, and security must be met. Beyond other basics like water and enough food for survival, optimal physical health includes nutritious food, an active lifestyle, sufficient rest and sleep, adequate health care, and perhaps physical touch and sex. You may also broaden your perspective to include your physical surroundings and the material things in your life. A healthy body and a comfortable physical environment are important because they give you the security and vitality to do what you need and want to do.

> **MINDFUL MOMENT:** You have more time and energy when you're not so consumed by food, eating, and weight. Where will you invest it?

Mind Challenge, growth, creativity, stimulation, and a sense of accomplishment are all important for optimal intellectual health. From a practical standpoint, your thoughts have a powerful impact on your feelings and actions and therefore your overall health.

Heart The area of emotional health includes your ability to accurately identify your feelings because they give you important information about whether what is happening is in alignment with what you really want. Optimal emotional health does not mean being perfectly happy; rather, it means embracing the full spectrum of emotions for the depth and richness they bring to your life. Other important aspects of emotional wellness include your ability to cope with your feelings, satisfying relationships with others, effective communication, healthy personal boundaries, and well-developed self-nurturing skills.

Spirit Spirituality is your sense of connection and purpose. For some this may include religion, but it really is much more than that. It is knowing that who you are is not defined by your possessions, your appearance, your accomplishments, or even your contributions. You are worthy of love just as you are. It is the awareness that there is something greater than yourself and that there's a purpose for your life.

Remember Tom and Angie from chapter 1? Tom shared these thoughts on what makes him feel healthy.

> I know that what I eat affects my physical health, but I can't imagine letting it rule my life. It's just food. What really makes me feel great is doing the things I love. I love spending time with Angie, laughing about our culinary disasters or sharing the challenges of our day. I love climbing to the top of

a mountain and looking out as far as the eye can see. In those moments I experience both a sense of awe and an incredible sense of peace. To me, that is optimal health.

Where Do You Invest Your Energy in an Overeating Cycle?

The Overeating Cycle can lead to unnecessary weight gain, decreased pleasure in eating, decreased metabolism, and physical and emotional discomfort. When you primarily eat in response to triggers other than hunger, or when food is your major source of pleasure or comfort, it will be difficult to build optimal health. Not surprisingly, experiencing a void or unresolved turmoil in one or more of these other areas of your life may make it more difficult for you to reach or maintain a healthier weight.

Body When hunger doesn't initiate your desire to eat, your body probably doesn't need the fuel. The result is that your body saves the extra as fat. When you eat for reasons other than hunger, you're more likely to choose foods based on availability and emotional appeal and less likely to choose foods that nourish your body. Furthermore, when you're not eating to satisfy your physical need for food, you're more likely to overeat. If you also have a sedentary lifestyle, you'll have less energy and your physical health will suffer.

Mind People with food or weight issues often eat mindlessly, so their eating seems illogical and out of control. They generally know they shouldn't eat so much but they find themselves thinking about food much of the time. They may have a constant negative little voice that feeds results they don't really want.

Heart Food and eating are sometimes used as a substitute for healthy coping skills and communication. For example, if you eat to stuff anger, your anger isn't expressed in a healthy manner, so it becomes destructive to you and your relationships. Or, if you eat half of a package of chocolate chip cookies because you're lonely, you'll still be lonely when you're finished eating—but you'll be stuffed, too. To make matters worse, you may feel bad about yourself when you eat this way, and that can trigger more emotional eating. Another important reality is that food can give only temporary relief from stress and difficult emotions. When emotions are not addressed in a healthy manner, they continue to feed into unhealthy coping mechanisms—so the Overeating Cycle perpetuates itself.

Spirit The spiritual part of you strives to find inner peace, unity, and a greater purpose for living. Overeating does not usually lead to inner peace or harmony and may distract you from fulfilling your higher purpose.

Think about Sarah and Paul from chapter 1. They were trapped in an Overeating Cycle but realized it wasn't bringing them optimal health. Here's what Sarah said.

> I was worried that my weight was starting to affect my health. I was tired and didn't have enough energy to exercise. My mind was on food most of the time; I either wanted to eat or felt bad because I had. And now I know when I eat because of stress or other feelings, I'm not meeting my emotional needs either. This endless cycle was zapping me of the energy I needed to live the life I deserve.

Where Do You Invest Your Energy in a Restrictive Eating Cycle?

Diets and other restrictive means of losing weight don't address your whole self either. You have essential intellectual, emotional, and spiritual facets of your life that are connected to your relationship with food. Any diet or weight-loss program that doesn't address these connections (or worse yet, attempts to sever them) will ultimately fail, simply because human beings are multidimensional creatures.

Think about your past attempts at weight loss. What went wrong? Did you feel like you were struggling to overcome your urges to eat? If a diet worked temporarily but failed to provide lasting results, what got in the way? Besides disrupting your body's physical balance, did your diet seem to clash with or completely ignore other important aspects of your life? Let's explore this idea a little further.

Body Most diet programs focus on your physical being through diet and exercise, but they deal with the rest by simply saying, "It has to be a lifestyle change," which usually translates to "You'll be on this diet for the rest of your life!" Sometimes the rules aren't even particularly healthy because they limit important nutrients. Ironically, chronic under-eating can have a detrimental effect on your metabolism and your energy level. There's also an excessive focus on appearance and numbers—external ways to measure your progress and worth.

Mind A narrow, dogmatic diet is counterintuitive to your sensible, grounded nature. After all, attempting to lose weight by doing things you know you can't continue for the rest of your life just doesn't make sense. Your intellectual nature seeks personal and professional growth, but overanalyzing and worrying about every eating decision limits your productivity and efficiency. Furthermore, overly restrictive diets rob you of the energy you need to maintain concentration, and endurance.

Heart Many people have strong emotional connections to food. Restaurants, holidays, and vacations are full of tempting so-called bad foods you aren't supposed to eat, so you have to make a choice—the diet or the fun. While dieting, you may feel sad or angry because you aren't allowed to eat the foods you enjoy. Sharing meals and food with others is more difficult, so you may start to dread gatherings because they conflict with the rules of your diet. When your family, friends, and coworkers don't have to follow the same rules, you feel awkward, resentful, or left out. You may reach a point when trying to lose weight doesn't seem worth it. Most important, since many of your urges to eat are triggered by your emotions, these urges don't go away simply by imposing a strict set of rules.

Spirit Dieting requires a tremendous amount of energy and often leads to inner turmoil, guilt, and a sense of disconnection from the way things were intended to be. What could feel less natural and further from spirituality than eating in a manner that leaves you feeling weak, depressed, and even angry? Using rigid rules to guide your eating sends a message of distrust in your innate wisdom.

> **MINDFUL MOMENT:** When you're focused on food (or not eating food), you can't focus on living your life. When you focus on living your life, food becomes much less important.

Trying to ignore these other aspects of living while dieting may have caused you to feel out of balance or out of sync with your own life. Karen from chapter 1, who was caught in a Restrictive Eating Cycle, felt this way.

> I thought I was just trying to be healthy and look better. Now I'm not so sure that what I was putting myself through was healthy at all. Most of my energy went toward trying to reach an arbitrary weight goal and hating my body. It hadn't dawned on me that I would never find happiness by reaching a certain dress size—and my life was passing me by while I tried.

INVEST YOUR ENERGY IN OPTIMAL HEALTH

Where is your energy going? Where would you like it to go? As you free yourself from overeating and restrictive eating, you can redirect your time and energy toward other more productive and satisfying pursuits. As you considered these four aspects of your health, perhaps you recognized areas in need of more of your attention and energy.

Here are a number of ideas for caring for your physical, intellectual, emotional, and spiritual health. Start with a few from each category that resonate with you.

Physical Self-Care

- Focus on improving your health rather than on losing weight.
- Make small changes rather than trying to overhaul your entire life.
- Be careful not to turn this process into a diet by trying to follow it perfectly or feeling guilty when you don't.

- Schedule regular checkups with your personal physician. Take care of your preventive health needs and don't ignore new, persistent, or unusual symptoms.
- Eat fresh, healthful, and interesting foods.
- Engage in regular, enjoyable physical activity.
- Instead of spending passive hours in front of the television or computer, do something active that restores your energy.
- Get plenty of rest and adequate sleep so you'll feel clear and refreshed.
- Give and receive physical affection.
- Treat yourself to a massage, manicure, pedicure, or facial.
- Take a hot bath or long shower to relax and unwind.
- Wear clothes that are comfortable and fit your current size and shape.
- Clear the physical clutter around you.
- Create a pleasant personal space for yourself. Include photographs, candles, music—whatever makes you feel happy and calm.
- Plant a garden and grow fresh vegetables, herbs, or flowers.
- Spend time in nature walking, hiking, camping, or just sitting.

Intellectual Self-Care

- Lay a firm foundation by examining your values and priorities.
- Give your brain a map to follow by setting inspiring short- and long-term goals. Frequently visualize yourself reaching your goals.
- Recognize that your thoughts lead to your feelings, actions, and results. Challenge yourself to think positively and powerfully.
- Learn something new—a skill, trade, hobby, language, or anything else you find interesting.
- Read often and experience new genres outside of your usual preferences.
- Visit museums or other novel places.
- Do brainteasers and play challenging games, alone and with others.

- Be creative, especially if you don't ordinarily have an opportunity to express yourself creatively. Experiment with art, crafts, and hobbies.
- Listen to music, sing, or play an instrument.
- Take classes online or at your local community center or college.
- Expand or deepen your knowledge in one of your areas of interest.
- Become an expert in something. Learn everything you can about an area and share that knowledge with others by writing, speaking, or teaching.
- Participate in stimulating discussion groups.
- Explore new occupational and career opportunities.
- Travel or explore areas close to home.

Emotional Self-Care

- Love yourself as you are right now.
- Spend quality time with your family and friends having fun and sharing.
- Build intimacy and emotional connections with your partner.
- Make new friends and renew old friendships.
- Identify your emotions through writing in a journal or talking with a trusted friend or counselor.
- Set appropriate boundaries in your relationships. Letting other people know how far into your emotional space they can go creates healthier relationships.
- Assert yourself to let others know how you feel, what you think, and what you need. Accept that beyond that, you can't control what other people think, feel, or do.
- Manage stress effectively. It's not possible or even desirable to eliminate stress, but you can learn to release and cope with it.
- Practice forgiveness. Harboring anger and hurt is harmful and eats up precious emotional energy.

- Be vulnerable. Let people you trust see your imperfections and fears. This can deepen intimacy and free you from the need to be perfect.
- Seek coaching, counseling, or therapy if needed for emotional support and to build coping skills.

Spiritual Self-Care

- Practice mindfulness. Be fully present in whatever you're doing—eating, talking, working, or playing—to experience the full pleasure and meaning.
- Renew and restore yourself through prayer and meditation.
- Schedule time for your inner work. Know yourself, your values, your dreams, and your purpose.
- Define your guiding principles so you'll have a clear path to follow.
- See your problems as opportunities for learning and growth.
- Reclaim your joy! Experiencing joy is possible even as you face challenges.
- Look for the good in others; it's there somewhere, just waiting to be discovered.
- Write in a personal journal to explore your deepest thoughts and feelings.
- Volunteer and give back to your community by helping others.
- Visit your place of worship—or find one.
- Read meaningful, inspirational works.
- Have an attitude of gratitude. Being thankful for even the smallest of things will remind you of all you have.
- Practice kindness without any expectation of receiving something in return.
- Remember, you already have everything you need to live an abundant life.

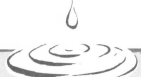

STRATEGIES: BALANCE, VARIETY, AND MODERATION IN ALL THINGS

As you think about where you invest your energy, there may be an aspect of your physical, intellectual, emotional, or spiritual life that you realize you've been neglecting. If you made a long mental To Do list, let it go. Ann had a new twist on it.

> As I raced around trying to get my house cleaned before we left on vacation, it dawned on me that the principles of "balance, variety, and moderation" don't just apply to food. They apply to life. Whether I am working, exercising, cleaning, playing, or socializing, I get myself in over my head, so I start to feel exhausted and frustrated. Instead, I'm going to seek balance in the way I spend my time, variety in my exercise and playtime, and moderation in my work, both at the office and at home.

Strive for balance, variety, and moderation—not just in the way you eat but also in the way you live your life.

RESTORE YOUR ENERGY

Instead of waiting for an energy blackout to force you to slow down, make a conscious, personal choice about how you'll deal with the multitude of responsibilities, stressors, and opportunities you face. Not just in the way you eat but also in the way you live your life. Make a conscious, personal choice about how you'll deal with the multitude of responsibilities, stressors, and opportunities you face. Self-care is not about spending an equal amount of time or energy in each area. It's about making the commitment to care for yourself and meet your true needs. It worked for Sarah.

> **MINDFUL MOMENT:** No matter how hard you work on one area of your physical, intellectual, emotional, or spiritual health, it cannot make up for the complete lack in another.

Up until now, I was eating constantly, never stopping long enough to get hungry. Last night I found myself staring into the refrigerator looking for something to fill me up. I remembered what you said, so I asked myself, "Am I hungry?" I had to admit I wasn't, so I knew there must be something I needed besides food.

Suddenly, I thought of my oil paints that I hadn't touched for months. I threw on an old shirt, turned on some loud music, and painted for three hours straight! The thought of food didn't cross my mind again the whole evening. I didn't need to eat; I needed to create! And for the first time in a long time, I truly felt full.

Decide where you'll invest your energy—body, mind, heart, and spirit— for optimal health. You'll finally break free from your eat-repent-repeat cycle when food serves its true purpose: fueling your full and satisfying life.

PART 2

NOURISH

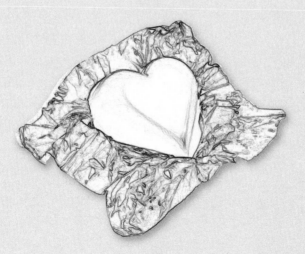

CHAPTER 9

DIETS DON'T WORK

Recently, a reporter posted a query for a story he was writing: "I need tips about new diet trends." I responded with, "Ironically, the biggest weight-loss trend is NOT dieting. We've been dieting for decades and look where it has gotten us. Instead, the trend is finally toward relearning how to eat instinctively again." I went on to describe the differences between restrictive eating and instinctive eating. He wrote back, "Thanks. 90% of the ideas I received were about not dieting. This is the most illuminating take I've had but not sure it's newsy enough." Needless to say, he didn't write about it.

CONSUMED

You've learned strategies for breaking free from your eat-repent-repeat cycle. Now you're in charge of making the best choices for yourself about what to eat. These chapters will provide you with nutrition guidance, not guidelines, but giving up rules may not be as easy as it sounds.

We live in a society obsessed with weight and dieting. We're constantly bombarded with the latest weight-loss scheme to "rid ourselves of those unsightly pounds." New fad diets scream at us from magazines and books, talk shows and news programs, commercials and testimonials, doctors' offices and health food stores. Americans spend billions of dollars annually on weight-loss products and services. Paradoxically, the more we diet, the heavier we become as a nation.

Medical research has proven that even a 5 percent weight loss can significantly improve health. You can reduce your risk of high blood pressure, diabetes, high cholesterol, heart disease, arthritis, and some types of cancers. Of course, many people diet to look better. There's nothing wrong with losing weight to improve your physical appearance and self-esteem, but many people have unrealistic expectations, which drives them to try to lose weight *regardless* of the cost.

No matter what your motivation, the striking reality is that diets are not very effective in the long run. Accurate statistics are very hard to come by, but it's widely quoted that 90 to 95 percent of dieters regain their lost weight. This is a difficult number to pin down since there are so many ways to lose weight, so many people trying it on their own, so few people studied for long periods of time, and so many people going off their diets before they lose a significant amount of weight in the first place. Whatever the numbers are, if dieting was truly effective, your problem would have been solved with the first one.

Diets Are Just Rules

The diet message is loud and clear: "You're out of control, so you need to follow our rules." The latest "expert" or authority may recommend counting calories, exchanges, points, grams, or ounces. The diet may require that you eat prepackaged food or meal replacements. There may be strict meal plans or complicated diets to follow. Some methods eliminate entire food groups—or solid

> **MINDFUL MOMENT:** At what point will society begin to doubt the wisdom of dieting rather than the fortitude of dieters?

food altogether. Diets may claim that there are magical food combinations or that some foods should be forbidden. And of course, the rules are changing all the time. No wonder so many people feel confused.

Most diets impose food rules that people do not, cannot, or should not follow for very long. When they can't stick to the rules, some dieters will resort to appetite suppressants to help control their hunger or dangerous thermogenics to boost their metabolism. Some people finally opt for weight-loss surgery to force changes in their eating.

Diets Consume Your Energy

Planning ahead and preparing nutritious meals are important for optimal health, but dieting takes this to the extreme. Since diets are based on rules, you have to learn and follow the regimen indefinitely if the diet is to be effective. You may wake up in the morning thinking about food, planning what you'll eat for the entire day—before you're even out of bed! You may find yourself counting out pretzel sticks, weighing chicken breasts, and measuring milk to make sure you're complying with the rules. You may carefully scrutinize every food label for calorie counts and forbidden ingredients. You may even avoid parties and your favorite restaurants so you're not tempted by the sinful pleasures you'll find there.

The irony is that overeating was the reason you started the diet in the first place, but now all you think about is food. Ultimately, this constant effort and vigilance may wear you out and cause you to return to your Overeating Cycle to escape.

Diets Cause Cravings

Most diets are based on limiting various foods in one way or another. At the beginning of a diet, you may be happy and relieved to have this structure and control over your eating.

When certain foods are forbidden, however, you start to value them more—as if they were on a pedestal, just out of reach—so food gains even more power over you. When certain foods are restricted, you may begin to feel deprived. These feelings of deprivation can cause strong cravings. Remember how you craved rich, creamy peanut butter when you weren't supposed to eat fat, or piping hot bread when you were on a low-carb diet?

When you finally give in to the powerful cravings for these presumably bad foods, you feel guilty and out of control. You give up the diet and even binge on the foods you've been missing.

Like most people, you probably become frustrated at how hard it is to stick to the diet's rules in the long run. You feel deprived so you break the rules, but then you feel guilty. This constant struggle leads to an endless eat-repent-repeat cycle and a painful love-hate relationship with food. Of course, most dieters blame themselves when the diet fails, but in reality, dieting itself is to blame.

Diets Miss the Point

Diets don't really address the reasons why most people overeat in the first place. Although substituting celery sticks for potato chips may temporarily decrease your calories, if you're eating potato chips because you're bored, celery sticks aren't going to fill the bill either. Consequently, when the diet is over (and it will be, sooner or later), you'll return to your previous eating habits because nothing really changed. You end up having negative thoughts and feelings about yourself because you believe you've failed.

Some people manage to stick with the rules but develop a Restrictive Eating Cycle in the process. They have to become experts at ignoring hunger and/or depriving themselves of foods they love in order to stay in control. This is a significant price to pay since it takes a lot of energy to eat only so-called good foods and avoid the bad ones. In the Restrictive Eating Cycle, eating leads to conflict and guilt, not pleasure.

Diets Are an External Authority

According to a growing anti-diet or non-diet movement, diets don't work because they're an external authority that teaches dieters to disregard their own internal authority. Some diets don't let you eat when you're hungry ("You are only allowed to eat 1,400 calories per day") or make you eat when you're not ("Eat every three hours").

You must follow the latest expert's rules about when, what, and how much to eat; dieting, therefore, disconnects you from your own body's innate cues of hunger and satiety. As a result, you move even further from your ability to know what your body really needs. Diets don't teach you about the importance of hunger as your natural guide for when, what, and how much food your body needs. When you diet, you have to be in control—but you are not in charge of your own eating.

Diets Are All or Nothing. Life Isn't.

Fueling your body is a natural response to hunger. When you are trying to lose weight, however, you may experience conflict between what comes naturally and what you think you're supposed to do.

When you stand in front of your open refrigerator at home, what goes through your mind? "I shouldn't eat that; it's too fattening." "Hmmm. I wonder how many carbs that has?" "I guess I should eat this because it's healthy, but what I really want is . . ." "Boy, I wish I was allowed to eat that."

This good food–bad food approach is common and contributes to your struggle with eating and weight. People often label foods to help them make healthier choices, but it takes a lot of effort to avoid all the bad foods and consume only the good ones. Even people who eat instinctively but need to make accommodations for health reasons may struggle with making significant changes in their diet.

Diets Decrease Your Metabolism

Your body is required to manage the difference between the number of calories you feed it and the number of calories it burns. When you take in more

STRATEGIES: DON'T MEASURE YOUR SELF-WORTH

Do you allow a number on your bathroom scale to determine your mood or ruin your morning? Many of the people I work with have discovered that weighing themselves sometimes backfires. Have you ever said to yourself . . .

- I did so well this week, I deserve a treat!
- I was so good, but I still didn't lose any weight. I might as well eat.
- I don't have to weigh in until next week, so I'll splurge now and make up for it later.
- I ate terribly this week, but I still lost weight. I guess I don't need to be as careful as I thought.
- I lost only half a pound. It wasn't worth it.

Your weight is simply a measure of the weight of your tissues (including your bones, organs, muscle, and fat) and substances that are just passing through (like water, food, and waste). Your weight can fluctuate dramatically depending on your hormones, when you last ate, and other factors—none of which have anything to do with your value as a person or the long-term benefits of the changes you are making.

In fact, you probably won't see significant changes in your weight from day to day, or perhaps even week to week. Further, when you exercise, you'll build muscle and lose fat, so although the numbers may not change, your body composition, metabolism, and health are improving. If you're depending on a needle on a scale to tell you how you're doing, you may feel discouraged and tempted to give up even though great things are going on inside.

TAKE THE WEIGHT OFF YOUR SHOULDERS

This time, focus on the process, not the outcome.

- Be honest about how the numbers affect you. If knowing your weight tends to backfire, put your scale under the sink or out in the garage. You can decline to be weighed at your doctor's office or ask that they record it without telling you the number.

- Decide how often you need to weigh yourself. Some people prefer to be weighed only when they go to the doctor, but for most people once a week or even once a month is a good interval. If you weigh yourself more than once a day you're playing games by measuring meaningless physiological fluctuations.

- Let go of old benchmarks. You may never again reach your wrestling weight or your wedding day weight, but you can live an active lifestyle and make conscious choices that will serve you now.

- Don't weigh yourself to confirm what you already know. When you've been mindful of your choices, don't take a chance that the scale will derail your confidence.

- Don't use the scale to punish yourself. When you know you are off track, focus on the changes you'll make rather than beating yourself up.

NO WEIGH

A man I met recently at a conference said, "I don't need a scale; I have pants." I smiled at the simplicity and accuracy of his method of monitoring himself. A few ounces won't make a difference, but a few pounds will determine how comfortable he feels. Look for other ways to assess your health and progress.

- Resting heart rate
- Blood pressure
- Cholesterol
- Fasting blood sugar
- Waist circumference
- How your clothing fits and feels
- Minutes of walking
- Number of steps on your pedometer
- Amount of weight you are able to lift
- Quality of your food choices
- Energy level
- Mood
- Stamina
- Progress on other goals

fuel than your body requires—typically by starting to eat or continuing to eat when you aren't hungry—you create a surplus. This excess is stored as body fat until needed (if needed). When you take in far fewer calories than your body needs, your body has some critical decisions to make.

When short on fuel, your body turns to its reserve tanks to utilize other energy sources. Initially, it uses up glycogen (stored carbohydrate) in your muscles and liver. When that's gone, it begins to break down certain tissues, specifically fat and muscle, to use for its energy supply.

In a state of ongoing fuel shortage or semi-starvation, your body must pick and choose which cells to continue supporting and which ones to drop. The cells that provide vital activities take top priority. Muscle cells require energy, so those not being used regularly will be given the pink slip. This loss of calorie-burning muscle is a blow to your metabolism.

When your food supply remains low, your cells must also become more efficient. They attempt to perform their jobs without burning as many calories, so they adapt to the lower energy intake by expending less energy. If this happened in your car, you'd be thrilled, but when it happens in your body, you're in trouble. After a period of energy deprivation, your body also becomes more efficient at storing body fat because fat is less metabolically active and provides a ready source of extra fuel. This makes it easier for you to gain weight and harder for you to lose weight, which may cause you to feel sluggish and weak.

When the diet is over and you return to your previous eating habits, your body quickly replaces its fat stores. Unless you are actively exercising, you will not rebuild the majority of the muscle tissue you lost during the diet. Ultimately, this may cause you to have a lower metabolic rate and thus gain weight more easily. Just as important, when you regain fat but not muscle, you will

MINDFUL MOMENT: The key to resolving your struggle with weight and food does not lie in a magical, or even logical, combination of eating and exercise.

have a higher body-fat percentage, and that puts you at higher risk for certain diseases. Ironically, many people end up less healthy than before they tried to lose weight by going on a restrictive diet.

For all these reasons, dieting usually just leads to pain and disappointment. Since it's proven that people do more of what brings them pleasure and strive to avoid what brings them pain, it's not surprising that diets are not an effective long-term solution for weight management.

IF DIETS DON'T WORK, WHAT DOES?

Although you've been bombarded with information about eating right and exercising, you and millions of others still battle with weight issues.

The real solution is relearning how to use your instinctive eating patterns and eat in a way that fuels your metabolism. As you address your relationship with food, you'll likely discover that you also want to take charge of learning how to nourish yourself rather than just working toward some arbitrary weight goal. Maggie said it best.

> Becoming more mindful about my eating made a big difference in the quantity of food I was eating. I feel so much better physically and emotionally. I think the natural next step is to become more mindful about the quality of the food I eat, too. It really isn't even about my weight anymore; it's about being healthy at the size I am right now.

As you read through the following chapters, you'll see that you have the freedom to eat foods you love and that it's possible to eat in a way that is enjoyable and nourishing. You'll learn how your food choices can fuel your body, mind, heart, and spirit.

CHAPTER 10

REDISCOVER FOOD

used to love watching my kids at Halloween because they taught me so much about instinctive eating. They were just as excited about their costumes, trick-or-treating with their friends, and sorting and trading their candy as they were about eating it. Don't get me wrong; they love candy. But the candy it was only a part of the whole experience.

When my children were small, I kept their Halloween candy out of reach and rationed it by allowing them to choose a couple of pieces each day from their separate stashes. I was still dieting in those days, so I never had any candy of my own. I would carefully steal anything chocolate that I didn't think they'd miss. Fortunately, they never found the wrappers I guiltily shoved to the bottom of the garbage. By the time they were old enough to figure it out, I was no longer trying to control them—or myself.

When they were older, their diets were healthier than most kids' (and adults' for that matter), and I knew they were capable of managing such things as their own Halloween candy. I marveled at how each one's individual personality showed up when they were in charge. Tyler loved the sugary kid-candy and would devour it within a few weeks. His usual intake of popsicles and other treats decreased accordingly. Elyse insisted on keeping her candy in her closet so her brother wouldn't eat it. Each day she would rummage through her bag to find a few perfect pieces. I'd like to think I taught her moderation, but I know she just loved to savor it. She'd eventually forget about the candy or lose interest when her favorites were gone, and I'd throw the rest away by Valentine's Day.

I usually have my own chocolate now. Not the leftovers my kids don't want, but the kinds I love. It takes weeks for me to finish a box or a bag, and on more than one occasion, I've been surprised by coming across some that I had completely forgotten about.

MASTERPIECE OR PAINT-BY-NUMBER

The blurring of the line between healthy eating and restrictive eating is the difference between a work of art and a paint-by-number. Either way, you end up with a nice picture—until you get up close to take a look.

Part of the challenge is that the "healthy eating requires restriction" message is so pervasive that it has become conventional wisdom; almost no one questions it. The "healthy equals restriction" message is spread vertically through advertising, television, magazines, books, the Internet, medical research—even the government. Marketers, models, celebrities, reporters, experts, bloggers, legislators, and academicians propagate this message. It is then spread horizontally from doctor to patient, dietitian to client, friend to friend, wife to husband, and parent to child. Sometimes people who spread this belief eat instinctively themselves, but they promote restriction for others.

Restrictive beliefs also are moving swiftly from the United States to the rest of the world. European countries seeing an increase in obesity rates are now being inundated with the same diet messages Americans have been hearing for decades. It hasn't helped us and it won't help people overseas. Mark my words: if they start dieting, French women *will* get fat.

MINDFUL MOMENT: When guilt is no longer a factor, common sense prevails.

There are subtle but important differences between eating well and eating restrictively. Is your picture of health constrained by rigid lines and predetermined colors? Or does it express your individuality, preferences, and lifestyles? Compare healthy eating to restrictive eating.

HEALTHY EATING	VS.	RESTRICTIVE EATING
In charge		In control
Nourishment		Diet
Fuel		Calories
Quality		Points
Healthy		Skinny
Aware		Preoccupied
Conscious		Consumed
Mindful		Vigilant
Information		Dogma
Guide		Rules
All foods fit		Good or bad
Balance		Perfection
Variety		Temptation
Moderation		Deprivation
Choosing		Earning
Deciding		Rationalizing
Flexible		Rigid
Hunger based		By the clock
Comfort		Portion sizes
Physical activity		Penance
Introspective		Smug
Effortless		Willpower
Trust		Fear
Learning		Failing
Self-acceptance		Condemnation
Enjoyment		Guilt
Pleasure		Shame
Freedom		Bondage

STRATEGIES: YOUR PICTURE OF HEALTH

Choose how you want to create *your* work of art by getting rid of "healthy eating is restrictive eating" thoughts. Here are ten specific steps you can take.

1. Let go of the belief that you are incapable of managing your weight without rigid rules. Find role models, health care providers, magazines, and support systems that don't propagate that belief.

2. Filter everything you read, hear, and say by asking, "Is this restrictive?"

3. Become more aware of your thoughts by using a Mind-Body Scan; it may also be helpful to keep a journal to capture the essence of your beliefs, thoughts, feelings, and choices. When you notice restrictive-eating thoughts on the previous page, gently replace them with true healthy-eating thoughts.

4. Remember, all foods fit into a healthy diet when you use balance, variety, and moderation to guide you.

5. Banish the words *good* and *bad* from your thoughts and words, as in "I was good at dinner last night" or "Fast food is bad."

6. Use nutrition information as a tool, not a weapon. Don't use it to deprive yourself of certain foods, restrict yourself from ingredients like fat or carbohydrates, force you to ignore your body's signals about what it wants and needs, or make you feel guilty.

7. Let go of the belief that you need to eat perfectly. Just make the healthiest choices you can *without* feeling deprived.

8. Accept that sometimes you'll regret certain choices you've made; that's part of healthy eating. When you don't get caught up in guilt and shame, you're able to learn from your experiences.

9. Repeat this thought frequently: "It's just food."

10. Apply all these ideas to your beliefs and thoughts about exercise, too!

ALL FOODS FIT

In the following chapters you'll learn why certain nutrients are important, what happens when you eat them, and how to optimize your intake (without deprivation, of course!). The nutrients we'll cover include:

- Water
- Macronutrients
  - —Carbohydrates
  - —Fats
  - —Proteins
- Micronutrients
  - —Vitamins
  - —Minerals
  - —Phytochemicals

Admittedly, this is an artificial way to explain nutrition because you don't consume isolated *nutrients*—you eat *food*. Therefore, you'll also find many practical strategies and tips in each chapter for implementing what you learn. Look for this symbol indicating that the recipes are found in part 4, Eat.

If you're looking for rules about what you should and shouldn't eat, you won't find them here. Think about people who eat instinctively. One distinguishing feature is that they eat whatever they want—when they're hungry. They don't obsess or worry about grams or calories. They may choose certain foods because they've learned about their health benefits, but they don't deprive themselves of foods they love. As a result, they're less likely to overeat their favorite foods since they know they can have them anytime they want.

MINDFUL MOMENT: While some foods are more nutrient rich than others, all foods can fit into well-balanced eating.

When you're hungry, instead of turning to a long list of restricted and allowed foods, use three simple but essential principles for effectively implementing this "all foods fit" approach to eating: balance, variety, and moderation.

Ken provides a good example of why balance, variety, and moderation are important.

> When I worked as a technician, I brought my lunch to work most of the time. Then I got a new position in sales, and my job became more stressful. I did a lot of business entertaining and had a lot of lunch meetings. My diet shifted to large-portion, high-fat restaurant meals, and I gained twenty pounds in the first year. I decided to try a high-protein, low-carb diet. It was easy at first since I could eat as much steak, bacon, and cheese as I wanted. To be honest, I think I just got bored with eating the same things all the time, so I ate less and lost twelve pounds. After a couple of months, I was really missing the foods I wasn't supposed to eat, like pasta and fruit. I decided I couldn't—and probably shouldn't—keep myself from eating all of those foods. Unfortunately, when I went back to my old eating habits, I regained all the weight I'd lost.

Principle One: Balance

Balance refers to the importance of providing your body with all its necessary nutrients while balancing eating for nourishment with eating for enjoyment. Whether Ken was on or off his diet, he was out of balance. Perfection isn't the goal here; you have the flexibility of adjusting your intake from one meal to the next (or even one day to the next) to achieve overall balance in your eating.

Principle Two: Variety

Variety refers to eating an assortment of different foods. As Ken discovered, eating the same foods all the time leads to monotony. Not only was it boring, it probably wasn't meeting all his nutritional requirements. It's important to eat from all the different food groups and to eat a variety of foods within each group since no single food has everything you need. Variety in eating promotes overall health and enjoyment.

Principle Three: Moderation

Moderation refers to how much and how often you eat certain things, but don't confuse it with weighing and measuring food. These extreme methods aren't necessary. The best way to determine if you've had enough to eat is to listen to your cues of hunger and satiety. Many people don't listen to these cues even when they're dieting. They continue to overeat the allowed foods, so when the diet is over, they're still in an Overeating Cycle, just as Ken was. When your goal is to feel comfortable after eating, however, you're more likely to eat in moderation. When you are listening to your instincts, you are also more likely to choose less-healthful foods in moderation.

As you can see, this approach doesn't rely on willpower, or more accurately, *won't power*. However, understanding more about the nutrient content of your food will help you make decisions about balance, variety, and moderation (look for a summary in the Bottom Line at the end of each nutrient chapter). As you let go of all the restrictive and complicated diet rules and build a solid foundation of nutrition information, you'll be in charge of making the best possible choices for yourself. Create your own masterpiece!

CHAPTER 11

DRINK AND BE MERRY

One day spent at a spa, and my view of fluids was forever changed. As I checked in, I noticed two beautiful glass jars filled with water and ice, lemon slices in one jar and cucumber slices in the other. I was led past trickling waterfalls to the locker room where I was given a robe, slippers, and a water bottle. In the lounge where I relaxed before my first treatment, a selection of hot herbal teas, more water, and fresh fruit were displayed. After my massage, the therapist urged me to drink lots of water to remove the toxins she had massaged from my tissues. My aesthetician recommended drinking plenty of fluids to keep my skin hydrated from the inside out. Near the end of my spa day, I sipped raspberry iced tea by a sparkling pool. In the middle of a busy day I can re-create that same feeling of nurturing and nourishing myself by taking a moment to slice a lemon for my water or relax with a cup of hot tea.

WHY IS WATER IMPORTANT?

Water is often overlooked and underconsumed. Approximately 60 to 70 percent of your body is comprised of water. That's about ten to fifteen gallons! It's found in every cell, tissue, and organ; nearly every life-sustaining body process requires water to function.

Water helps your body:

- Maintain your blood pressure and blood flow
- Digest the food you eat
- Transport nutrients throughout your body
- Eliminate waste products from your body
- Decrease constipation
- Protect and lubricate your organs and tissues
- Regulate and maintain your body temperature
- Metabolize fat
- Give you a feeling of fullness

What Happens in My Body?

In order to ensure that these important functions are carried out, your body attempts to keep this delicate system in balance at all times. When you consume far too little water, your body must work very hard to maintain this system. Your body secretes a hormone called aldosterone in order to conserve water by holding on to all the water (and sodium) it can. This can lead to fluid retention in your tissues and suppression of thirst.

When you drink enough water most of the time, your body's production of aldosterone decreases and the extra fluid and sodium are released. When this "breakthrough point" is reached, you may notice a sudden loss of several pounds, a decrease in your symptoms of fluid retention such as puffiness and swelling, and a return of normal thirst.

Many people are chronically, mildly dehydrated but don't realize it. If you continually struggle with fatigue and lack of stamina, you may be living in a state of slight dehydration. Imagine being able to let go of extra water weight and boost your energy level just by drinking enough water. Try it and see.

MINDFUL MOMENT: Imagine being able to boost your energy level just by consuming enough fluid.

Severe dehydration can be very serious—even deadly. Significant dehydration occurs with prolonged fluid restriction or when you don't drink enough fluid during hot or humid weather, exercise, or illness such as vomiting, diarrhea, or fever. Symptoms of serious dehydration include irritability, moodiness, fatigue, headaches, dizziness, muscle weakness, cramping, nausea, diarrhea, and confusion. These symptoms require immediate medical attention.

How Much Do I Need?

You've probably heard that you should drink eight to twelve 8-ounce glasses of water daily. Since there's a lot of variation among individuals, paying attention to the color of your urine is a more practical method to determine just how well hydrated you are. When you drink enough water, you'll pass plenty of very light yellow or pale urine. When you don't drink enough water, your body must hold on to as much fluid as possible by making your urine more concentrated. Therefore, you'll pass smaller amounts of urine, and the urine will look deeper yellow. (Some vitamins and some medications can also affect the color of your urine.)

A number of important factors affect your fluid needs.

> **Temperature:** Water helps regulate your body temperature by perspiration through obvious sweating and imperceptible evaporation; higher temperatures will cause you to lose more water. This is especially important when you're in a hot climate.
>
> **Activity:** Any increase in activity will result in more perspiration and loss of water. You must increase your water intake before, during, and after physical activity to avoid dehydration. Be especially mindful of the symptoms of dehydration in yourself and others during exercise.
>
> **Age:** Children and the elderly are more prone to dehydration and the effects of fluid shifts, especially during illness and hot weather.

Body Weight: The more you weigh the more fluid you need.

Medical Conditions: Vomiting, diarrhea, high fever, hyperventilation, certain medical problems, and various medications can lead to the loss or retention of fluid. Medications such as diuretics, commonly known as water pills, should be used strictly under medical supervision.

Hormones: Women may experience marked fluid shifts as a result of their menstrual cycles, pregnancy, or use of hormonal medications.

Dietary Intake: That initial impressive weight loss on some diets is actually due to fluid loss. Since food is composed of an average of 70 percent water, a sudden decrease in the amount of food you eat can result in a temporary loss of water weight. Low-carbohydrate diets also cause a remarkable loss of water weight at first. However, your goal should be a loss of fat, not fluid.

HOW DO I OPTIMIZE MY FLUID INTAKE?

Fluid is essential for weight management and optimal health. Here are some specific strategies for increasing your water intake.

Set goals for improving the quantity and quality of your fluid intake. Whenever you want to change something, first create a plan and break it into small, specific steps. This works much better than just saying, "I'm going to drink more water." Start by jotting down the amount and type of fluid you are taking in.

Increase your water intake gradually. If your urine is not consistently light colored, then every day or two, add an additional cup (8 ounces) of water to what you're already drinking.

MINDFUL MOMENT: Some fluids are really food.

Make it appealing. If drinking water is difficult for you, try very cold, bottled, or filtered water. For more flavor and interest, try sparkling water or flavored bottled water over ice cubes. You can also add wedges or slices of lime, lemon, orange, cucumber, raspberries, cranberries, mint leaves, or sprigs of fresh rosemary to enhance the flavor. Make beautiful ice cubes by adding any of these to your ice cube tray before freezing.

Spread your fluids throughout the day. The initial inconvenience of increased trips to the bathroom will improve over time. You may decide to stop drinking fluids well before bedtime if you find you have to get up at night to urinate.

Keep water within easy reach. If water is handy, you're more likely to drink it. Some helpful ideas:

- Keep a 16- or 24-ounce water bottle at your desk, in your car, and with you at home, setting a goal to drink and refill it every two to three hours.

- Drink an 8-ounce glass of water every couple of hours or before and between each meal.

- Keep a half-gallon jug of water in the refrigerator and commit yourself to finishing it before the end of the day.

- Make a trip to the water cooler every time you take a break from work.

- Never pass a water fountain without taking a drink.

- Add ice to your beverages so that as it melts, you'll get even more fluid.

Drink before you eat. Thirst can be mistaken for hunger. If your fluid intake has been below par, try a glass of water before eating, especially when you're not sure if you're hungry.

Watch your sodium (salt) intake. Excessive salt intake can lead to more water retention. For some people, this can even lead to elevated blood pressure and other medical problems. The recommended daily intake of sodium is no more than 2,400 milligrams (about a teaspoon).

STRATEGIES: THINK BEFORE YOU DRINK

Some fluids are packed with nutrients. Others are loaded with calories, so you get more than you bargained for. Consider the following advice to achieve balance, variety, and moderation.

The deal on dairy. Low-fat or fat-free milk is a great source of fluid, calcium, protein, and other nutrients. Some studies have shown that three servings a day may help with weight management. Try our **Fresh Fruit Smoothie** recipe in part 4, made with skim milk, yogurt, and fruit, as a satisfying breakfast or snack.

Some foods are high in fluids. Although water is your best source for staying hydrated, many foods like fruits, vegetables, salads, and soups have high water content. Try one of our soup recipes: **Harvest Vegetable, Chicken and Rice**, or **Southwestern**.

Some fluids are loaded with calories. Popular specialty coffee drinks and commercial smoothies often have a lot of fat and sugar in them, and a chocolate shake is really just liquefied ice cream. Some of these beverages have more than 400 calories—as much or more than a meal. Don't overlook this significant source of calories.

Keesha figured this one out.

I used to be one of those people who was always drinking something: juice and a large coffee drink in the morning, one or two of those garbage-can-sized sodas during the day, and once in a while a smoothie or a shake in the afternoon. The problem was that it didn't seem like eating to me. I mean, there's no chewing involved, right? Now I'd rather eat an orange and drink a glass of water than drink orange juice. I discovered that I like to eat my food, not drink it.

Some drinks contain a lot of sugar. Soft drinks and fruit-flavored drinks may have 150 calories or more per serving. Keep in mind that soft drinks may also have a lot of sodium, which can cause fluid retention, and carbonation, which can lead to gas and bloating. Gradually cut back by replacing sugary drinks with water. Drinks sweetened artificially may also be a good substitute and are safe in moderation.

Sports drinks are for strenuous sports. It's best to consume sports drinks only during intense exercise that lasts more than an hour since they provide fluid, electrolytes (including sodium), and sugar. They're not recommended for rehydrating during average activity.

Watch the extras. Since sugar, sweetener, creamer, flavorings, and other extras you add to your beverages can add up quickly without really satisfying hunger, consider whether they really add to your enjoyment.

What about alcohol? On a positive note, some studies have shown that moderate alcohol intake (particularly red wine) may have health benefits. Moderation means two drinks a day for men and one for women. Don't start drinking if you don't drink already or if you're prone to problems with alcohol. Remember that the risks outweigh the benefits if you drink too much.

Alcohol won't help hydrate you because of the way your body processes it. In fact, it has a mild diuretic effect that causes water loss. Alcohol also contains a significant number of calories: seven calories per gram as compared to protein and carbohydrates, which have four calories per gram, and fat, which has nine. It can also interfere with your ability to make mindful decisions about your food choices. As always, moderation is the key.

Be aware of too much caffeine. Caffeine is considered safe in moderation for most adults: about 300 milligrams, or three 8-ounce cups of coffee per day. (Tea, soda, and chocolate generally have less caffeine than coffee does.) Because large cups and mugs are popular, it's a good idea to watch your portion sizes. If you decide to cut back, begin to decrease gradually to avoid caffeine-withdrawal headaches. Every few days, try cutting out one serving or replacing it with a caffeine-free version.

Drink more water before, during, and after you exercise. Increase your water intake to replace fluid losses as you increase your activity level.

Water weight is temporary. Don't be discouraged by fluctuations in your weight that may be due to hormonal cycles and fluid retention. If this is an ongoing problem for you, seek medical advice.

THE BOTTOM LINE FOR FLUIDS

BALANCE

Create a plan for improving the quantity and
quality of the fluids you drink.

VARIETY

Water satisfies thirst best. If drinking water is difficult, try it over ice
or with a slice of lemon. Consume foods that are high in fluids, like
vegetables, salads, fruit, soup, and nutrient-rich fluids like milk.

MODERATION

Be aware of extras, particularly sugar, salt, caffeine, fat, and alcohol.

CHAPTER 12

CLEARING CARB CONFUSION

held my breath as I approached the conference breakfast buffet. All too often, just Danish pastries and coffee are served—or some variation on that theme. There's nothing inherently wrong with Danish, but I like to start most days with a good foundation. Luckily, at this meeting there were other options including fresh fruit, hard-boiled eggs, and cereals with low-fat or nonfat milk. Lunch was equally good: a garden salad with fresh veggies and grilled chicken on top, served with balsamic vinaigrette, whole wheat rolls with butter, and dessert. Still, it was more than I usually have for lunch, and I had to stay mindful. Sitting through long meetings can give me a sense of entitlement ("I earned it"), and I can easily become distracted by socializing or networking during the meal and eat too much. I don't want to turn over the responsibility for what I eat and how I'll feel all day to the meeting planner who selected the menu.

WHY ARE CARBS IMPORTANT?

Carbohydrates have gotten a lot of attention during the last several years. Sometimes the information you hear is confusing, contradictory, or difficult to follow. In short, carbs are an important family of nutrients that provide your body with energy. In addition, many carbohydrate-containing foods provide fiber and important vitamins, minerals, and phytochemicals that have been shown to improve health. Carbohydrates are found in bread and other grain products, legumes, vegetables, fruit, dairy products, and sugar.

Carbohydrates are important for many reasons:

- They are the preferred source of energy for your body. One gram of carbohydrates provides your body with four calories to use or store as energy.
- Many foods that contain carbs are nutrient rich and high in vitamins and minerals such as B vitamins (thiamin, riboflavin, niacin), vitamin E, iron, zinc, calcium, selenium, and magnesium.
- Many carbohydrate-containing foods have naturally occurring phytochemicals, which may have protective effects.
- A diet high in fruits, vegetables, whole grains, and fiber has been shown to reduce the risk of cardiovascular disease and cancer.
- A high-fiber diet promotes smoother digestion, aids in preventing constipation, and helps prevent certain diseases of the colon.
- High-fiber foods help increase fullness and regulate blood sugar levels.
- Research supports the beneficial effects of fiber in whole-oat, barley, and rye products in reducing blood cholesterol levels.

What Happens in My Body?

At some point you may have heard someone say, "Carbs just turn to sugar in your body." The word *sugar* refers to glucose, an important form of energy for your body. Therefore, the majority of carbohydrates do turn into "sugar" during digestion, but that's what they're supposed to do. Since many people think of sugar as "bad," they also think of carbohydrates as "bad." To understand why they're not, however, a brief science lesson is in order. (If you trust me that glucose is not a bad thing and you're not up for a science lesson, skip to the section titled "What Are Carbohydrates Anyway?")

When carbohydrates are eaten and digested, they are broken down to glucose, which floats in your bloodstream (hence the term *blood sugar*), where it's ready to be used for energy or stored. Under normal circumstances, your body closely regulates your blood glucose (blood sugar) levels.

Your blood glucose level rises after you eat, causing your pancreas to release insulin. Insulin is the key that opens the cell's door to let glucose in. Insulin has two main jobs: (1) to stimulate your brain, muscle, fat, and other cells to use glucose for fuel, and (2) to stimulate the liver to make glycogen, the storage form of glucose. This process helps keep the level of glucose in your blood stable, providing adequate fuel for your body. About one to three hours after you eat, your blood sugar and insulin levels both return to baseline.

When you haven't eaten in a while, your blood sugar levels begin to fall and you start to feel hungry. Since red blood cells and brain cells depend on glucose to function, you may experience moodiness, irritability, fatigue, nausea, headaches, and difficulty concentrating. If you don't eat, your pancreas releases a hormone called glucagon, which breaks glycogen back down into glucose to keep your blood sugar levels from falling too low.

With chronic overeating, inactivity, and weight gain, many individuals develop insulin resistance: their tissues ignore the insulin signals. In other words, the key doesn't work as well, so the blood glucose levels remain too high. The body tries to compensate by making more keys—producing even more insulin—which results in hyperinsulinemia. These high insulin levels promote fat storage and inhibit fat burning. Hyperinsulinemia contributes to the development of Metabolic Syndrome, which increases the risk of developing diabetes and heart disease. (To read more about this serious problem, see the Health Notes about "Metabolic Syndrome" in the appendix.)

Although it may not seem like it, this explanation is actually a bit of an oversimplification. The main point is that carbohydrates are an important and significant source of fuel for your body. Understanding how your body functions and uses this fuel will help you make the best possible decisions for yourself.

What Are Carbohydrates Anyway?

Plants manufacture most of the carbohydrates found in foods, except for in dairy products, the only animal source of carbohydrates. There are two basic types of carbohydrates: simple and complex. Both are made up of glucose molecules, but the molecules are arranged differently.

Simple Carbohydrates Also known as simple sugars, simple carbohydrates are small packages of glucose that are broken down easily and rapidly by your body. Simple carbohydrates include fructose found in fruits and honey, lactose found in dairy products, and sucrose found in table sugar, corn syrup, and some vegetables. (See table on page 181.) Eating a piece of fruit, drinking a glass of juice, or eating candy when you're hungry will give you a quick but short burst of energy because simple carbohydrates can be quickly digested. Just be prepared for hunger to return a short time later! (See tables on pages 181–183.)

Complex Carbohydrates These carbohydrates are made of long chains of hundreds to thousands of glucose molecules. Complex carbohydrates fall into two main categories: starch and fiber.

Starches can be broken down into glucose molecules by your body and used for energy. Starches are found in grains (such as wheat, rice, barley, and oats), products made from grain (such as bread, pasta, tortillas, and cereal), legumes (such as beans, lentils, and nuts), and vegetables. High-starch vegetables include potatoes, corn, and peas. Low-starch vegetables include lettuce, green vegetables, peppers, onions, and many other vegetables. Although it takes longer to digest complex carbohydrates than it does simple carbohydrates, starch eventually breaks down into glucose that can be used by your body for energy.

Fiber is the term used for indigestible complex carbohydrates. The human body can't break down the chemical links between the glucose molecules in fiber, so fiber helps fill you up, increases satiety, and helps with digestion, but doesn't provide energy in the form of calories. Fiber is found in fruit, whole grains, legumes, and vegetables (some processed foods are fortified with fiber, too). The recommended fiber intake is about 25 to 30 grams a day. (See table on page 182–183.)

Simple Carbohydrates at a Glance

TYPES	SOURCES	EXAMPLES	SERVING SIZES	GRAMS FIBER
Fructose	Fruit	Apples, citrus, peaches	1 medium piece of fruit or ½ cup chopped	1–5
		Banana	1 small	2
		Berries	¾–1 cup	3–5
		Melons, tropical fruit	¾–1 cup	1–2
		Fruit juice	¾ cup (6 oz.)	0–1
	Honey	Table honey	1 tablespoon	0
		Honey added to foods	Varies	0
Lactose	Dairy	Milk	1 cup (8 oz.)	0
		Soft cheeses (i.e., cottage)	½ cup (4 oz.)	0
		Hard cheeses (i.e., cheddar)	1½ to 2 oz.	0
		Yogurt	1 cup (8 oz.)	0
		Ice cream	½ cup	0
Sucrose	Sugar	Table sugar	1 teaspoon	0
		Corn syrup, table syrup	1 tablespoon	0

How Much Do I Need?

Most dietary guidelines recommend that the majority of your food intake be carbohydrates, with the recommended percentage of total caloric intake from carbohydrates ranging from 45 to 60 percent (depending on the authority).

Complex Carbohydrates at a Glance

CARBS	SOURCES	EXAMPLES	SERVING SIZES	GRAMS FIBER
Starch	Whole Grains (Unrefined) and Grain Products	Whole grains (i.e., brown or wild rice, barley)	½ cup	2–5
		Whole-wheat pasta	½ cup	2–5
		Whole-wheat bread	1 slice	2–5
		Whole-wheat or corn tortilla	1 6-inch tortilla	2–5
		Whole grain crackers	6 crackers	2–5
		Whole grain cereal	1 ounce (¾ cup)	3–7
	Refined (Processed) Grains	White rice, pasta	½ cup	½–1
		White bread	1 slice	1
		Flour tortillas	1 6-inch tortilla	1
		Cereals (refined)	1 ounce (usually ¾ cup)	½–1
	Legumes	Beans, lentils	½ cup	5–7
		Nuts	¼ cup	2
		Nut butters (e.g., peanut butter)	2 tablespoons	2
	High-starch Vegetables	Peas	½ cup	5
		Corn	½ cup	2
		Potatoes	1 small (with peel)	2
		Winter squash	½ cup	6
	Low-starch Vegetables	Raw or cooked	½ cup	1–3
		Leafy vegetables	1 cup	1
		Juice	¾ cup (6 oz.)	0–1

CARBS	SOURCES	EXAMPLES	SERVING SIZES	GRAMS FIBER
Fiber	Fruit	See fiber content in *Simple Carbohydrate at a Glance*		
	Grains	See fiber content above		
	Legumes			
	Vegetables			

Following this recommendation, Tonya had an Aha! moment.

> I finally understand the Food Pyramid. When I'm eating all the stuff they recommend, I'm not hungry for as much of the junk I used to eat.

Here are the general guidelines for how much to eat each day to provide your body with adequate carbohydrates, fiber, and certain vitamins and minerals.

- At least six servings of grains or grain products; three of these should be whole grains
- Three to five servings of vegetables
- Two to three servings of fruit
- Two to three servings of dairy products

HOW DO I OPTIMIZE MY CARBOHYDRATE INTAKE?
Go for Grains

- Strive to eat three servings of whole grains each day.
- Look for whole wheat, whole grain, or bran as the first ingredient in bread, cereal, and other grain products.
- When you choose bread, tortillas, crackers, pasta, rice, or cereal, check the nutrition label for fiber content: the higher the better. When foods have been highly processed or refined, the fiber content may be reduced or even eliminated. (For more details about reading nutrition labels, see the Health Notes in the appendix.)

STRATEGIES: MAKING HEALTHIER CHOICES

Keep it simple. Generally, the closer a food is to its original form the better. Focus on foods that haven't been highly processed and that have a short ingredient list. You can't get any shorter than "apple."

Make it convenient. The best way to encourage these food groups is to keep them on hand, ready for snacks and meals. If you can't eat fresh, frozen is the next best thing for maximum nutrient content.

Experiment with new flavors. On your next visit to the grocery store or local farmers market, pick up fruits, vegetables, and grains you've never had or try preparing your favorites in new ways.

Think "plant-based diet." A plant-based diet is packed with nutrients and helps fill you up and boost your fiber intake. Look for whole grains and whole grain products. Go for fruits and vegetables with deeply colored flesh such as mangoes, blueberries, cantaloupe, tomatoes, red peppers, and dark leafy greens since they generally have more micronutrients. Eat edible skins and peels (thoroughly washed) to increase your fiber and nutrient intake.

Practice moderation. Because they are generally less nutritious, eat refined and sugar-containing products in moderation.

Be aware of portion sizes. Carbs are important nutrients, but it's essential to pay attention to the size and number of servings you eat. A bagel may be three to five servings of bread, and a large plate of spaghetti may be three or more servings of pasta. Pay attention to your hunger and fullness levels; your body knows when it has had enough.

Be mindful of how carbs are prepared. Toppings, sauces, and condiments boost flavor, but be aware that they can also add significant calories and fat.

- High-fiber and whole grain foods may have a coarser texture and are often darker in color. Don't be misled by dyes or molasses added by the manufacturer to darken a product.

- Try brown rice and whole-wheat pasta. Many people say they prefer the flavor and texture once they try them. You can mix them with the traditional white version to get used to the different flavor, if necessary. Our recipe in part 4 for **Whole Wheat Pasta with Basil and Cherry Tomatoes** is simple and tasty.

- For variety, try one of the many exciting and flavorful grains available in the market. Look for wild rice, basmati rice, jasmine rice, barley, bulgur, couscous, quinoa, polenta, and kasha. Cook according to package directions or use vegetable or chicken broth in place of water. Add fresh or dried herbs, a small amount of olive oil, flavored vinegar, and diced vegetables for a hot side dish or cold salad. Our recipe for **Confetti Quinoa** is good hot or cold.

- Look for high-fiber cereals; a pretty good guide is five or more grams of fiber per serving. If you aren't used to it, try mixing high-fiber cereal with your usual brand for a while.

- Top high-fiber cereal with fresh fruit, fat-free milk, or low-fat yogurt.

- Fill a whole-wheat or corn tortilla with beans, grilled or fresh vegetables, lean meats, fish or chicken, and **Salsa Fresca** (see our Fiesta Night menu).

- Replace all or part of the white flour with oat bran or wheat flour when baking. Our **Whole-Wheat Pizza Crust** makes a great base for **Rustic Grilled Pizzas**.

- Choose whole-wheat toast, bagels, and English muffins; just watch your portion sizes. Top them with all-fruit spreads, lower-fat

> **MINDFUL MOMENT:** When shopping for foods with a short list of ingredients, you can't get any shorter than "apple."

cream cheese, fancy mustards, and other low-fat alternatives. Pastries, croissants, doughnuts, and muffins contain less fiber and more fat.

- To increase satiety and provide more sustained energy in the morning, include peanut butter, an egg, low-fat dairy, or other lean protein sources with your cereal, toast, fruit, and other carbohydrates.

Value Your Veggies

- Keep precut raw vegetables crisp in water in the refrigerator.
- Add chopped broccoli, mushrooms, squash, colorful peppers, or other veggies to rice, pasta, and stuffing.
- Add extra frozen vegetables to a frozen entrée for added nourishment and a more filling "fast" food.
- Fresh spinach, sprouts, shredded carrots, and sliced cucumber or zucchini will liven up your sandwich.
- Try our **Salsa Fresca**, made with fresh ingredients like tomatoes, onions, herbs, and even fruit, for serving over chicken and fish.
- Keep a pot of homemade vegetable soup on hand for a satisfying meal. You can freeze handy-to-use portions for later. Try one of our easy recipes.
- Add vegetables and beans to your stews, soups, or pasta sauce.
- Spinach is great in meatloaf, and the kids will never notice shredded carrots in the spaghetti sauce.
- Choose darker green leafy and other types of lettuce because they have more flavor, fiber, and micronutrients than iceberg lettuce.
- Try mashed cauliflower in place of mashed potatoes for variety.
- Roasted vegetables such as potatoes, carrots, onions, and sweet potatoes are wonderful with meat and poultry. Try our recipe for **Roasted Roots**, a family favorite.
- Fresh sweet corn is delicious with a little salt and pepper—no butter needed.

- Make flavorful **Grilled Vegetables**. Just marinate asparagus, sliced peppers, eggplant, portobello mushrooms, zucchini, or onions in a dressing and grill or broil to serve as a gourmet side dish. Use leftovers in sandwiches, salads, pizzas, and pastas.

- Try low-fat sour cream, ricotta, steamed vegetables, or good old salt and pepper in place of butter, sour cream, cheese, and bacon on baked potatoes (or just use less!).

- A glass of tomato or vegetable juice is a great pick-me-up. It also makes a nice base for a spicy gazpacho with finely chopped onions, peppers, cucumbers, and tomatoes.

- Use fresh herbs, spice blends, seasoned vinegars, or lemon juice as flavorful seasonings.

Focus on Fruit

- Keep ready-to-eat fruit on hand—fresh whole fruit or dried fruit—as a convenient, sweet, high-fiber snack that will often satisfy a sweet tooth.

- Freeze seedless grapes, bananas, strawberries, or peach slices for an icy treat.

- Try our **Fresh Fruit Smoothie** recipe for a refreshing snack or breakfast.

- Use apple or banana slices instead of jelly on a peanut butter sandwich.

- Top pancakes with sliced fruit like berries, peaches, or bananas instead of syrup.

- Top a scoop of frozen yogurt or sherbet with your favorite fruits like berries or peaches.

- Baked fruit is a great dessert; I think you'll love **Cinnamon Apple Packets** and **Blueberry Peach Almond Crisp**.

- Whole fruit has more fiber than juices that have been strained. If you drink juice, look for 100 percent juice instead of fruit-flavored drinks, and check the label for added sugar (or better yet, make your own juices from fresh fruit, leaving the peels on whenever possible).

Do Three Dairy

- Aim for three a day. Dairy products are nutrient rich: they contain protein, calcium, vitamins A, D, B12, and riboflavin, phosphorous, and magnesium.

- Sample our simple **Yogurt Parfait, Fresh Fruit Smoothie,** or **Brunch Oven Eggs**.

- Experiment with different types and different brands of lower-fat versions of dairy products to find the ones that balance good flavor with good health.

- Gradually taper from regular (full-fat, or 4 percent) milk to 2 percent, then 1 percent, then fat-free. You can even mix two types together to adjust to the switch more gradually.

- If you think you're lactose intolerant, experiment with consuming dairy in small amounts with meals rather than by themselves. You may also find that you do better with certain types of dairy products such as yogurt or cheese. Lactose-reduced or lactose-free milk is available or you can try lactase tablets or drops, and products supplemented with lactase to assist your digestion of dairy.

Sweet as Sugar

What about sugar? Some people refer to sugar as empty calories because it doesn't provide nutrients like vitamins, minerals, or fiber. However, since it's a source of calories that can be used for energy, and it provides pleasure for those who like it, sugar is really not "empty." There's room in a balanced diet for a little sugar if you enjoy it.

Some people say they're addicted to sugar because they crave it or feel out of control when they eat it. There is a lot of research and controversy about sugar addiction, but for many people, simple and refined carbohydrates bring a brief feeling of a boost in energy followed by an energy drop, leading to increased hunger and cravings. Further, if you're in the habit of eating sugar in response to emotional triggers or thinking of sugar as something bad that should be avoided (there's that "should" again), you're setting yourself up for cravings. When you resist your cravings for sugar and then give in and eat it anyway, you may feel guilty, weak willed, and out of control, which can reinforce the feeling of being addicted.

In part 4, I've included a few of my family's favorite dessert recipes including **Bitter Sweet Chocolate Soufflé, Toasted Angel Food Cake with Strawberries,** and **Chocolate Chip Cloud Cookies**. Adopting an all-foods-fit approach and observing your body's responses to various foods allows you to enjoy sugar guilt free. Your cravings will lessen and you'll find it's easier to practice moderation when you eat mindfully.

THE BOTTOM LINE FOR CARBOHYDRATES

BALANCE

Focus on whole grains, fruits, vegetables, and fat-free or low-fat dairy.

VARIETY

Select a variety of grains (eat mostly whole grains). Choose fruits and vegetables that are deeply colored, and eat edible skins after washing.

MODERATION

Use moderation when eating refined carbohydrates and sugar.

CHAPTER 13

FAT FACTS

Years ago, I stopped eating salads. I had eaten them all the time while I was dieting, and perhaps I associated them with restriction. It seemed strange, though, since I love vegetables. As I thought about it, I realized that I used only fat-free dressings, a holdover from my diet days. Most didn't taste very good to me, so I just didn't bother anymore. When I switched to regular dressings in moderation I fell in love with salads again.

WHY IS FAT IMPORTANT?

For many people, fat-containing foods are high on their forbidden food list, a leftover from the low-fat diet craze. More recently, numerous studies and reports have improved our understanding about fat. It's time to separate fact from fiction so you can make the best choices for yourself (without deprivation, of course!), like Kelly.

> I always thought that eating fat made me fat, but when I tried to cut the fat out of my diet, my food didn't taste as good and I just didn't feel satisfied. I was thrilled when I heard that I didn't need to cut out fat completely but instead shift to eating healthier fats, which were actually good for me. Now, most of the fat in my diet is from the foods we ate when we were in Italy: olives and olive oil, fish, and nuts. And I switched from margarine back to real butter; I don't eat as much, but I like it a lot more.

Fats are important for many reasons:

- One gram of dietary fat provides your body with nine calories to use or store as energy.
- Fat is essential for growth and development (especially brain development during childhood).
- Fat is necessary for the absorption and transportation of vitamins A, D, E, and K.
- The omega-3 fatty acids decrease the risk of heart disease, stroke, and overall mortality.
- Fat helps maintain healthy skin and hair.
- Fat increases satiety (satisfaction and fullness).
- Fats give food flavor and texture.

What Happens in My Body?

Certain types of fat are beneficial, as you'll see. Where did fat get its bad rap, then? Well, the calorie content of fat is more than twice as high as in carbohydrates or protein, which can make it easier to consume more calories than you need. Since dietary fat is already in the chemical storage form your body prefers, you can easily store any excess as body fat. It's important to recognize, however, that an excess intake of calories from any source will be converted to body fat for storage.

Excessive intake of certain types of fat is also associated with heart disease, cancer, and other medical problems. Once again, knowledge about nutrition will help you make the best choices for yourself.

What Is Fat Anyway?

Different types of fats have different effects on your health. It will be easier to remember which is which when you understand that they are named for their chemical bonds. Fats (also called fatty acids) are made of long chains of carbon atoms. These carbon chains like to bond with hydrogen atoms. When a chain has all the hydrogen bonds it can handle, it's saturated. When it's missing one or more hydrogen bonds, it's unsaturated. Unsaturated fats are either mono-unsaturated (one unsaturated bond) or polyunsaturated (multiple unsaturated bonds). The fats in food are made up of a mixture of these three different types of fatty acids (saturated, monounsaturated, polyunsaturated) and are named by the type of fatty acid they have the most of.

Saturated Fat Saturated fat is typically solid at room temperature because all its carbon atoms have hydrogen bonds. The hydrogen bonds are like railroad ties that make the rails more stable. Saturated fat is found in animal products including meat and meat products, dairy products, egg yolks, and butter. Tropical oils like palm, palm kernel, and coconut oils are also saturated and may be found in candy, snack products, and movie popcorn. Saturated fats raise blood cholesterol, which increases the risk of heart disease. An easy way to remember this is:

Saturated fats are Solid at room temperature and Sit in your arteries.

Unsaturated Fat Unsaturated fat is liquid at room temperature because one or more of the hydrogen bonds are missing.

- Polyunsaturated fat is primarily found in these oils: safflower, sunflower, corn, sesame seed, flaxseed, soybean, and cottonseed. Fish is also an excellent source.
- Monounsaturated fat sources include canola oil, olive oil, and peanut oil. A helpful way to remember these is Good COP (canola, olive, peanut). Avocado, nuts, olives, and peanut butter are also good sources of monounsaturated fats.

Substituting unsaturated fats for saturated fats can improve overall heart health and help reduce total cholesterol.

Omega Fatty Acids Omega-3 and omega-6 fatty acids are types of polyunsaturated fats.

- Good sources of omega-3 fatty acids include cold-water fish, flaxseed and flaxseed oil, canola oil, walnuts and walnut oil, and soybeans and soybean oils. Health benefits from omega-3 fatty acids include lowering of triglyceride levels, slowing the buildup of plaque in the arteries, slight lowering of blood pressure, and reduction in risk of death from heart disease.
- Good sources of omega-6 fatty acids include safflower, sunflower, corn, and soybean oils, nuts, and seeds.

The ratio of these two fatty acids is important, and since the typical American diet is relatively high in omega-6 fatty acids, most people would benefit by shifting their intake toward more foods that contain omega-3.

Trans Fat Another type of fat, called trans fat, primarily results from man-made processes that alter unsaturated fats. Food manufacturers make trans fat by bubbling hydrogen gas into liquid vegetable oils, which causes hydrogen bonds to form, making the liquid solid or semi-solid. Trans fats raise the risk of heart disease.

Fats at a Glance

TYPES	EFFECTS ON HEALTH	SUBTYPES	EXAMPLES	TYPICAL SERVING SIZES
Saturated Fats (Solid)	Raise cholesterol		Butter	1 teaspoon
			Lard	1 teaspoon
			Palm oil	1 teaspoon
			Palm kernel oil	1 teaspoon
			Coconut oil	1 teaspoon
			Cocoa butter	1 teaspoon
			Cream cheese	1 tablespoon
			Cream	2 tablespoons
			Half & half	2 tablespoons
			Sour cream	2 tablespoons
			Mayonnaise	1 teaspoon
			Cream-based salad dressings	1 tablespoon
			Fatty meats	Varies
			Egg yolks	Varies
			Dairy products	Varies
Unsaturated Fats (Liquid)	Lower cholesterol	Polyunsaturated	Corn oil	1 teaspoon
			Cottonseed oil	1 teaspoon
			Flaxseed oil	1 teaspoon
			Safflower oil	1 teaspoon
			Sesame seed oil	1 teaspoon
			Sunflower oil	1 teaspoon
			Soybean oil	1 teaspoon
			Margarine	1 teaspoon
			Oil-based salad dressings	1 tablespoon
			Fish	Varies
		Monounsaturated	Canola oil	1 teaspoon
			Olive oil	1 teaspoon
			Peanut oil	1 teaspoon
			Avocado	$\frac{1}{5}$ of a whole
			Nuts	1 oz., ¼ cup
			Nut butters	½ tablespoon
			Olives	11 large

- Trans fats might be found in margarine, shortening, chips, snack foods, crackers, baked goods, and fried foods.
- Trans fats are listed on the nutrition label when there is half a gram or more per serving. They will also be found in the ingredient list as hydrogenated or partially hydrogenated oils. The closer to the beginning of the list an ingredient appears, the more of it the product contains. For more on reading nutrition labels, see the Health Notes in the appendix.

It's recommended that no more than 1 percent of your total daily calories come from trans fats.

Cholesterol Cholesterol is not a fatty acid; rather, it is a cousin of fat in the lipid family. Cholesterol plays an important functional role in your body, but too much cholesterol can contribute to your risk of heart disease. Cholesterol comes from two sources: it's made in your liver and it's consumed in your diet—for example, meat and eggs. Your cholesterol levels, therefore, are primarily hereditary and partly dietary. Authorities recommend a cholesterol intake of less than 300 milligrams daily. If you have a personal or family history of elevated cholesterol levels, heart disease, or diabetes, you'll want to be even more cautious about eating high-cholesterol foods and saturated fats. (See the Health Notes about "Cholesterol and Heart Disease" in the appendix for more details.)

HOW DO I OPTIMIZE MY FAT INTAKE?

Decrease your intake of saturated fat.
- Use liquid oils instead of solid fat whenever possible.
- Cut back on animal products such as fatty red meats, poultry with skin, whole-fat dairy, and butter.
- Select leaner cuts of beef and pork (these often have the words *round* or *loin* in the name), trim visible fat, and remove the skin from chicken before cooking.
- Choose ground beef labeled lean (ideally less than 10 percent fat). Drain excess fat carefully. Drain excess fat (or rinse with hot water in a colander) before adding additional ingredients.

- Chill soups and stews made with poultry or meat and skim off the solidified fat before reheating to serve.

- Eat fish in place of meat at least twice a week.

- Enjoy your vegetables without butter by seasoning with lemon juice, salt and pepper, or herbs and spices.

- Try meatless meals using vegetable sources of protein like beans and soy.

- Use low-fat or nonfat (skim) versions of your favorite dairy products.

- Use small amounts of cheese; grate and sprinkle for flavor rather than using large chunks or sauces.

- Eat snack foods made with tropical oils in moderation.

Choose unsaturated fats.

Though they're still calorie dense, substituting polyunsaturated and monounsaturated fats for saturated fats is beneficial for your heart.

- Buy or make salad dressings with vegetable, olive, or canola oil. Use these oils in place of butter or lard when cooking. You'll love our **Balsamic Vinaigrette** recipe in part 4.

- Use a thin spread of avocado or our **Guacamole** in place of mayonnaise or butter on a sandwich.

- Olives add a flavorful and beneficial dose of fat to pastas, salads, and other dishes. My favorite is our **Olive Tapenade** served on **Bruschetta** (French bread brushed with olive oil and toasted).

- Peanut butter is an old standby; again, it's high in fat but satisfying in small amounts.

- Tree nuts like almonds and walnuts have additional health benefits. They can make a great snack and add nice flavor to pasta dishes and stuffing. We like them in salads. Toasted or candied nuts are delicious paired with fruit, like strawberries or oranges, in a salad.

MINDFUL MOMENT: Eat more healthful fats (fish, nuts, oils) in place of saturated and trans fats.

Eat more omega-3 fatty acids.

- The omega-3 fatty acids in fish oil decrease the risk of heart disease, stroke, and overall mortality. Try to eat at least two four-ounce servings of fish each week. (If you have a history of coronary heart disease, the American Heart Association recommends one serving of fish daily.)

- Fatty fish such as salmon, tuna, rainbow trout, herring, mackerel, and wild oysters have the highest levels of omega-3 fatty acids. Our recipe for **Grilled Salmon** is a good place to start.

- If you don't like fish, consider taking fish oil capsules (one gram daily) and increasing your intake of flaxseed, canola oil, and walnuts.

Watch trans fat.

- Look for trans fat on the Nutrition Facts label and check the ingredient list for hydrogenated or partially hydrogenated oil. (For more on reading labels, see the Health Notes in the appendix.)

- Ask whether your favorite restaurants use trans fat for frying, cooking, or baking.

Reduce your total fat intake.

Consuming too much fat, even the more beneficial types, can make it more difficult to manage your weight. Look for easy ways to decrease the amount of fat you eat. Here are some examples.

- Prepare or order foods that are grilled, roasted, baked, boiled, or braised instead of fried or sautéed.

- Use less butter, oil, mayonnaise, cream cheese, and other condiments.

- Use less than the usual amount of salad dressing, sauces, and toppings.

- Ask for your salad dressing and sauces on the side. Dip the tip of the tines of your fork in the dressing before you spear your salad; you'll get a little flavor with every bite, but a lot less fat than you would if the dressing was poured over the salad.

- Spray your pans with cooking spray instead of coating them with fats and oils.

- Add bouillon cubes, broth, or minced garlic in place of butter or oil for an extra touch of flavor when preparing rice or mashed potatoes.

- Use less fat than a recipe calls for when you're cooking. This is more challenging with baking, but it's possible to substitute applesauce or pureed prunes in some recipes for baked goods.

- Try lower-fat versions of your favorite foods. Be sure to read the label, though; low fat doesn't necessarily mean low calorie.

- Our **Baked Tortilla Chips**, **Crisp Pita Triangles**, and **Bruschetta**, or thinly sliced baguettes are great for healthy dips and toppings in place of higher-fat chips and crackers.

- Choose red or tomato sauces in place of white or cream sauces on your pasta. Try our **Roasted Roma Tomato Sauce** (great on pizza, too).

- Use less butter, cream, cheese, or oil when you make your own sauces; use high-fat sauces in moderation on your pasta. A little goes a long way.

- Use moderation when eating those higher-fat foods you love.

Make healthy substitutions.

For many practical and delicious ideas to decrease your overall fat intake see "Strategies: Fat—Making Healthier Choices" on page 200.

How Much Do I Need?

Numerous health authorities recommend that your total fat intake be in the range of 20 to 35 percent of your total calories. For example, for a person requiring 2000 calories a day and striving for 30 percent of calories from fat, 600 calories or less of his daily intake should be from fat (approximately 65 grams or less). The majority of your fat intake should be unsaturated fat. The American Heart Association recommends that you limit your intake of saturated fat to less than 7 percent and trans fat to less than 1 percent of your fat intake.

STRATEGIES: FAT—
MAKING HEALTHIER CHOICES

A HEALTHIER CHOICE	USE MODERATION
FATS AND OILS	
Soft tub margarine made with safflower, corn, or sunflower oil	Butter or stick margarine made with partially hydrogenated oil
Canola, olive, or peanut oil	Lard, shortening, meat fat, coconut oil, or palm oil
Nonstick pans or cooking spray	Cooking with butter or lard
Flavored vinegar and salad dressing made with oil	Regular salad dressing made with tropical oils, cream, or cheese
Dressing and sauces on the side	Dressings poured over the top
Broth	Butter, lard, or margarine
Mustard	Mayonnaise
Baked potato with low-fat toppings	French fries
PROTEINS	
Grilled, broiled, boiled, baked	Fried
Skinless chicken or turkey	Poultry with skin
White meat poultry	Dark meat
Lean beef trimmed of visible fat	Prime, heavily marbled cuts, or organ meats
Lean ground beef, drained	Regular ground beef
Lean pork (loin, shoulder, leg)	Pork ribs or roast, hot dogs, bacon, sausage
Fish	Shellfish
Egg whites (2)	Whole egg
Low-fat egg substitute	Eggs
Meatless: beans, tofu	High-fat protein sources

A HEALTHIER CHOICE	USE MODERATION
BREADS AND CEREALS	
Whole grain bread, bagels, or English muffins	Doughnuts, pastries, muffins, or croissants
Brown or white rice	Fried rice, crispy noodles
Pasta with tomato sauce	Pasta with cream- or butter-based sauces
Hot or cold whole grain cereals	Granola
DAIRY PRODUCTS	
Skim or 1% milk	Whole milk
Evaporated skim milk	Cream or half and half
Reduced or fat-free sour cream, cream cheese, and yogurt	Regular sour cream, cream cheese, and yogurt
Low-fat cheeses (skim mozzarella, cottage cheese, or ricotta cheese)	American, cheddar, Swiss, Brie, and other high-fat cheeses
Frozen yogurt, ice milk, sherbet	Ice cream, shakes
SNACKS AND DESSERTS	
Pretzels, light popcorn, flatbread, whole grain crackers, melba toast, nuts (in moderation)	High-fat or fried snack foods made with butter, cheese, or partially hydrogenated oils (trans fats)
Angel food cake, graham crackers, fruit, gingersnaps, real fruit popsicles, sherbet	High-fat cakes, cookies, candy, chocolate, desserts

Remember, eat what you love—and use these suggestions to help you balance eating for nourishment with eating for enjoyment.

THE BOTTOM LINE FOR FATS

BALANCE

Balance your intake of higher-fat foods with lower-fat
foods in the same meal or throughout the day, shifting the
balance toward more beneficial unsaturated fats.

VARIETY

Eat a variety of nutrient-rich fat-containing foods.
Increase your intake of omega-3 fatty acids by eating
more fish, flaxseed, canola oil, and walnuts.

MODERATION

Enjoy fats in moderation rather than all or nothing. For those foods
you love that are higher in less-healthful fats and cholesterol, use
moderation in how much you eat and how often you eat them.

CHAPTER 14

PROTEIN POWER

When I was seeing patients in the office, I had breakfast every morning around 6:30. My favorite was (and still is) cereal and skim milk with blueberries when they're in season. Once in a while for a change of pace, I'd share a toasted bagel with a little bit of butter on it with my daughter. Like clockwork, I was hungry by 10:00 a.m., so I had to plan to write chart notes around that time so I could have a snack. One day, 10:00 came and went with nary a hunger pang, and I remembered that I had had peanut butter on my bagel that morning instead of butter. Finally, around 11:00, I was ready for my snack, but I decided to wait until lunch instead. That little bit of extra protein with my breakfast staved off hunger for an hour. Since then, I have learned to purposefully adjust the type and amount of food I eat according to my plans for the day.

WHY IS PROTEIN IMPORTANT?

Protein is found in every cell in your body, and it plays a role in basic bodily functions ranging from walking to digesting food. It is critical for building muscle and vital for optimal health. Eating protein also promotes the greatest satiety of the three macronutrients. The satiety that comes from eating protein made a big difference for Leigh Ann.

> As I became aware of when, what, and how much I was eating, I saw a strong connection between the things I ate and my hunger levels. For example, I loved to eat an apple for my afternoon snack, but most of the time I'd have to have another snack before dinner. If I put a little peanut butter on it, I could make it through the rest of the afternoon. Now I keep nuts, string cheese, slices of turkey, and other high-protein snacks on hand so I'm not running back to the kitchen all afternoon.

Protein is important for a number of reasons. It:

- Builds, repairs, and maintains healthy muscles, organs, skin, and hair
- Manufactures enzymes, hormones, and blood-clotting factors
- Maintains water balance, transports oxygen, regulates acid-base balance, and supports immune function
- Provides your body with four calories of energy per gram, if necessary
- Contributes essential nutrients: for example, dairy products are a significant source of calcium; beef is an excellent source of iron. Dairy products and meat also provide zinc as well as vitamins B6 and B12.
- Increases satiety so you feel fuller, longer

MINDFUL MOMENT: Protein-containing foods help you feel fuller, longer.

What Happens in My Body?

During digestion, proteins are broken down to provide amino acids and nitrogen for your body. During starvation (as we discussed in the carbohydrate chapter) your muscle tissue can be broken down to provide amino acids and energy for your body to use.

What Is Protein Anyway?

Protein is made up of nitrogen-containing building blocks called amino acids. Just as the letters of the alphabet are arranged in different ways to make words, the twenty amino acids are arranged in different ways to build proteins with specific forms and functions.

Amino acids are classified as essential and nonessential. They're all important, but you must eat the nine essential amino acids in order for your body to make the protein it needs. Your body can manufacture the other eleven nonessential amino acids with the nitrogen it gets from amino acid.

Animal protein sources such as meat, poultry, fish, eggs, and dairy products, and plant sources such as soybeans and quinoa contain all of the essential amino acids. Grains, beans, lentils, nuts, and seeds contain various essential amino acids, so by eating a variety of these foods, you can consume all of the amino acids necessary to make the proteins your body needs.

How Much Do I Need?

Based on recommendations from various authorities, your protein intake should fall in the range of 10 to 35 percent of total calories per day. On average, healthy women between the ages of 19 and 70 need approximately 46 grams of protein a day; healthy men between the ages of 19 and 70 need approximately 56 grams of protein a day to avoid deficiency. In general, healthy adults should consume 0.8 grams of protein for every kilogram of lean body weight (1 kilogram = 2.2 pounds).

A woman could easily consume 46 grams of protein by drinking an 8-ounce glass of milk in the morning, eating a sandwich made with a 3-ounce chicken breast for lunch, having 1 ounce of nuts as a snack, and eating half a cup of beans at dinnertime. A man could add 3 ounces of beef or fish to dinner to meet his protein requirements. Of course, these examples don't include the proteins in grains, vegetables, or additional dairy products, which would further increase their intake. The point is that your daily protein needs can be easily met without consuming a large amount of food.

Protein requirements are greater during childhood, to support growth and development; during pregnancy and breast-feeding; when recovering from malnutrition, illness, surgery, or trauma; and during athletic training. These protein needs can generally be met through increased dietary intake; protein and amino acid supplements aren't usually needed.

Protein at a Glance

SOURCE	TYPE	AMOUNT OF PROTEIN PER SERVING	SERVING SIZE
Dairy	Milk	8 grams	1 cup (8 oz.)
	Soft cheese (cottage or ricotta)	14 grams	½ cup (4 oz.)
	Hard cheese	5–7 grams	1½–2 oz.
	Yogurt	6–8 grams	8 oz.
	Ice cream	3–5 grams	½ cup
Eggs	Egg	6 grams	1
	Egg white	3.5 grams	1
	Egg substitute	5–6 grams	¼ cup
Meat, Poultry, or Seafood	Cooked lean meat, poultry, or fish	6–9 grams per ounce	2–3 oz.
Soy	Soy, cooked	14 grams	½ cup
	Tofu	10 grams	½ cup
Legumes	Beans or lentils	6–8 grams	½ cup
Nuts	Assorted nuts	6 grams	1 oz.; ¼ cup
	Peanut butter	8 grams	2 tablespoons

STRATEGIES: THE VEGETARIAN CHOICE

Vegetarians do not eat meat, fish, poultry, or their derivatives, such as gelatin, lard, or fish oils. Lacto-ovo vegetarians consume dairy products and eggs, whereas vegans do not eat or use any animal products. People choose vegetarian lifestyles for ethical, religious, or health reasons.

With education and planning, a vegetarian diet can meet all your body's protein and nutrient needs. The key to a healthy vegetarian diet, as with any eating style, is to eat a wide variety of foods, including fruits, vegetables, leafy greens, whole grains, nuts, seeds, and legumes. Learning about alternative sources of nutrients commonly found in animal protein will help you eat an adequate amount of essential and nonessential amino acids, micronutrients, and calories to meet your body's needs. It can be challenging to eat enough iron and B12 on a vegetarian diet, so a multivitamin with iron is generally recommended.

Even if you're not interested in a total vegetarian lifestyle, there are many advantages to going meatless sometimes. It's a healthful move because it's been shown to reduce the risk of heart disease, stroke, obesity, some forms of cancer, and adult-onset diabetes. It can be as easy as choosing pasta with tomato sauce, meatless chili, or a vegetarian stir-fry. You can be more adventurous and incorporate exotic grains, new varieties of rice and vegetables, and tofu. Striking the right balance depends on your taste preferences and lifestyle, so you may want to try the "Be aware. Be different. Be prepared." approach.

BE AWARE

- When do I eat meat? When do I enjoy it the most: breakfast, dinner, weekends, while dining out?
- When would it be easiest for me to forgo meat?
- Which meats do I most enjoy? Which could I live without or eat only on occasion?

BE DIFFERENT

- Designate certain meals as vegetarian meals.

- Designate a certain number of days or specific days of the week as vegetarian, such as "meatless Mondays."

- Experiment with different meatless foods and recipes. You'll love our vegetarian recipes, such as **Brunch Oven Eggs** or **Tuscan White Beans with Garlic**. Try a soy product or meat substitute in meatloaf, spaghetti sauce, tacos, or our **Lettuce Wraps**.

- At a restaurant, try a vegetarian item or ask for vegetarian substitutions. Ask the restaurant staff about the ingredients; some items appear to be vegetarian but may contain such animal products as chicken broth or lard.

BE PREPARED

- Keep fast-cooking grain products on hand, like pasta, couscous, quinoa, and rice. You can easily add sauces and vegetables for a quick meal like our **Confetti Quinoa**.

- Stock up. Keep an assortment of canned beans such as pinto, kidney, or garbanzo beans on hand. Enjoy bean burritos or tostadas and bean soups or salads. Try our **Un-refried Beans**, **Southwestern Soup**, and **Roasted Red Pepper Hummus**, a delicious dip made with garbanzo beans, served with **Crisp Pita Triangles**.

- Dried beans are easy to cook: just throw them in the Crock-Pot with plenty of water and seasonings and they're ready when you get home.

- Stock your freezer and pantry with vegetarian entrées and stir-fry mixes.

- Make meals like vegetarian lasagna and chili ahead of time and freeze for later use.

HOW DO I OPTIMIZE MY PROTEIN INTAKE?

Go lean.

Select round and loin cuts of beef and pork. Our **Pork Tenderloin with Pears and Cranberry Sauce** is great for special occasions. Select the leanest available ground beef; a family favorite is **Lettuce Wraps** made with lean ground beef. Use skinless chicken or turkey breast. Try the recipes for **Chicken and Rice Soup** and **Chicken Fajitas,** or add chicken or turkey to **Southwestern Stew** or to **Whole-Wheat Pasta with Basil and Cherry Tomatoes.**

Be selective.

When possible, select low-fat or fat-free dairy products such as skim or 1 percent milk, buttermilk, 2 percent or less cottage cheese, low-fat yogurt, and low-fat cheeses. For those dairy products where the lower-in-fat version doesn't make the cut for your taste preferences, be selective in how often and how much you use them.

Up your omega 3s.

Aim for two 4-ounce servings of fish each week.

Experiment with plant-based proteins.

Such plant-based proteins as beans and legumes are low in saturated fat and contain other important vitamins, minerals, and fiber. Add flax seed, walnuts, and soy to your diet.

Preparation is important.

Choose items that are grilled, broiled, baked, or poached instead of fried or served with heavy butter- or cream-based sauces. For flavor, marinate meats, poultry, and fish in low-fat dressings, sprinkle with a special seasoning mixture, or rub with a flavorful blend of herbs and spices.

THE BOTTOM LINE FOR PROTEIN

BALANCE

Balance your intake of other macronutrients with protein;
protein helps you feel satisfied sooner and longer.

VARIETY

Consume protein from a variety of animal and plant sources for
optimal nutrients; for example, red meat is high in iron, fish is
high in omega-3 fatty acids, dairy is high in calcium, legumes are
high in fiber, and nuts are high in beneficial unsaturated fats.

MODERATION

Limit animal sources of protein that are high in saturated fat.

CHAPTER 15

IT'S THE LITTLE THINGS

A s a doctor who is married to a professional chef, I know I have an advantage. You might think that we eat fancy exotic meals, but the truth is, it's the simple things that our family enjoys the most: homemade salsa and guacamole, whole-wheat pasta with fresh basil strips and cherry tomatoes, crisp green beans with almonds and a hint of butter. We experiment with flavors like lemon juice, fresh herbs, and exotic spices to add depth to the simplest ingredients. The more mindful I've become, the less I prefer processed foods that bear no resemblance to their origins in taste or form. I didn't need to go to medical school or marry a chef to discover the value and pleasure of nourishing my body with healthful, delicious foods.

WHY ARE MICRONUTRIENTS IMPORTANT?

You now have a better understanding of the macronutrients in your diet: carbohydrates, protein, and fat. Now it's time to turn our attention to micronutrients: that is, vitamins and minerals, as well as phytochemicals and other small but important compounds found in the foods you eat.

Micronutrients perform hundreds of vital functions in your body:

- Each vitamin and mineral serves a unique and essential role in your body. The "Vitamins and Minerals at a Glance" Health Notes in the appendix outline each one, including major functions, common food sources, and recommended intake.
- Phytochemicals found in plants may offer protective benefits that reduce the risk of certain diseases.
- Vitamins (except for vitamin D) and minerals cannot be made by your body in sufficient amounts and therefore must be eaten.

In general, it's not necessary to know exactly how much of each nutrient a food contains or even exactly what each nutrient does, as long as your diet reflects balance, variety, and moderation.

What Happens in My Body?

Food is your best source of micronutrients. These micronutrients, unlike those in supplements, occur in a natural form that can be easily absorbed and used by your body. Since nutrients are found in varying amounts in different foods, it's important to focus on variety when planning your meals and snacks. If your choices are excessive in one macronutrient (protein for example), but lacking in another (carbohydrates for example), you risk missing out on critical micronutrients, too. It's also important to eat a variety of foods *within* each category because no one food provides all the essential micronutrients.

MINDFUL MOMENT: Nutrient-rich foods are the cornerstone of a balanced diet.

What Are Micronutrients Anyway?

Vitamins and minerals are small compounds required for certain reactions in your body. (For details, see "Vitamins and Minerals at a Glance" in the appendix.) Although much is known about vitamins and minerals, new research continues to identify other naturally occurring compounds in food. Small chemical compounds called phytochemicals are found in a variety of flavorful plants, including grains, beans, fruits, and vegetables. There is some evidence that phytochemicals may reduce the risk of cataracts, cancer, and heart disease. Presently, thousands of phytochemicals have been identified, and more are being discovered all the time. Among them are carotenoids, lycopene, sulforaphane, flavonoids, and isoflavones.

It is often difficult to attribute the beneficial effects of certain foods to an individual component; instead, a food's components may work together, just as they are found in nature. In fact, the health-protective benefits seem to come from eating food rather than from taking supplements.

HOW DO I OPTIMIZE MY MICRONUTRIENT INTAKE?

Consider nutrient density.

Some foods pack a powerful nutritional punch compared to the number of calories they contain. These nutrient-rich foods should become the cornerstone of your diet.

Go for color.

The more deeply colored the flesh of fruits and vegetables, the more phytochemicals they're likely to have. Our **Spinach Salad with Oranges** recipe is loaded with micronutrients and fiber.

Fresh is best.

Storing fruits and vegetables for a prolonged time will cause them to lose some of their nutrients. If you can't buy and eat your produce at the freshest possible stages, fresh frozen is the next best thing.

STRATEGIES: CHOOSING SUPER FOODS

Some plant foods are packed with nutrients and healthful phytochemicals. Here are representative examples of these "super foods." By consuming some of these every day, you may increase your nutrition considerably.

VEGETABLES	FRUITS
Broccoli	Blackberries
Carrots	Blueberries
Chili peppers	Grapes
Kale	Guava
Legumes (beans, lentils)	Mango
Pumpkin	Melon
Soybeans or tofu	Oranges
Spinach	Strawberries
Sweet potatoes	Tomatoes

GRAINS/NUTS	HERBS
Almonds	Cinnamon
Barley	Garlic
Brown rice	Ginger
Flaxseed	Green tea
Oatmeal	Oregano
Quinoa	Parsley
Walnuts	Rosemary
Whole wheat	Thyme

Eat 'em whole.

Eat the skins and peels whenever possible, but remember to wash them thoroughly before cooking or eating. Our **Roasted Roots** recipe uses potatoes unpeeled.

Don't overcook.

Cook vegetables just to the tender-crisp stage so they look and taste their best and retain more nutrients. Use a minimum amount of water so you don't lose the vitamins when they're drained. Better yet, steam them using a steamer or colander in a covered pot with a small amount of boiling water. Stir-frying is another quick and easy method to cook vegetables with relatively little fat, and it preserves the crisp texture, bright color, and maximum nutrient content of the vegetables.

Know your options.

Organic foods are more readily available than ever. Organic doesn't necessarily mean more nutritious or more safe; it is often an option, however, when making your selections.

Experiment with new recipes.

Try flavorful recipes with fresh ingredients like our **Mango Salsa** on fish or chicken. Your friends will also love our **Bruschetta** topped with our **Roasted Garlic**, **Basil Pesto**, or **Olive Tapenade**, sliced tomatoes, fresh basil leaves, and goat cheese or low-fat mozzarella.

Drink wine (in moderation, of course).

If you drink alcohol, red wine in moderation may provide some benefits. It's possible these same benefits can be found in other alcoholic beverages and certain juices.

Do I Need to Take a Vitamin/Mineral Supplement?

Because of our busy lifestyles today, it's sometimes difficult to make sure we are getting all the nutrients we need. Perhaps you can relate to Joleen's dilemma.

It is amazing to me that now that I can eat whatever I want, I want to eat more nutritious foods. My challenge is finding the time to shop, prepare, and eat all the nutrients I think my body needs every day.

Taking a single daily multivitamin/mineral supplement can help fill in the gaps of a less-than-perfect diet under less-than-perfect circumstances—as in real life! Choose a brand or generic brand with USP (which stands for United States Pharmacopeia) on the label to ensure that it contains the amount of the ingredients listed and will dissolve properly. Look for a multivitamin with about 100 percent of the daily value for most nutrients, and take it with a meal for maximal absorption.

There may be specific reasons why your health care professional will recommend additional supplementation—calcium with vitamin D, for example—but taking megadoses of vitamins and supplements is not necessary for most people.

THE BOTTOM LINE FOR MICRONUTRIENTS

BALANCE

Balance your diet with plenty of nutrient-rich foods that support your health goals; a single daily multivitamin and mineral supplement will help fill in the gaps.

VARIETY

Eat a variety of nutrient-rich foods.
Choose "super foods" regularly for meals and snacks.

MODERATION

Use moderation when eating less nutrient-rich foods. It's not necessary to take megadoses of vitamin and mineral supplements.

CHAPTER 16

A FLEXIBLE
APPROACH TO
SELF-CARE

I was a perfectionist. It was apparent in my dieting behaviors, and it showed up in other areas of my life, too. I once heard someone say, "Expecting yourself and others to be perfect guarantees that you'll never be satisfied." Ouch. Letting go of the need to get it right and, instead, approaching my eating with flexibility and self-acceptance was the beginning of a transformation that rippled through all aspects of my life.

MINDFUL MOMENT: Don't expect yourself to be perfect. It isn't possible and it isn't necessary.

WHAT TO DO WHEN YOU GET OFF TRACK (Hint: That's Normal!)

At this point you may be asking yourself, "What now?" You may even be a little concerned that you'll go back to your previous habits since that's what happened when you went off your diet in the past. But this isn't a diet, so there is nothing to "go off." This process is about learning to be in charge of the choices you make.

Unlike dieting, which gets harder and harder over time, learning to eat instinctively again becomes easier with practice. Simply choose to use every opportunity to understand more about yourself and why, when, what, how, and how much you eat—and where you invest your energy.

MEASURING CHANGE

Take a look at how far you've come. On a sheet of paper, draw a vertical arrow. At the top write "Flexible" and at the bottom write "Rigid." Then draw a horizontal arrow intersecting the vertical arrow through the middle. On the right side write "Self-care" and on the left write "Neglect."

Using the following explanations, think about where you were when you started this process and place yourself in one of the four quadrants. See how you answered the questions in "Recognizing Your Eating Cycle" in chapter 1 to help you remember your thoughts and feelings about eating. Now think about where you are at this moment and again place yourself in a quadrant.

Self-Care vs. Neglect

Think about how the decisions you make affect your health and well-being. At one end of the horizontal spectrum is self-care. Decisions that promote

STRATEGIES: GETTING BACK ON TRACK

Don't expect yourself to be perfect. You're in charge. Whenever you recognize that you are off track, notice which decision point you're at in your Eating Cycle and return to eating instinctively with the next decision you make. Take a look at the following examples to see how this works.

BACK TO INSTINCTIVE EATING

Learning Opportunity #1: In the middle of eating, I notice I'm eating too fast.

Why? I've been conscious about eating instinctively to meet my needs for nourishment and enjoyment. I was in my Instinctive Eating Cycle when I started eating.

When? I was a "2" on the Hunger and Fullness Scale when I decided to eat.

What? I chose tasty, healthy food that I really wanted.

How? I paused when I hit my speed bump and noticed how fast I was eating. I'm reading my mail while I eat. I'm distracted, so I'm not eating with intention or attention.

Back to Instinctive Eating I'm going to stop reading my mail until I'm done eating. I'll slow down and focus on enjoying my food.

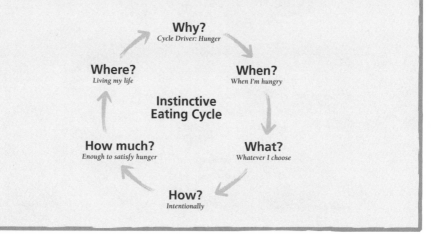

Learning Opportunity #2: I've been overeating snacks and sweets all week at work.

Why? I'd been losing weight gradually for several months. I have a vacation to Hawaii next month, so I decided I needed to lose about ten pounds to look better in a bathing suit. Against my better judgment, I started a new diet, and before I knew it, I had slipped back into my Restrictive Eating Cycle.

When? I was trying to eat only when I was hungry, but after a week on my diet, I was craving foods I thought I had stopped having problems with.

What? I was trying to avoid sugar and high-fat foods—but that seems to be all I think about now.

Back to Instinctive Eating Clearly, trying to follow a rigid low-fat/no-sugar diet increased my desire for those foods. Instead of restricting myself, I started to focus on *How Much?* by making sure that I eat to a "5" most of the time and *Where?* by adding more exercise. My cravings decreased almost immediately.

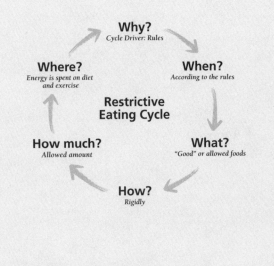

Why?
Cycle Driver: Rules

Where?
Energy is spent on diet and exercise

When?
According to the rules

Restrictive Eating Cycle

How much?
Allowed amount

What?
"Good" or allowed foods

How?
Rigidly

Learning Opportunity #3: I noticed that my clothes are getting tight.

Why? I'm in an Overeating Cycle and gaining weight.

When? I haven't been asking myself "Am I hungry?" because I know that most of the time the answer will be "No," but I want to eat anyway. I guess something is out of balance and driving my overeating, but until now I haven't taken the time to think about it or do anything about it.

Back to Instinctive Eating I remembered how good it felt when I was really listening to my body and practicing good self-care. I started asking "Am I hungry?" whenever I wanted to eat. When I wasn't, I tried to "FEAST"—Focus, Explore, Accept, Strategize, and Take action. It quickly became clear that I feel stretched too thin and I've been rewarding myself with food. Instead of beating myself up for gaining weight, I made a list of things I can do to nurture myself—read an article from a favorite magazine, say a prayer, take a hot bath, ask for help, start planning my next vacation. I already feel better and less like overeating.

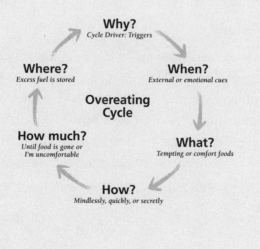

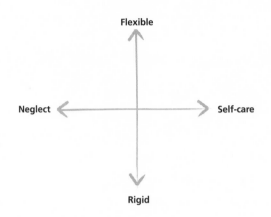

self-care will have the most desirable effects on your physical, intellectual, emotional, and spiritual health. Obvious examples include eating a healthy diet and exercising regularly, but also consider other ways you care for your body, mind, heart, and spirit.

On the other end of the spectrum is neglect. You're neglecting yourself when your decisions ignore or disregard your best interests. Examples of neglect include eating an excessive amount of saturated fat–containing foods even though you have a history of heart disease, or eating too much before bed even though it gives you heartburn. In the extreme, neglect can even be abusive.

Flexible vs. Rigid

Think about how you make your day-to-day decisions. At one end of the vertical spectrum is flexibility. Flexibility allows you to adapt to any situation. Another way of thinking about flexibility is freedom, meaning that you can make any decision you choose at any given time.

At the other end of the spectrum is rigidity. Rigid decision making is strict, with no room for error or unexpected detours. When you try to rigidly follow a diet, for example, you strive to be perfect, not allowing yourself to make any mistakes or to ever go "off the plan."

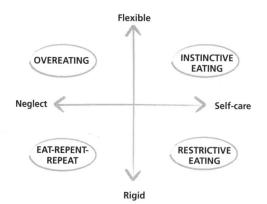

Where Are You Now?

The flexibility or freedom to do whatever you want without regard to your best interests or self-care can lead to overeating and inactivity (Overeating Cycle). On the other extreme, rigid adherence to a food or exercise plan may improve your health, but it comes at a high price (Restrictive Eating Cycle).

Since it's nearly impossible to rigidly adhere to any plan that feels harsh or restrictive, you shift back and forth in an eat-repent-repeat cycle. This neglects your physical, intellectual, emotional, and spiritual well-being and leads to guilt, shame, and ultimately, defeat.

On the other hand, when you're in your Instinctive Eating Cycle, you strive to take good care of yourself while giving yourself the flexibility to adapt your eating and exercise patterns to fit your personal preferences and allowing yourself to adjust to changing circumstances.

Where do you want to be in the future? What do you need to work on to achieve that vision of yourself?

A LIFELONG APPROACH

By practicing flexible self-care, you create a pattern of eating and living that you can maintain for life.

- You listen to your internal cues of hunger and satisfaction instead of trying to follow strict or arbitrary rules about your eating.

- You build a strong foundation of nutrition information and freely choose from all foods to meet your needs instead of trying every fad diet that comes along.

- You eat foods you really enjoy without guilt instead of depriving yourself or bingeing.

- You eat mindfully in a manner that nourishes your body, mind, and spirit instead of eating unconsciously or obsessing over every bite of food.

- You're physically active because it gives you energy, stress relief, and an active metabolism instead of exercising to punish yourself or earn the right to eat.

- You become aware of your thoughts, feelings, and actions and how they affect you instead of judging yourself because you didn't follow a program rigidly.

- You create a self-care buffer zone and meet your true needs instead of eating too much or neglecting yourself.

Mitzi and Brad are well on their way to lifelong weight management.

We both love to eat and always thought that was keeping us from getting to a healthier weight. But now we're healthier and enjoying food even more. Mitzi took a Chinese cooking class at the community college and makes amazing stir-fry dinners with unusual vegetables. Not to be outdone, I built a barbecue, and Mitzi loves my grilled salmon with papaya salsa. I'm not saying we don't still love chocolate cake, but now we go out to dinner and share an entrée and one piece of cake between the two of us and it's plenty. I think the greatest difference is in our awareness of why we're eating and how the food we choose affects not only our weight but also how we feel.

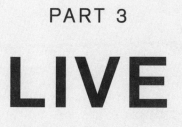

PART 3

LIVE

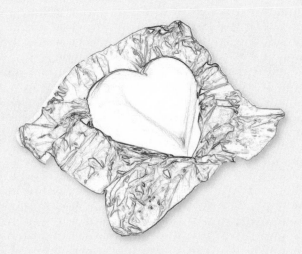

CHAPTER 17

BORN TO MOVE

When my son was in grade school, he did a project for a science fair using pedometers (step counters) to compare how active each of his family members were. Tyler, his younger sister, and his mom, dad, grandma, and grandpa took turns wearing the pedometer to record the number of steps we took as we went about our days. Tyler then graphed the number of steps on a large poster board using colorful feet stickers—little ones for his preschool-aged sister, large ones for his father and grandfather.

When I slipped the pedometer on my waistband in the morning for my turn, it felt like a little power pack. Knowing that every step counted, I parked a little farther away from my office, took extra trips down the hall, and paced while I talked on the phone. At the end of what felt like a very busy day in the office, I had taken only about half the steps each of my kids had taken on their turns. I knew that Tyler's poster would be on display for all of my neighbors and patients to see, so I went for a long walk when I got home and doubled my steps for the day.

INSTINCTIVE MOVEMENT

You were born with the instinctive ability to eat to meet your body's needs—and you were born to move. As soon as they're able, babies move around to experience and explore their environment. Young children run, jump, play, and move their bodies spontaneously and joyfully. Most adolescents think nothing of walking over to a friend's house or hopping on their bikes to go to the store. Some teens love to dance, others compete in sports, and still others would walk around the mall all day if their parents would let them.

Movement is instinctive. And just as you have the internal wisdom to feed your body, your body naturally adapts to your activity patterns. In the distant past, movement was critical for survival. But modern society has developed ways to do almost everything more efficiently, automatically, and effortlessly. While these conveniences may save time, they also save energy—your energy, which may result in weight gain. Even more significantly, less movement and a low level of physical activity result in decreased fitness, so you may not have the stamina, flexibility, or strength to live your life to the fullest.

YO-YO EXERCISING

Just as you may have learned to overeat, you may have learned to under-move. Ask yourself these questions: "Am I active or sedentary? Do I enjoy being physically active? Do I avoid doing things that require movement or effort? Do I wish I felt more energetic and fit? Am I able to do everything I want? Does my current level of fitness limit me?"

As in overeating, under-moving can be a vicious cycle. You may have negative thoughts about physical activity that leave you feeling unmotivated or powerless. You may have found that the less you move, the more challenging it is to get going. This adds to the negative feelings and can sap your inspiration. For some people, exercise feels like punishment: either physical—because of aches and pains—or psychological—because you've linked it to the number of calories you eat. To compound the problem, the less active you are, the easier it is to gain weight, which only makes it harder to move.

On the other hand, some people develop exercise habits that mirror restrictive eating. Ask yourself these questions: "Do I use exercise to earn the right to eat or to punish myself for eating? Do I have rigid exercise patterns? Do I do things I enjoy? Am I fearful of what would happen if I didn't exercise a certain amount on a specific schedule? Do I dismiss the value and benefit of just being active because I don't believe it's strenuous enough?"

Although you may justify a strict exercise regimen as healthy, your thoughts may be number driven: minutes, calories, reps, and pounds. You may be focused on the end result rather than being mindful of the movement itself. You pass up activities you might enjoy because you have a limited view of what "counts." You may be disconnected from an awareness of what your body wants or needs in order to feel and function at its best.

Or perhaps you've started an aggressive exercise program in the past but then quit it altogether when it felt too hard or boring. It's the same pendulum that swings wildly between being in control and being out of control with your eating.

Just as you learned to take a less rigid, self-care approach to your eating, you can learn to take that same approach to your activity. As you begin to move more, you'll discover increased energy, function, and vitality. As you develop a fitness program that is flexible and enjoyable, you'll benefit from the process rather than focusing on the numbers. You'll nurture a positive, self-perpetuating cycle you can live with.

MASTERING YOUR METABOLISM

You learned about the negative effects of the Overeating and Restrictive Eating cycles on the way you think and act. They also have negative effects on your metabolism. Jennifer is a perfect example of this.

I swear I eat less than my sister, but she's always been skinny. I feel like I gain weight from just smelling food! It wasn't always this way. I remember when I was a kid I played all the time and I could eat anything I wanted. But then I gained sixty pounds with my first pregnancy, and I still haven't lost my "baby weight" even though my baby is now twelve! Actually, I've lost weight a bunch of times, but each time I've gained back even more. I know I'm not nearly as active as I used to be, but it just seems to get harder as I get older.

Jennifer is describing a common pattern that I see with people who have a history of switching between Eating Cycles. Your body has the amazing capacity to adapt to your fuel supply and activity level; as a result, yo-yo dieting and inactivity may lead to a decrease in your metabolism. Understanding your metabolism and how it works is essential if you're going to break out of this frustrating pattern and make your metabolism work for you.

What Is Metabolism Anyway?

The word *metabolism* is thrown around a lot these days. People often complain about having a slow or sluggish metabolism. Many products promise to boost your metabolism. But what is metabolism anyway?

In a nutshell, metabolism simply refers to the amount of fuel or energy, measured in calories, that your body burns each day. When most people think of burning calories, images of treadmills and aerobics classes come to mind. However, you're burning calories right now just reading this book. In fact, how you live your life determines your metabolism—it is "where" your energy goes.

Your Basal Metabolism

Think of your metabolism as the amount of fuel your body needs, pictured here as a fuel can. The largest part, called basal metabolism, is the number of calories your body needs to support your basic bodily functions. These vital functions include your heartbeat, breathing, brain function, and numerous other important but invisible activities going on inside of you at all times. Even eating, digesting, and processing food contribute to your metabolism.

In fact, every little cell in your body is like a tiny engine that burns fuel continuously in the process of doing its job. These tiny engines never shut off—at least while you're living. Even when you're sleeping or sitting still, your body's cells are still actively working to keep you alive. It's just like your car; when the engine is running, it's burning fuel—even if the car is just sitting in the driveway.

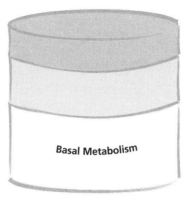

BOOST YOUR METABOLISM WITH ACTIVITY

Your activity level is another important part of your fuel needs, and it's the one you have the most influence over. Your body's workload increases with any type of activity, from brushing your teeth and taking a shower to walking around your home or office. This extra work boosts the number of calories your cells burn because the labor of those cells increases. For instance, your lung cells must work to take in oxygen and release carbon dioxide, but they work harder when you're walking at a brisk pace than when you're sitting in a chair. The more you demand from your body, the more calories each tiny cell burns while doing its job.

Anything you do above your basal metabolic level constitutes activity. This includes lifestyle activities—all the things you do throughout your day-to-day existence. In fact, many people who seem to have a high metabolism are actually just more active throughout their day. A few added steps here and there and a little extra effort during everyday work and play really add up.

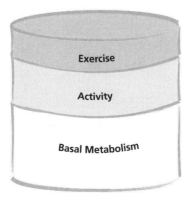

Another great way to boost your metabolism, in addition to being active, is by exercising regularly. Exercise not only burns more calories while you're doing it but also slightly increases the amount of fuel your cells burn for a short time afterward. Obviously, a person who walks two miles a day will burn more calories and will be more fit than someone who doesn't exercise at all.

Muscle Burns Calories

Another piece to this metabolic puzzle is your body composition. Your body is composed of water, adipose tissue (better known as fat), and lean tissue, which is everything else (muscle, bone, hair, and other tissues). Muscle is called "metabolically active tissue" because the tiny engines of muscle cells burn more energy than less-active cells. That is why people say "a pound of muscle burns more calories each day than a pound of fat."

Not only do muscle cells require more energy to do their work, they also require energy for maintenance. Whenever you do more than your body is accustomed to, your body will build more muscle to accommodate the new workload. Building this new muscle tissue requires even more fuel. Of course, once you build additional muscle tissue, it takes more energy to maintain it. In short, the more you increase the number of active cells you have, the more calories you'll burn. It's like a factory; as the number of workers increases, the productivity, or output, goes up.

But I Hate to Exercise!

If you're not currently doing any activity or you have negative thoughts and feelings about exercise, the idea of becoming a person who actually looks forward to exercise may seem unlikely. However, the majority of people I've worked with who were inactive report that they significantly increased their

MINDFUL MOMENT: Forget all or nothing. Become more active by starting wherever you are and increase gradually, step by step.

STRATEGIES: EVERY LITTLE BIT COUNTS

Whether you're already active or not, even a few added steps here and there and a little extra effort during everyday tasks can add up to big benefits. In fact, many people who've conquered health and weight challenges have made increased activity a way of life. Look at some simple ways to boost your lifestyle activities and check the ideas you'll try. Remember to have fun!

AT LEISURE

- Play actively with your children or grandchildren. They love to play tag, ride bikes, or practice sports—don't be surprised if you strengthen your relationships, too.
- Walk your dog, play fetch, or chase him around the backyard.
- Join an adult sports league like softball or bowling.
- Sign up for a walking, hiking, or jogging club.
- Walk the golf course and carry your own golf clubs instead of renting a cart.
- Take up tennis or learn another sport.
- Take a swim to cool off and relax in the summer or find an indoor pool in the winter.
- Reconnect at the end of the day with your partner or a friend on an evening walk.
- Plan a hike or a walking tour when you have out-of-town visitors.
- Instead of always going out for a meal, choose dancing, bowling, or other active pursuits with friends.

AT HOME

- Housework such as vacuuming, scrubbing floors, making beds, and washing windows keeps both your house and your body in shape.

- Balance on one foot while you're cooking, washing dishes, or brushing your teeth.

- Instead of piling things at the bottom of the stairs, make a trip upstairs every chance you get.

- Stretch while you're reading your mail.

- Do some floor exercises while you watch television, or stand up and stretch during the commercials. Even standing while you watch TV will burn more calories and build more muscle than just sitting.

- Tape your favorite daytime show to watch in the evening while you use a treadmill or stationary bike. Better yet, turn the TV off, turn on some music, and dance.

- Yard work like mowing your lawn, weeding, and gardening are great.

- Wash your car, walk to the mailbox, get up to change the channels, and walk to the next room to talk instead of yelling.

- If the gym setting doesn't work for you, check out websites that offer exercise videos.

AT WORK

- Get off the bus or subway a stop or two early, or park in a distant parking space and walk the rest of the way.

- Consider walking or riding your bike to work.

- Use the stairs instead of the elevator; start with one flight once a day and gradually increase until you hardly use the elevator at all.

- Walk down the hall to your coworker's office instead of using the intercom, phone, or e-mail. Contract and relax your muscles while you're sitting at your desk.

- Fidget. Fidgeting like tapping your foot or bouncing your leg requires energy—just don't drive your coworkers crazy!

- Stand and stretch or walk around when you need a break.

- Walk to your meetings and to lunch. Take a walk during your lunch hour or use a nearby gym. Even better, ask a coworker to join you.

- See if your employer offers any fitness benefits like an on-site exercise facility or discounts to local clubs. If these aren't presently available, ask for them; everyone benefits from healthier employees.

WHILE OUT

- Whenever possible, do your errands on foot. (They don't call it running errands for nothing!)
- Park your car in a central location and walk to all your destinations.
- Walk through the mall briskly. In fact, many malls open early so you can walk in a temperature-controlled environment; take a few laps and window-shop before the stores open.
- Take the stairs instead of the escalator or elevator.
- Stretch and tighten your muscles while waiting in lines or sitting at stoplights.

WHILE TRAVELING

- Walk around the airport or conference center instead of sitting around waiting.
- See the local sights by foot or walk to attractions.
- Take advantage of the hotel's gym or the resort's exercise classes, or use the Internet for workouts you can do right in your hotel room.
- Use the stairs and walk to meetings and restaurants.
- Plan a vacation that includes lots of opportunities to rejuvenate your body as well as your mind.

AT REST

- Stretch when you wake up and after sitting for a long time.
- Learn basic yoga or tai chi and practice daily.
- Try deep breathing exercises, relaxation techniques, and meditation.
- Give yourself time to relax at the end of the day.
- Get enough sleep so you'll have plenty of energy for your more active lifestyle.

activity by the end of the workshops. I think the reason for this change is that they've developed a whole new attitude toward physical activity by taking the approach you're about to learn. Let's hear how this happened for Leslie.

> I never thought I would be a person who actually enjoys exercise. It always seemed so hard and uncomfortable. I would rather sit at my kitchen table and pay bills than go out for a walk! At first I started out just by looking for ways to do a little more at work and at home. Now, instead of using the intercom system at my office, I just get up and find the person I need. I don't dread vacuuming anymore—I just look at it as a chance to burn a little extra fuel. Once I saw how easy it was to be more active, I decided to start a fitness program. I started by walking fifteen minutes about three times a week. By the second week I was doing twenty minutes. In the third week I increased my walks to four times a week. I also added some stretching exercises and some push-ups and sit-ups. I even have a hill near my home that I just added to my walks, and I'm thinking about pulling the bike I bought a few years ago out of the garage and giving it another try. I actually look forward to exercise now!

In the following pages, you'll learn strategies for developing a positive attitude and increasing your motivation to be more active. You'll see how you can boost your metabolism, increase your energy, and enhance your sense of well-being by increasing your exercise and lifestyle activity. We'll also explore ways for you to steadily and comfortably build your stamina, strength, and flexibility. Ultimately, the real purpose is to help you reconnect with your body and rediscover that you were born to move and live your life to the fullest.

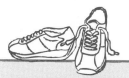

FITNESS Rx
Moving More

You're in charge of how active you are each day. If you've been inactive, any additional movement is a positive step in the right direction. If you're already exercising regularly, congratulate yourself and use the information in these chapters to make sure you're getting the optimal benefit for your effort.

What are you going to do, starting today, to move more and increase your metabolism?

CHAPTER 18

CHANGE YOUR MIND

When I was dieting, I'd look at those charts that showed how many calories I'd burn if I did 30 or 60 minutes of various activities. I also knew how many calories were in just about everything I ate. Exercise had become a way to earn the right to eat or to punish myself for eating something "bad." No wonder it felt like a chore.

When I stopped dieting, I stopped looking at those charts and started exercising for the way it made me feel: energetic, flexible, and strong. No wonder I love it now!

ARE YOUR THOUGHTS ON YOUR SIDE?

Although exercise is one of the most powerful tools available for improving your health and boosting your metabolism, for many people the word *exercise* conjures up negative thoughts and feelings.

Julie, for example, realized her thoughts weren't helping her.

> Whenever I saw someone who looked really fit I thought about how long it would take me to get to that point. It seemed so unreachable that I felt totally overwhelmed and paralyzed. Needless to say, I just never seemed to get started. Then one day I thought, "No matter how long it will take me to get in shape, that time will pass anyway. I'll either be closer to my goals—or still right where I am right now. It's up to me." That was the day I got moving.

Thinking ineffective thoughts is a habit, and a habit can be broken with awareness and practice. For example, if you believe that fitness is important but you're not very active or exercising regularly, it's likely you have some negative and limiting thoughts that keep you from doing it. With practice, you can change your thoughts about physical activity, eating, and just about everything else to thoughts that help you reach your goals.

MORE POWERFUL THOUGHTS

Let's look at the following to compare common limiting thoughts with more powerful ways of thinking.

Negative vs. Positive

I know I should exercise, but I hate it, so I just can't seem to make myself do it. The negative thoughts and feelings can be heard in the words *should*,

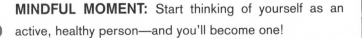

MINDFUL MOMENT: Start thinking of yourself as an active, healthy person—and you'll become one!

STRATEGIES: APPLYING TFAR

Think about exercise for a minute and write down everything that comes to mind. I'll wait.

Now take a look at what you wrote.

- Are your thoughts about exercise positive or negative?
- What feelings do those thoughts stir up?
- What do you do (or not do) as a result of those thoughts and feelings?
- What results do you get?
- How do you end up proving your thoughts right?

Whether we're talking about exercise, eating, or any other aspect of your life, remember that your *thoughts* lead to your *feelings*, which lead to your *actions*, which lead to your *results*.

For example if you think, "I'm not athletic," you'll probably have feelings of incompetence and dislike exercise. Because of your negative thoughts and feelings, you may be less likely to exercise or try new types of physical activities. As a result, you won't build new skills, discover hidden talents, or have the opportunity to find joy in movement. Indeed, you won't become more athletic and you'll end up proving yourself right!

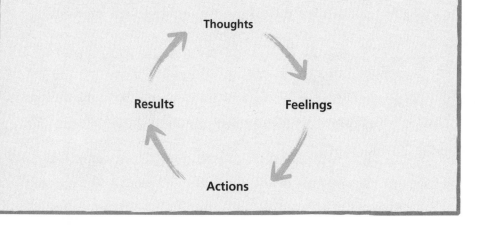

hate, and *make myself*. Even *exercise* has become a dirty word to many people; I call it the "E-word." These thoughts and feelings come from negative past experiences like being chosen last for teams, boring exercise routines, and discomfort or pain from doing too much, too fast. Some people exercise just when they are trying to lose weight, so they have come to think of exercise as a punishment for their overeating. However, the past does not predict the future. In other words, are your negative thoughts about the "there and then" or the "here and now"?

I enjoy becoming more physically active each day. This time focus on all the great things physical activity does for you and how wonderful you feel instead of focusing on how much weight you think you should lose. Find fun physical activities that suit your personality and lifestyle. Most important, start slowly and allow your body to adjust gradually and comfortably. It will be different this time if you think it will be.

Limiting vs. Encouraging

I don't know if exercise is really worth the effort. Most people know physical activity is very important, yet many people choose to lead sedentary lives—and even more find it difficult to start an exercise program or stick with it.

I deserve all the amazing benefits I get from being physically active. Exercise really does make a difference. Studies have shown that more than 90 percent of people who lose weight—and keep it off—exercise on a regular basis. Even more significant, exercise has many well-documented health and psychological benefits. It lowers blood pressure and blood sugar levels, improves cholesterol and energy levels, enhances mood and the sense of well-being, and helps people live longer. If you could buy all that in a pill, everyone would want a prescription.

Exercise also helps you reconnect with your physical body. This is important since many people who struggle with their weight are disconnected from the neck down because they feel their body has betrayed them. Becoming more active will help you see that your body does serve you well and that it's capable of becoming more fit when you challenge it even a little. There's great joy to be found in simply moving your body. Exercise is not a means to an end but an end in and of itself.

Scarcity vs. Abundance

I don't have time. Time is a real issue for many people, but the reality is we all have exactly the same amount of time but differ in the way we choose to spend it. In truth, it will take just 1/48th of your whole day to exercise for thirty minutes. Most people waste a lot more time than that on unproductive activities like watching TV or surfing the Internet.

When you say, "I don't have enough time to exercise," you simply won't recognize opportunities for physical activity because your brain doesn't believe they exist. On the other hand, you probably make time for other grooming routines, like bathing, putting on makeup, and washing your clothes, because you decided to. You could also make time for physical activity, and it'll do even more for your appearance, not to mention all the psychological and health benefits.

I make time for my health and well-being. You have time for the things that are the most important to you. If you're too busy for exercise, you're just too busy! Being physically active is more important for your health and well-being than most of the other things you think must get done each day. The key is giving activity the priority it deserves. You could ask your husband to watch the kids so you can go to the YMCA, or you could walk on a treadmill while you sort your mail (speaking from personal experience, that requires a little practice!).

If it's easier or more convenient for you, studies have shown that breaking your exercise sessions into smaller chunks throughout the day is just as beneficial as one longer session. You could do ten minutes in the morning, ten minutes after lunch, and ten minutes in the afternoon and it would still "count."

Self-defeating vs. Affirming

I don't have the energy. This thought becomes a self-fulfilling prophecy because if you don't exercise, you'll continue to have low energy.

I feel myself becoming healthier and more energetic each day. Have you ever noticed that fit people seem to have more energy than others? It turns out exercise increases your strength and stamina and helps you sleep better, so you'll become more productive and feel great.

No matter how you feel when you start exercising, you're likely to feel better within just a few minutes of starting. These good feelings usually last long after the exercise is finished. Therefore, even when you feel tired, commit to exercising for at least ten minutes. Promise yourself you can stop and try again another day if you still aren't feeling any better. If you don't want to continue, that's okay. But most of the time you'll feel so good you'll want to keep going.

Powerless vs. Powerful

I'll start exercising when I've lost some of this weight. Rather than taking charge of the situation, you wait for something to happen. If you don't exercise while you're losing weight, however, you'll lose valuable muscle. It can become gradually harder to lose weight, and almost impossible to keep it off.

I support my weight-loss efforts and metabolism with regular exercise. Doing any kind of extra physical activity uses additional calories and makes it easier to lose weight in the first place. In addition, physical activity reduces cravings and curbs your appetite by raising your endorphins (feel-good chemicals) and serotonin levels (calm chemicals). Besides, cardiorespiratory exercise and strength training will minimize your loss of lean body mass during weight loss, which prevents a decrease in your metabolism.

Outdated Thinking vs. Forward Thinking

Exercise is too hard for me. If your past experience with exercise has led to severe discomfort or pain, there's a good chance you may have been working out at an intensity that was too great for your level of fitness at the time.

I have more stamina, strength, and flexibility every day. Physical activity doesn't have to be hard or hurt to be beneficial. It's important to find activities that are comfortable, convenient, and fun so you'll stick with them. Even if you have physical limitations, it's always possible to find some way to increase your activity level. If you've been very inactive, start by increasing your lifestyle activity as we talked about in the last chapter and then work toward a regular exercise routine. You'll be amazed at how your body adapts to whatever challenges you give it.

Judgmental vs. Unconditional

I'm too embarrassed to be seen exercising. When you judge yourself harshly, you may assume that other people judge you in the same way. Ironically, most other people are so focused on themselves, they're not going to notice you anyway. Those that do will likely admire you for making an effort to take care of yourself.

I exercise to take care of me. Eventually you'll feel less self-conscious, but in the meantime, find activities and places that make you feel comfortable so you can focus on all the wonderful benefits. One option might be to exercise in the privacy of your own home using DVDs or fitness classes on the Internet. Remember, you're doing this for yourself—to feel better and become healthier.

Shaming vs. Accepting

I'm so out of shape, I don't even know where to start! There's no such thing as instant fitness. If you don't choose to start somewhere, don't be surprised when you're still out of shape months from now.

I have to start somewhere! If you choose to start this week by increasing your movement and physical activity, little by little you'll become leaner, stronger, more energetic, and healthier.

If you haven't been physically active at all, you may need to check with your doctor before you start. Review the "Exercise Clearance" Health Notes in the appendix to see if that's necessary. Once you've been medically cleared, you have to start somewhere, so start right where you are.

Black and White vs. Shades of Gray

I can't do what they recommend so why bother? This is your all-or-nothing voice talking. Get rid of the notion that you have to exercise for thirty to sixty minutes, four to five days a week, or not at all. That's ridiculous!

I do what I can to become more fit and healthy. Increased activity throughout the day really adds up. Taking the stairs, walking a little faster, and working or playing more actively every day can accomplish this. Every bit of activity over your usual level counts, so be on the lookout for opportunities to "just do it."

Ineffective vs. Effective

I have a strenuous job, so I don't need to exercise when I get home. Your activity level, both at work and at home, definitely contributes to your overall health, but few jobs provide all the elements of a great fitness program.
I am building a great overall fitness plan for myself. Your fitness program should include lifestyle activity, cardiorespiratory, strength training, and flexibility for prevention of disease and optimal energy and health.

Perfectionistic vs. Realistic

I was doing pretty well until I got sick (or busy, or company came, or I went on vacation . . .). To quit your exercise program because you missed a day, a week, or even longer makes as much sense as eating the whole bag of cookies because you ate three. No person and no schedule are ever perfect, but thinking you have to do it perfectly will derail you every time.
I have a flexible, consistent exercise program. In order for physical activity to become part of your life, try to be as consistent but as flexible as possible. Many people have found that writing their exercise schedules on their calendars helps them stay on track. If they miss a session, they simply reschedule it, the way they would any other important appointment.

Outwardly Focused vs. Inwardly Focused

I started exercising but I quit because I wasn't seeing the weight loss I expected. You won't see a change on the scale if you lose a pound of fat and build a pound of muscle, but your metabolism will be higher and your body will be firmer. Besides, when you focus only on weight loss, you lose sight of the most important goal—living an active, fulfilling, and healthy life.

I feel so good when I move my body. Fitness is a process, and whether you're losing weight or not, you're becoming healthier. Instead, set goals based on the many other benefits of exercise, like having the stamina to play with your grandchildren and not feeling winded by just walking to the mailbox.

Weight Focused vs. Health Focused

I already exercise but I am still overweight. You'd likely weigh more if you didn't exercise, and you'd certainly be less healthy and have less stamina. I've also found that some people get stuck in the rut of doing the same exercise all the time, so they aren't getting as much out of their program as they could.

I challenge my body to become healthier and more energetic no matter what I weigh. Overweight people who exercise are generally healthier than "ideal" weight individuals who are inactive. Gradually increase the frequency, intensity, and time you exercise, and try new types of activities to keep your body challenged and your exercise plan from becoming boring.

Hypercritical vs. Gentle

I used to be so athletic in high school; now I'm just a fat, lazy bum! It's easy to measure yourself against what you used to be able to do, but that only leads to negative self-talk. When you set the bar too high, the fear of failure will prevent you from trying to jump.

I'm not trying to compete in sports; I just want to get comfortable in my skin again. Think about what is most important to you now instead of focusing on what used to be. When you're gentle with yourself, you'll make a lot more progress.

Problem Oriented vs. Solution Focused

I can't exercise because it's too cold (or hot) outside. Waiting for the perfect weather to exercise rules out the majority of the year in most places. It makes more sense to have different activities for different seasons and moods.

I have a lot of options for staying active even when circumstances aren't ideal. Dress in layers and head out at the best time of day depending on the weather. If the weather just isn't cooperating, there are lots of options for exercising in a climate-controlled environment. Think about videos, classes, a treadmill, a stationary bike, dancing, and mall walking.

Effective thinking is a habit, and new habits take practice. For example, instead of saying, "Exercise is boring," practice saying, "Being active gives me the opportunity to relieve stress and feel better." Repeat more encouraging thoughts frequently and you'll begin to notice more-positive feelings, more-effective behaviors, and more-powerful results.

This all applies to other areas of your life too, of course. If you don't like your results, ask yourself what you were thinking first. What other negative thoughts, attitudes, and feelings do you have that might be limiting you? Imagine how having more-realistic, positive, and powerful thoughts could lead to feelings and actions that would give you the results you desire. Now that's good food for thought!

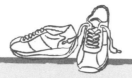

FITNESS Rx
Exercise: The Best Medicine

People often secretly wish for a miracle to make them healthier and end their struggles with weight, but so far, none exists. However, if you could bottle exercise, you would have the closest thing there is to a wonder drug.

BRAND NAME: EXERCISE

Numerous effective generics available: aerobics, basketball, bike riding, body sculpting, dancing, hiking, housework, jogging, jump roping, playing with children, racquetball, rowing, stretching, swimming, tennis, walking, walking the dog, weight lifting, working out, yard work, yoga, and many others.

   Indications: Shown to be very effective for weight management and relief of fatigue, stress, low self-esteem, insomnia, boredom, and symptoms of depression and anxiety. May prevent, improve, or delay the onset of the following conditions: overweight/obesity, diabetes, high blood pressure, high cholesterol, heart disease, some types of cancer, some forms of arthritis, fibromyalgia, premenstrual syndrome, constipation, addictions, and many other health problems.

   Benefits: Increased energy and productivity, increased metabolism, weight loss, improved sense of well-being and appearance, better sleep patterns, improved sex life, improved appetite regulation, lower blood sugar, lower heart rate and blood pressure, higher HDL (good) cholesterol, improved blood sugar control, and reduced risk of cancer.

   Side Effects: Patients report feeling stronger, healthier, energetic, and more youthful.

   Precautions: You should consult with your physician first, especially if you have any chronic medical conditions, heart problems, or unexplained symptoms. If you develop unexpected shortness of breath; chest, jaw, neck, or arm pain or pressure; rapid or irregular heart rate; lightheadedness; pain or any other unexplained symptoms—stop and seek immediate medical advice and attention. (See the "Exercise Clearance" Health Notes in the appendix for additional information.)

   Dosage: Start with small doses taken most days of the week and increase gradually as tolerance develops. Dosage may be adjusted if necessary to accommodate other responsibilities. Due to the many beneficial effects, however, consistent usage is very important. Choose among the numerous generic brands available and alternate brands as needed to improve overall level of fitness and maintain interest and motivation.

   WARNING: Likely to become habit-forming when used regularly.

CHAPTER 19

LAY YOUR FOUNDATION

As a teenager in New Zealand, my husband, Owen, played rugby and ran nearly 10 miles a night, delivering milk in glass bottles. However, in the last couple of decades his exercise had consisted of walking the dog a few times a week and intermittently working out at the YMCA. I was surprised when he announced that he had set a goal to run a half-marathon and signed up with a team to train for it.

At first he could just "wog" (alternately walk and jog) a mile at a time, but he stuck to it. He found that he enjoyed the structure of the training schedule, the camaraderie of running with his friends twice a week, the challenge of training for a long-distance event, and the opportunity to raise money to introduce children to the joy of running. During his five months of training, Owen progressed from wogging a mile to running all 13.1 miles on race day. I was proud of him, but more important, he was proud of himself.

WHAT MOVES YOU?

Have you ever felt inspired to exercise, eat better, lose weight, or make other positive changes, only to feel your enthusiasm slip away as time passes or the going gets tough? Although motivation seems elusive at times, when you understand how to tap into your personal motivators, you'll feel more in charge of your attitude and know what to do to maintain and restore your drive and inspiration.

First, clearly identify your personal reasons for making a change. Although you may know why you want or need to become more active, it's important to peel away the layers to make sure you get to the heart of your motivation. Some sources of motivation are internal: thoughts and feelings like fear or longing. Others are external: events, people, situations, or rewards that inspire you. Both internal and external motivators can fuel the process of change, especially when you tap into those that create strong emotion for you. These powerful motivators will keep you moving in the right direction.

Mary was surprised to discover that her source of motivation was more significant than she initially thought.

> For months I've been saying that I wanted to start exercising to get healthier. I hadn't given much thought to why, other than the fact that I'm not getting any younger and the longer I wait, the harder it will be. Somehow that just didn't motivate me. After some reflection, I realized that what is really important to me, in addition to improving my health, is feeling good, physically and emotionally. I want to feel confident, attractive, and vibrant. Now it's more important than ever because my husband and I will be retiring next year and I want to be full of energy and able to do everything we've planned. Now that inspires me!

In order to identify your own powerful motivators, take out a piece of paper and answer these two questions:

- Why is it important to me to make a change (for example, become a more active person)?
- Why do I want to make this change *now*, at this point in my life?

MINDFUL MOMENT: Why this? Why now?

When you're done, think about what you've written and challenge yourself to dig deeper to uncover even more meaningful answers. Ask yourself the two questions again: So why is that important to me? And why now? You may need to ask the "why" questions a few times to peel back the layers and get to the personal motivators that feel like powerful fuel for change. You'll know you've hit on something when you feel a strong emotion.

MOTIVATION TOP 10

It's human nature to experience varying levels of enthusiasm for exercise. Keep in mind that your goal is not perfection. Rather, strive to increase your activity most days of the week and accept that there will be days when it's more challenging than others. Here are some tried-and-true ways to get started and keep your fitness plan alive.

1. **Start Small.** One of the greatest sources of motivation is achieving your goals, no matter how small. If you're having a hard time getting started, ask yourself, "What is the least amount of physical activity I could do consistently?" and start there.

2. **Set Goals.** You wouldn't start out on a trip without knowing where you're going, would you? Knowing your end point helps you decide on the path for getting there. Read "Strategies: Setting Powerful Goals" to help you create a detailed map for your brain to follow.

3. **Be Consistent.** Consistency is one of the keys to improving your fitness and creating a habit. It's helpful to write down your plan on your calendar or on your To Do list and then treat it like any other important commitment. You'll be surprised at how soon regular exercise becomes a part of your routine, much like brushing your teeth. You'll actually miss it when you can't fit it in.

4. **Be Flexible.** Too often, people wait for the perfect time to get more active. It's unlikely the perfect time will ever come—and it won't last anyway—so make fitness fit into your life just the way it is today. When life gets in the way (and it will), adjust your routine so you can still fit in fitness. Even if it's not the type or time you planned, anything is always better than nothing.

5. **Be Patient.** One of the things I hear most frequently from people I work with is that although it takes time, they eventually reach a point where they actually look forward to being active. The challenge is that it may not feel that way right away, so you may have to operate on faith that it will get better.

6. **Reward Yourself.** Since it takes time to see results, come up with both small and large incentives to motivate yourself to reach your short- and long-term goals. Perhaps you could give yourself points for the minutes you spend exercising then trade them in for time to do other things you enjoy, too. You could pay yourself a quarter or a dollar every time you complete a session and later spend it on exercise clothing, music, a massage, or a manicure. Of course, the greatest reward is in knowing that you've done your best.

7. **Use Reminders.** Your motivation can fade simply because you've lost touch with why you wanted to change in the first place. Create reminders to keep your source of motivation top of mind. For example, if you're motivated to get physically fit because you want to keep up with your children, have them draw a picture of you playing with them, put a photo of them on your screensaver, or have them call you at work to encourage you to hit the gym before you come home.

8. **Surround Yourself.** Set yourself up for success by removing barriers and making physical activity more convenient. One workshop participant was having trouble meeting her goal of walking three evenings each week. She made a mental commitment to the idea each morning, but by the time she got home from work, it was too much effort to get ready to go. Her solution? She took her exercise clothes to work and changed before she left so she'd be ready to walk as soon as she got home. Other ideas:

keep basic fitness equipment in your living room, put a sign up at the elevator at work to remind you to take the stairs, or set regular exercise appointments with a friend or personal trainer.

9. **Team Up.** When you're not feeling motivated, you can borrow some motivation from others around you. Find an exercise buddy, someone who will make exercise more fun; besides, you won't want to let them down by not showing up! Join a walking club or walk with a coworker during your breaks. Sometimes a little friendly competition will do the trick. Hire a personal trainer for support and optimization of your fitness plan. An online community can help you, too; just make sure it is a positive, supportive group.

10. **Have Fun!** Remember what it was like to play when you were a kid? Keep your exercise enjoyable, interesting, challenging, and rewarding.

    - Don't let boredom derail your plan. Join a team, take some lessons, or practice a new skill. Tape your favorite show to watch while you exercise. Spend time with your children playing or take your dog (or someone else's) for a walk.

    - Don't let your routine get routine. Try a different time of day, two shorter sessions instead of one longer one, new equipment, new music, a new route, or even your usual route backward.

    - Mix it up a bit by trying new activities once in a while. If you usually walk, try a gentle hike; if you ride a stationary bike, ride outside; if you do ballet, try yoga; if you do aerobics, take a dance class; if you do Pilates, lift weights.

    - Vary your activities during the week; try walking, swimming, stretching, and strength training, for example. This will keep you from getting bored and will give your body the benefit of a complete fitness program.

MINDFUL MOMENT: Powerful written goals give your brain a clear map to follow.

STRATEGIES: SETTING POWERFUL GOALS

Whether you're setting goals for better health or any other area of your life, the key to success is to create inspiring and achievable goals and a strategic plan to achieve them.

The following steps will guide you through the goal-setting and achievement process:

Assess your starting point: Take an accurate and detailed assessment of where you are now relative to the goal you'd like to achieve. Don't beat yourself up; the gaps represent your opportunities to make a change.

Consider your values: Goals based on your core principles and values will form a passionate attitude. For example, if you value spending time with your family and advancing your career, then your goal to lose weight must be aligned with those priorities. If your goal is healthier meals with your family and increased productivity and confidence at work, you're more likely to stay on track and motivated.

Dream: Project yourself into the future and imagine the possibilities. Focus on the areas that challenge and inspire you. How will you feel? What will your life be like? Picture yourself taking the necessary steps and successfully building new habits into your lifestyle.

Set yourself up for success: Break your goals into small, specific steps that you feel confident you can achieve. Ask yourself, "On a scale of 1 to 10, with 10 being the highest, how confident am I that I can really do this?" If your answer is less than an 8, rework your goal until you feel very confident that you can achieve it.

Make your goals measurable: Set specific exercise goals using the FITT Formula: Frequency, Intensity, Time, and Type (for more details, see the "Fitness Prescription" at the end of this chapter). Here's an example: I walk five days a week for thirty minutes, and I take the stairs every day at work without feeling breathless.

Write them down: Write your goals in positive, present terms using detailed words or pictures. Make them so clear that you can see them, feel them, and measure them; put your written goals or pictures in a place where you'll see them often. You might set them on your bedside table, write them on your mirror in felt-tip pen, or tape them to your computer monitor. Your written action steps give your brain a map to follow.

Develop a plan: Set long- and short-term goals, including a time line with deadlines. Be flexible and open to new opportunities and paths to your goals, but watch out for detours.

Identify obstacles and possible solutions: Think about possible obstacles, such as time constraints, inclement weather, and family obligations. Jot down at least one realistic strategy you could use if this obstacle arises. And of course, expect the unexpected! The difference between achieving your goals or not is how you recover from the inevitable challenges.

Frequently assess your progress: Check in often to assess your progress toward your goals, adjusting your approach as you learn what works for you. If you're having difficulty reaching a particular goal, break it down into smaller steps.

TOP PRIORITY: YOU!

You deserve to feel great, so make physical activity a top priority. Remind yourself that regular exercise is more important than just about anything else you can do with your time. An active lifestyle will make you healthier and happier; as a result, you'll be even more productive and energetic.

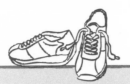

FITNESS Rx
The FITT Formula

Use the FITT Formula to tailor a fitness program to your personal health needs, preferences, lifestyle, and goals. FITT stands for Frequency, Intensity, Time, and Type. Write your own Fitness Prescription:

- Frequency—How often you're going to be active

- Intensity—How much effort you'll use during activity

- Time—How much time you'll invest in being active

- Type—What kinds of activities you'll do

CHAPTER 20

INCREASE YOUR STAMINA

live in Phoenix, just minutes from great hiking trails. Unless I'm the first one in or the last one out, I cross paths with other hikers who are a familiar and welcome part of my hikes.

First Timers: They carefully gaze at the map at the base of the trail. I overhear them saying, "It doesn't look too bad." And it's really not; the first mile is sort of flat. It's that last half mile that gets you. They'll just skip it the first few times.

Alone But Not Lonely: These hikers appear to be either deep in thought or scaling the mountain to whatever their iPod is pumping out. Either way, they seem to be enjoying what may be the only hour to themselves all day.

Gabbing Girlfriends: These women hike early before work or after their kids are safely on the school bus. Beats spending four bucks on coffee.

Couples Connecting: Stealing away to plan the day, or catch up when it is over, these pairs have found a perfect way to keep their relationship and their bodies in shape.

Fitness Buff: Easy to spot, wearing sports bras and expensive heart-rate monitors, these are runners rather than hikers. They gracefully fly down the mountain, barely skimming the rocks as they rush to make it to their 7:00 a.m. spin class.

Senior Warriors: These gray-haired marvels in wide-brimmed hats ward off advancing age with their regular treks up the mountain. They always say hi, and I silently promise myself that I'll still hike when I'm their age, too.

As for me, I'm the one with the dog, gabbing with my girlfriend, connecting with my husband, or by myself with my iPod on. If you say hi, I'll say hi back.

ESSENTIALS OF CARDIORESPIRATORY FITNESS

I hope that at this point you're already convinced of the benefits of exercise for good health and well-being. Now let's focus on the ways that specific types of exercise will help you, beginning with building your stamina through cardio-respiratory fitness.

Simply put, cardiorespiratory exercise, commonly called cardio, is any activity that strengthens your heart, lungs, and vascular system and improves circulation throughout your body.

Why Bother?

Cardiorespiratory activity will provide you with numerous health benefits. It:

- Conditions your heart, lungs, and vascular system
- Lowers your blood pressure and resting pulse
- Raises your level of HDL cholesterol—the good kind of cholesterol
- Lowers your risk for cardiovascular diseases such as heart attack, stroke, and atherosclerosis (hardening of the arteries)
- Increases your stamina
- Helps you lose excess body fat
- Strengthens your major muscles and creates a more-toned appearance
- Improves your sense of well-being
- Improves your sleep
- Boosts your energy level

What Do I Need to Know?

There are many cardiorespiratory activities to choose from: they include walking, cycling, water aerobics, swimming, dancing, low-impact aerobics, hiking, jogging, skating, stair-stepping, tennis, rowing, cross-country skiing, trampolining, jumping rope, basketball, soccer, and more. Even gardening

> **MINDFUL MOMENT:** Live longer, look better, and feel great—the perfect prescription.

and housework can be a good workout. As you can see, the list includes a variety of activities for all fitness levels, so there's something for everyone. For instance, I recently met someone who loves to jump on a pogo stick for fun and exercise!

No matter which activity you choose, the goal is to keep your heart rate up without completely losing your breath. Since each person is at a different fitness level, an activity that is comfortable for one person may be too much for someone else. For example, jogging might be a perfect activity for a person who exercises regularly, while a person who's just getting started might feel totally winded within a short period of time and have to quit. That individual would benefit far more from walking and would get just as good a workout for his or her current level of fitness. The point is, start wherever you are.

HOW DO I GET STARTED?

Once your doctor has cleared you, if necessary, to begin to exercise (see the "Exercise Clearance" Health Notes in the appendix), plan a cardiorespiratory exercise program that meets your needs.

Walking is an ideal activity for almost any fitness level, at just about any weight. You can walk almost anywhere, anytime, with minimal equipment—just a comfortable pair of shoes. Before you take your first step, however, make sure you're prepared to enjoy it.

Shoes: Wear comfortable shoes with flexible thick soles—preferably, shoes that have been designed for walking. You don't have to spend a lot of money, but it's helpful to speak to an experienced salesperson or doctor if you tend to have foot problems. And remember, the support inside your walking shoes wears out long before they look worn-out on the outside.

Clothing: Comfortable, light cotton clothing will absorb sweat and allow evaporation in the summer. Wear layers of clothes in the winter because you'll quickly warm up with activity. Don't be too concerned with how you look; the goal is to feel good.

Sun Protection: Don't forget to wear a hat, sunscreen, and sunglasses with UVA and UVB protection during the peak hours of the day, even during the winter.

Location: If possible, your neighborhood is the best place to start since it will be the most convenient. Having a treadmill at home also makes it convenient to walk anytime. For variety and interest, walk to, or in, other nearby neighborhoods, parks, malls, and trails. Look for smooth, even surfaces if you are not very sure-footed. Surfaces softer than concrete may be more comfortable. Try a track at the local high school or walk on the asphalt rather than the sidewalk, being very mindful of traffic, of course.

Safety: Walk in the daytime or in well-lit areas. Wear reflective clothing or shoes if you walk at night. Stay aware of your surroundings. Let others know your route and expected time of return, and take a mobile phone with you, if possible. Consider carrying pepper spray and a whistle or another type of alarm to use in case you are in danger. Walking with a partner provides additional security.

Proper Walking Technique: Walk with your head and chin up, your shoulders held slightly back, and your stomach pulled in. Touch your heel to the ground first then roll your weight forward. Make sure your toes point straight ahead. Swing your arms as you walk, either down at your side or with your elbows flexed to 90 degrees, with your fist swinging up to the level of your breastbone.

Partners: If you like the idea of sharing your walk with someone else, choose one or more partners who can walk on the same schedule and who are at about the same level of fitness or higher. This is a great chance to spend quality time with someone, and it definitely makes the time go faster. Sometimes pets or children on bikes or in strollers make good partners, too. I used to load my two young children into a double stroller after work to explore our neighborhood and nearby park to see if we could find "yub-yubs" (which is what my daughter called the bunnies we saw).

One Step at a Time

Many people choose to start with walking, so we'll use that as our example. However, if walking is not a good activity for you, choose something else you're likely to enjoy. No matter what you choose to do, start slowly, be consistent, and keep it interesting.

Walking three days a week will improve your cardiorespiratory health, but you'll want to walk more often if your goal is to lose weight. Deciding to walk "most days of the week" will give you the flexibility to adjust your frequency depending on your schedule that week.

The "best" time to exercise is whenever you'll do it most consistently. Many people find it easier to be consistent when they exercise first thing in the morning, before other distractions get in the way. Of course, the bonus is increased energy and less stress throughout the rest of the day. You can also break your walk into several shorter sessions if you're too busy or not used to exercising; you'll still get the benefits.

At the beginning of the week, schedule your walks and write them down on your calendar. Once you've committed yourself to those times, give them the priority they deserve. If you have to cancel, reschedule just as you would any other important appointment.

Each walking session should be made up of four parts:

- Warm-up: Walk slowly for five minutes and allow your muscles to warm up by increasing your circulation. Please note that warming up is not the same thing as stretching. Stretching is best after the muscles are warm, usually after your warm-up and again at the end of your walk.

- Brisk Walk: Gradually increase your intensity as you begin to feel more energetic. You should be able to carry on a conversation, but if you can sing, go a little faster. As you become more fit, increase your intensity and time by walking a little faster and adding a few extra minutes to challenge yourself.

- Cool Down: Walk slowly for five minutes to allow your muscles to cool down and your circulation to return to normal.

- Stretch: Stretching after your warm-up and again at the end of your walk will help prevent injuries. (Chapter 21 provides the details to get you started.)

This sample schedule is one way to build your cardiorespiratory fitness with walking. If you haven't been exercising regularly, start at the top of the schedule and gradually work your way up from fifteen minutes. If you're already exercising, simply choose the starting point that matches your current fitness level and go from there. This is just a sample, so make adjustments to meet your needs. You can also use this sample chart to build activities other than walking.

Sample Walking Schedule

WEEK	WARM-UP	BRISK WALK	COOL DOWN	TOTAL TIME	STRETCH
1	5 min	5 min	5 min	15 min	After walk
2	5 min	7 min	5 min	17 min	After walk
3	5 min	10 min	5 min	20 min	After walk
4	5 min	12 min	5 min	22 min	After walk
5	5 min	15 min	5 min	25 min	After walk
6	5 min	18 min	5 min	28 min	After walk
7	5 min	21 min	5 min	31 min	After walk
8	5 min	24 min	5 min	34 min	After walk
9	5 min	27 min	5 min	37 min	After walk
10	5 min	30 min	5 min	40 min	After walk
11	5 min	33 min	5 min	43 min	After walk
12	5 min	35 min	5 min	45 min	After walk

Walking is a fun and effective way to get fit and increase your energy level. By adjusting the Frequency (how often), Intensity (how much effort you use), Time (how long you walk), and Type (alternating walking with other cardiorespiratory activities, such as hiking, swimming, dancing, or bike riding), you can create a program that's just right for you.

KEEP IT INTERESTING

Make small changes to your regular routine frequently.

- Don't get stuck in a rut. Try a longer session once in a while, a different time of day, a new path, or a walking partner.

- Vary your walking environment: try walking on a treadmill, outdoors on pavement, through a wooded trail, up and down hills— even in water.

- Continually challenge yourself so your fitness level will continue to improve. You can increase how long, how far, or how frequently you walk. Increase the intensity of your walk by going faster, moving your arms, pushing a stroller, walking uphill, jogging for short periods of time, or using the fitness programs on your treadmill.

- Listen to an audio walking program that uses music to set your pace; some also give you instructions, like "Walk as fast as you can for one minute" to vary your routine.

- Try new cardiorespiratory activities. This keeps you from getting bored and utilizes different muscle groups to improve your overall fitness. Try activities like swimming, cycling, hiking, dancing, jogging, rowing, cross-country skiing, tennis, exercise classes, and others.

- Check with your local community education departments, community colleges, and fitness facilities for additional cardiorespiratory offerings.

- Try meditative walking to clear your mind while you are exercising your body. For example, inhale slowly for four steps, hold your breath for one step, exhale slowly for four steps, and then hold your breath for one step. Repeat.

STRATEGIES: HOW TO USE A PEDOMETER

Using a pedometer is a fun way to measure your activity level throughout the day, both during routine activities and while exercising. It's a small device that measures the number of steps you take, making it easy to set small goals for yourself. It's really motivating to see those steps add up—and to see your energy level rise as your fitness improves.

Pedometers are available just about anywhere you purchase fitness and sports equipment. They are available in a wide price range, but get the kind that counts steps since that's the best way to see small improvements.

Wear your pedometer on your waist, attached to your belt, skirt, or pants (even your underclothes, as long as it fits snugly against your body). Place it in line with the seam of your slacks or over the center of your kneecap, parallel to the ground. It will not give accurate readings if it is tilted to one side. Try it out in different positions along your waist, counting the number of steps you take and then comparing that number to what the pedometer actually reads.

STEP IT UP

First, get an idea of your baseline activity level by recording the number of steps you take in a day without changing your normal routine. Once you know your baseline, set step goals for yourself each day or each week. For example, you could decide to increase by five hundred steps. The most important thing is for the overall trend to be an increase in your total daily steps.

The great thing about a pedometer is that it helps you see what a difference increasing your lifestyle activity makes. Watch the steps add up when you pace while you talk on the phone, walk a flight of stairs, skip a half hour TV program to walk the dog, walk instead of drive, park farther away, or window-shop with friends instead of sitting to talk. Of course, not all activities can be counted in steps (for example, swimming or yoga), but they still count toward your fitness. You'll find that using a pedometer for simple, accurate feedback will motivate you to take a step in the right direction.

Building your cardiorespiratory fitness has many benefits for your health, weight, stamina, and energy. Choose activities you think you'll enjoy, create a plan, and keep it interesting. By taking it one step at a time, you'll find yourself on your way to optimal health.

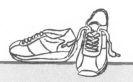

FITNESS Rx
FITT Formula for More Stamina

The FITT Formula—Frequency, Intensity, Time, and Type—can also be used to help you build more stamina.

- Frequency—Exercise most days of the week.

- Intensity—Use enough effort to challenge yourself.

- Time—Aim for anywhere between 10 to 60 minutes, either continuously or broken into shorter sessions.

- Type—Any activity that elevates your heart rate and makes you breathe harder.

CHAPTER 21

INCREASE YOUR
FLEXIBILITY

Like most people who try yoga, I was looking for increased flexibility and stress relief. What I discovered on my mat was a series of meaningful lessons that I apply in my life every day.

Mountain Pose: An outside observer would assume that I am simply standing still. They can't tell that I am focused on my foundation, making sure that I'm firmly rooted to the earth and "hugging my muscles to the bone," as one of my teachers would say. I visualize myself strong and solid—like a mountain. In my life, I occasionally remember to stand still and make sure that my foundation is firm, centered, and strong.

Tree Pose: From the solid foundation of Mountain pose, I slowly bend one knee and move my foot to rest on the inside of my opposite thigh. When I started yoga, I often toppled sideways as I tried to balance on one leg. My first instructor reminded me that this was part of the process so I need not become frustrated or discouraged. I have since learned to find a focal point, concentrate, and stay calm. Balance comes much easier to me now, in yoga *and* in life.

Forward Fold: The simple act of bending over at the waist sometimes causes my back, hamstrings, and calves to cry out, "Hey, you're going the wrong way! We're used to sitting in a chair in front of the computer!" Forcing them only makes it worse. Letting go and relaxing allows gravity to gently lengthen the tissues. When things feel too hard in my life, I find that it's better to stop struggling and allow the forces of nature to work things out.

Warrior Poses: From these poses, I learned that yoga is as much about strength and perseverance as it is about flexibility. In Warrior One, I am ready for battle: my arms raised overhead, my body facing forward, my feet spread wide with my front knee deeply bent. As I flow into Warrior Two, I lower my arms to shoulder height, expand them outward in opposite directions, and turn my body to face sideways. As I begin to feel fatigued, I focus and breathe. By reaching for my edge in everything I do, my limits have expanded far beyond what I ever thought possible.

Sun Salutation: During this graceful but challenging flow of postures, my breath is rhythmically timed to the movements. I find it calming yet incredibly energizing. Many times I move through a challenging day gently reminding myself to breathe.

Head Stand: I was never able to stand on my head as a kid, so I certainly didn't believe it was possible in my forties. I initially approached this pose with self-doubt and skepticism. When I changed my attitude and stopped judging myself, I was able to break the process into small steps and "feel" my way through it. Now, whenever my little voice says, "I can't!" I remember to change my attitude and take it one step at a time.

Corpse Pose: With my body pleasantly fatigued, I'm able to completely relax on my mat for the last pose of every yoga practice. It's not so easy to get my brain to quiet down, however. I hear my teacher say that yoga is not about going through the motions. The purpose of the first hour of class was to quiet my mind for this moment. She's right. When I can chase my mental To Do list out of the way, I experience a deep spiritual connection and a profound sense of peace and joy. On my mat, I realize that life is not about going through the motions either. The purpose is to experience more moments like this.

ESSENTIALS OF FLEXIBILITY

Stretching feels good. Animals, including humans, stretch instinctively. You've probably seen dogs or cats stretch spontaneously, almost lazily, naturally tuning up all their muscles. Infants will arch their backs and stretch their arms when you pick them up after a nap. After sitting in one position too long, you naturally stretch to relieve stiffness. If this spontaneous stretching can feel that good, imagine how good it will feel to stretch all your muscles regularly as part of your overall fitness program.

Flexibility is a key part of a complete and balanced fitness program. Flexibility is the ability of your joints to move through their full range of motion. Stretching exercises increase your flexibility by using gentle, stretching movements to increase the length of your muscles and connective tissues around your joints. Francine gives us a great example of why this is so important.

> I swear—all I was doing was wrapping Christmas presents. I reached for some ribbon and strained my back. How do you explain that to your friends without feeling ridiculous?

Why Bother?

Increased flexibility has many benefits. It:

- Optimizes your ability to function in your daily life
- Enhances physical and mental relaxation by decreasing tension and stiffness in your muscles
- Maintains and increases the range of motion in your joints by increasing the length of your muscles and tendons
- Offsets age-related stiffness and may slow the degeneration of the joints
- Helps you develop body awareness and improved coordination
- Improves your posture and muscular balance. Stretching the muscles of the lower back, shoulders, and chest will help keep your back in better alignment and improve your posture.

- Decreases your risk of lower-back pain. Improved flexibility in the hamstrings, hip flexors, quadriceps, and other muscles attached to the pelvis will relieve tension on the lumbar spine and reduce the risk of lower-back pain.
- Makes you feel good

What Do I Need to Know?

Everybody benefits from stretching. The methods are gentle and easy, and they apply regardless of your age, natural flexibility, or fitness level. You don't have to get into shape to stretch, but even athletes rely on flexibility training for peak performance. Before beginning any exercise program, consult with your doctor if you've been sedentary or have had any recent physical problems (see the "Exercise Clearance" Health Notes in the appendix).

The best time to stretch is when your muscles are warm. Like taffy, a warm muscle is more elastic and relaxes more easily. Overstretching a cold muscle can cause injury. Therefore, if you're going to stretch before you exercise, warm up first by walking or doing your planned cardiorespiratory activity at a light intensity for five to ten minutes. This will increase the elasticity of and circulation to the muscles. Remember, stretching is not the same thing as warming up.

Before Exercise: When you stretch before your workout (but after your warm-up, of course), gently stretch all the muscles you'll be using. For example, if you're going to ride a bike, lightly stretch the muscles in the front and back of your thighs and your lower legs.

During Exercise: Take a moment to stretch during cardiorespiratory activities when you stop to rest or take a drink. While strength training, you can stretch the muscles you're using between each set. (There's more on strength training in the next chapter.)

MINDFUL MOMENT: A few minutes of gentle stretching during a busy day will relax your body and your mind.

After Exercise: An important time to stretch is after you finish exercising. This will lengthen your muscles again and release the tightness that exercise may produce. Be sure to stretch all the muscles you used during your workout.

Anytime: Gentle stretching can be done anytime you feel like it: in the morning to begin your day, while sitting in a car, at your desk, after a warm bath or shower, or while you're just relaxing. Stretching is beneficial whenever you feel muscular stiffness or need to release nervous tension.

HOW DO I GET STARTED?

Stretching feels good when it's done correctly. It's important to listen to your body; you shouldn't experience any pain. Stretching should be peaceful, relaxing, and noncompetitive. Here are the basics of stretching.

Warm up: Make sure your muscles are warm before stretching: for example, walk at a comfortable pace for five to ten minutes.

Breathe: Exhale as you begin the stretch. Continue to take slow, rhythmical breaths throughout the stretch. Don't hold your breath.

Listen to your body: Start by slowly stretching to the point of mild, comfortable tension. Do not stretch to the point of pain.

Relax: Relax as you hold the stretch. The feeling of tension should subside as you hold the position. If it does not, ease off slightly and find a degree of tension that's comfortable. As you inhale, release the stretch slightly; as you exhale, relax further into the stretch.

Hold: Hold the stretch for 10 to 30 seconds. As you feel the tension decrease, you can increase the stretch until you feel a slight pull again.

No bouncing!: Bouncing activates the stretch reflex that causes tightening of the muscles; it is counterproductive and can cause injury.

Repeat: When time allows, repeat each stretch two or three times for optimal benefit.

STRATEGIES: SIMPLE STRETCHES

Use the flexibility exercises that follow to stretch the specific muscle you've used during a cardiorespiratory or strength-training session. For example, after a walk, cycling, or a lower-body strength-training session, do the lower-back and lower-leg stretches. After swimming, tennis, or upper-body strength training, do arm, chest, and upper-back stretches. By doing the entire sequence, these flexibility exercises will provide a good head-to-toe stretching session.

NECK STRETCH

Muscles: The neck and upper back (trapezius)

Relax your neck muscles, bend your head, and bring your chin toward your chest. Hold for 10 to 30 seconds. Lift your chin and look up; hold. Bring your head back to neutral and turn your head to one side as though you are looking over your shoulder. Repeat on the opposite side. Return your head to center and slowly lean your head to one side, bringing your ear toward your shoulder. You can place one hand on the side of your head to gently stretch the neck muscles further. Repeat on the opposite side.

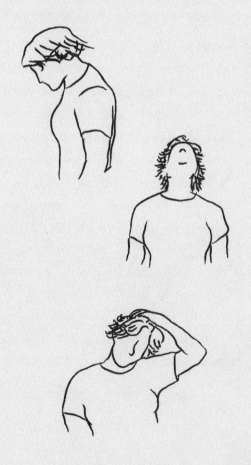

SHOULDER STRETCH

Muscles: The shoulders and upper back

Reach your right arm out in front of your body. Place your left wrist on your right elbow and pull your right arm across your chest. Keeping your right arm extended, use your left wrist to gently pull your right arm as close to your body as possible. Relax your shoulders down away from your ears. Hold for 10 to 30 seconds. Repeat on the opposite side.

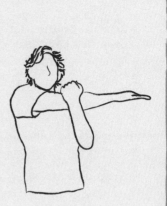

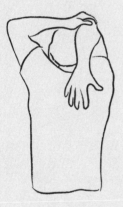

TRICEPS STRETCH

Muscles: The triceps (located on the back of your upper arm) and shoulders

Raise your right arm toward the ceiling then bend your elbow and touch your neck or upper back with the palm of your right hand so that your right elbow points to the ceiling. Grasp your right elbow with your left hand and pull it gently to the left until you feel a stretching sensation at the back of your upper right arm. Hold for 10 to 30 seconds. Repeat on the opposite side.

CHEST STRETCH

Muscles: The chest, shoulders, and back

Lace your fingers behind your back so your palms are facing in toward your spine, thumbs pointing down at the ground. Hold your chin up and lift your chest as high as you can. Pull your shoulders back and lower your linked hands slightly toward the ground. Hold for 10 to 30 seconds. Release the tension and relax for a few seconds. Now slowly raise your linked hands up toward the ceiling, keeping your neck and back relaxed until you feel a gentle stretching sensation in the front of your chest and shoulders.

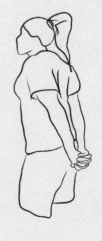

CAT STRETCH

Muscles: The entire back including the cervical, thoracic, and lumbar spine

Position yourself comfortably on your hands and knees with your back level. Inhale as you lift your head and allow your back to sag. Slowly exhale as you contract your stomach muscles and curve your back upward toward the ceiling, allowing your head to drop down and your tail to curve in. Hold for 10 to 30 seconds. Inhale as you slowly return to the starting position. Slowly exhale then repeat.

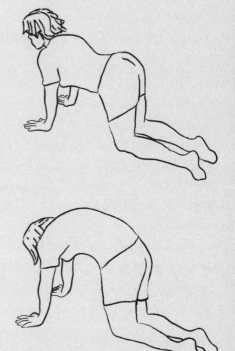

LOWER-BACK EXTENSION STRETCH

Muscles: The abdominal and supporting muscles of the lower back (lumbar spine)

Lie on your stomach and rest on your forearms with your elbows positioned under your shoulders. Gently raise your head and chest off the floor and look straight ahead, leaning comfortably on your forearms. You should feel a gentle stretch in your lower back and along the front of your body. Hold for 10 to 30 seconds. Repeat.

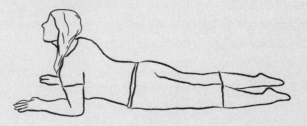

LOWER-BACK FLEXION STRETCH

Muscles: The supporting muscles of the lower back (lumbar spine)

Lie on your back, with both legs extended straight out. Bend your right knee and clasp it with both hands, then slowly pull the knee toward your chest. Hold for 10 to 30 seconds then switch legs. Alternatively, you can pull both knees in at the same time.

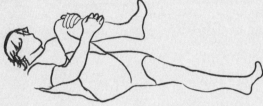

SPINAL TWIST

Muscles: The entire back and the sides of your trunk

While seated on the floor, extend your left leg in front of you. Bend your right leg and place your right foot on the outside of the left knee. Extend your right arm behind you and place your right palm on the floor to support your body. Use your left arm to gently twist your torso to the right until you feel the stretch along your left side and back. Hold for 10 to 30 seconds. Repeat on the opposite side.

INNER-THIGH STRETCH

Muscles: The inner thigh and groin muscles

While seated, pull both feet in toward your body with the soles facing each other. Grasp your feet with your hands and press down slightly on your knees with your elbows. Hold for 10 to 30 seconds.

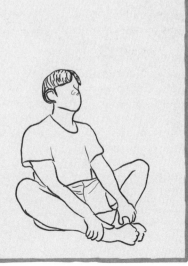

HAMSTRING STRETCH

Muscles: The hamstrings, located in the back of the upper legs

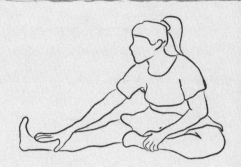

Sitting: Sit comfortably on the floor with your right leg straight and your left leg bent, so that the sole of your left foot rests flat against the inside of your right leg. While keeping your lower back straight, slowly reach toward your right foot until you feel a gentle stretching sensation in your right hamstring. During this stretch, keep your right foot pointing upward. Hold for 10 to 30 seconds. Repeat on the opposite side.

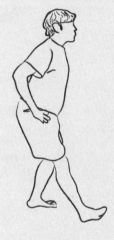

Standing: Place your right foot about 12 inches in front of the left foot. Lift the ball of the right foot and keep your leg straight. Bend the back leg and lean forward into the front leg. Place your hands on your left thigh for balance. Hold for 10 to 30 seconds. Repeat on the opposite side.

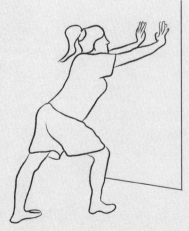

CALF STRETCH

Muscles: The calf muscles, located at the back of the lower leg

While standing, place your hands or forearms on a wall. Place your right foot near the wall and, keeping your left foot flat on the floor, move your left leg back until you feel the stretch in the left calf muscle and the back of your ankle (Achilles tendon). Hold for 10 to 30 seconds. Repeat on the opposite side.

QUADRICEPS STRETCH

Muscles: The quadriceps (quads), located in the front of the upper legs (thighs)

Stand tall and support your body with your left hand against a wall or solid object for balance. Raise your right heel toward your buttocks then grasp your toes or ankle with your right hand. Gently pull your heel up to your buttocks until you feel the stretch in your thigh. Hold for 10 to 30 seconds. Repeat on the opposite side.

Modification: If you are unable to reach your toes or ankle, pull on your pant leg to raise your foot. Alternatively, you can rest your ankle on the seat of a chair placed behind you if that provides enough of a stretch for the front of your thigh.

STRETCH YOUR LIMITS: YOGA

Some people think that yoga is just for flexible people. Actually, yoga is a great form of exercise for everyone—particularly people who need to increase their flexibility!

Yoga is a wonderful way to improve your flexibility, and it will improve your strength, stamina, and mindfulness, too. People of all ages and all levels of fitness can benefit from the physical practice of yoga. Many of the stretches listed in "Strategies: Simple Stretches" are yoga postures.

Numerous styles of yoga and classes are available for all levels. Look for level 1, introductory, gentle, or beginners' DVDs or classes if you're new to yoga. If you don't like a particular class, try a different one. A yoga mat is essential because it provides a nonslip surface to keep you steady as you move in and out of postures. A yoga strap provides extra length when you're extending your arms or legs. A yoga block can be placed under your hands in certain postures until you can reach the floor without it. A blanket provides extra cushion and lift when needed.

Personally, I've experienced significant benefits for my mind, body, heart, and spirit through the practice of yoga. In fact, the word *yoga* means "union" or "yoke"; it is the integration of all these parts into a unified whole. It has taught me how to slow down, focus, and listen to my body. In the process, I've become better able to listen to my heart and soul, too. It has definitely helped me stretch literally and figuratively!

KEEP IT INTERESTING

As with any exercise, varying your flexibility program will help you stick with it.

- In addition to stretching after exercising, periodically set aside time for a head-to-toe stretching session. It will feel so good.

- Listening to music and focusing on your breath can help you relax. When you're relaxed, your body is more responsive to flexibility training.

- Use towels, straps, large balls, and other accessories to add diversity and effectiveness to your stretching.

- Try a stretching class. These are available on DVD or may be offered by your local fitness facility, community center, or community college. Some focus exclusively on flexibility; others combine cardiorespiratory and strength training with stretching.

- Yoga and Pilates are great additions to your regular fitness program. They'll increase your flexibility and strength while teaching you how to focus and calm your mind.

Stretching regularly is a wonderful way to relax while you build your flexibility. It will help you tune up while you tune in to your body.

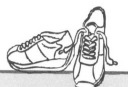

FITNESS Rx
FITT Formula for More Flexibility

Remember to consider the four aspects of the FITT Formula when you're working toward becoming more flexible.

- Frequency—Plan to stretch at least two to three times per week.

- Intensity—Gently stretch to the point of comfortable tension.

- Time—At first, hold each stretch for 10 seconds; gradually increase your hold to 30 seconds. For optimal benefit, repeat each stretch three or four times.

- Type—Stretch specific muscle groups after exercise and/or try a stretch class, yoga, or Pilates.

CHAPTER 22

INCREASE YOUR STRENGTH

For several years, I enjoyed walking for exercise. When I learned about the benefits of strength training, I decided to add some floor exercises to my routine. The first time I tried to do a push-up, I couldn't even do one. I felt discouraged and gave up. Later, it dawned on me that because I couldn't do a single push-up was exactly why I needed to try!

Every other day I would try to do push-ups again. I imagined my muscles saying, "For some reason she wants us to lift her off the floor instead of just lying here. We better get to work." On the opposite days, I could imagine my muscle fibers getting stronger. If I gave up and said, "I can't do push-ups" and never tried again, my muscles would go back to the way they were. Eventually I was able to do push-ups—but I was even happier when I realized that I could easily lift my own luggage in and out of the overhead bin. Now I often share "Dr. May's One Push-up Principle" in my workshops to motivate people to get started. Strength training isn't a matter of can and can't. It's a matter of if and when.

ESSENTIALS OF STRENGTH TRAINING

For a small investment in time, strength training will help you function better in your daily life and will increase your metabolism. Fortunately, you can maintain and even gain muscle at any age, even while losing fat.

Why Bother?

Building muscle tissue and increasing your strength has many benefits. It:

- Increases your ability to function in your daily life
- Enables you to lift a heavy object and lift a lighter object repeatedly
- Maintains or boosts your metabolism by increasing your muscle mass
- Helps you lose body fat
- Minimizes the loss of lean body mass when you lose weight
- Improves your physical appearance by creating a leaner, firmer body
- Helps prevent age-related decreases in your muscle mass and increases in your body fat
- Reduces the risk of overuse injuries by balancing the strength of opposing muscle groups
- Decreases lower-back pain by strengthening the core of your body
- Increases your bone mineral density to prevent or treat osteoporosis
- Improves your glucose metabolism
- Lowers your blood pressure and cholesterol levels
- Helps you appreciate the capacity of your body to meet the demands you place on it

What Do I Need to Know?

Strength training, also called resistance training, is exercise that makes your muscles work harder than they're accustomed to. As a result, the muscle fibers become larger and stronger. To build your muscles, you can lift your own body weight against gravity (like doing sit-ups or push-ups), work against resistance (like pushing an immobile object or pushing and pulling rubber tubing), or lift weights (like using free weights or exercise equipment designed for that purpose).

About 25 percent of your metabolism (your daily caloric need) is driven by the amount of muscle tissue you have. Muscle is more metabolically active than fat; the more muscle you have, the more calories you burn, even when you are at rest.

In fact, most of the age-related slowing of metabolism is due to lack of physical activity and loss of muscle tissue. Studies have shown a 5 percent decline in metabolism each decade throughout adulthood and a 25 percent decline in muscle function by age 65. This is why you may feel like you eat the way you did when you were younger but gain weight more easily.

The effects of yo-yo dieting compound this problem. Every time you drastically decrease your caloric intake, you lose muscle, not just fat, if you aren't exercising regularly. Once you abandon the diet and resume eating the way you previously did, you'll quickly regain fat but not the muscle you lost. As a result, your metabolism will be even slower. This often leads to even more weight gain and a higher body fat percentage. That makes you more prone to diabetes, atherosclerosis, and other chronic diseases.

Be Strong, Be Healthy

There are really two ways to look at muscle fitness. *Muscular strength* is the ability of a muscle to exert maximal force for a brief period of time. This is how much weight a person is able to lift once (for example, lifting a bag of dog food out of the trunk of your car). *Muscular endurance* is the ability of a muscle or group of muscles to perform many repetitions against resistance (for example, lifting a small child into the air repeatedly while playing). Resistance training will help you build both muscular strength and muscular endurance.

MINDFUL MOMENT: Make time for your health and well-being. If you are too busy for exercise, you are too busy.

If you're trying to lose weight, strength training will help prevent muscle loss that would otherwise occur as your body weight decreases. This is important because maintaining your muscle mass is crucial for maintaining an active metabolism. In addition, resistance exercise such as weight training burns calories during exercise and even continues to burn a few extra calories immediately after your strength-training session is over.

Since there are remarkable changes going on in your muscles, you'll notice your strength improve fairly quickly. However, it generally takes six to twenty-four weeks to notice significant changes in your appearance. Keep in mind that while the changes may or may not be evident on the scale, as your ratio of muscle to fat increases, you'll burn more calories, lose body fat, feel more comfortable in your clothes, and most important of all, become stronger and healthier.

Even people who already do strenuous physical activity will benefit from strength training. They need to do specific exercises to balance the opposing muscles, to build the muscles neglected in their usual activities, and to improve their efficiency and performance. For example, a person who digs trenches or lifts patients presumably has strong back muscles but should also do abdominal exercises. Someone who hikes regularly would also need to build upper-body strength. A tennis player would do strength training to increase the power behind his or her stroke.

You don't need to be concerned about getting too bulky or muscle-bound from strength training. Most people don't have the genetic capability or the time required for the intense training needed to gain that much muscle. Women have a relative lack of the male hormone testosterone, so it's very unlikely they will bulk up. In fact, as muscle mass increases and body fat decreases, you'll look leaner and lose girth, even if your weight doesn't change.

HOW DO I GET STARTED?

Consult with your physician prior to beginning an exercise program, if necessary. (See the "Exercise Clearance" Health Notes in the appendix.) Consider seeking the advice of an exercise professional for a specific fitness prescription and instruction. Follow proper technique and form to decrease the chance of injury and to maximize your results. This really helped Marcus and his wife, Gina.

We joined our local YMCA, but I just used the treadmill and Gina only took group classes at first. We finally arranged a session with a personal trainer who showed us how to use all of the equipment and designed strength-training programs for each of us. I feel like now we are really getting our money's worth from the gym.

It's important to prepare your muscles for strength training by performing a brief warm-up first. It's preferable to warm up the muscle groups you'll be working, rather than doing a generalized cardiorespiratory warm-up such as walking. For example, if you're going to do an upper-body strength-training workout, warm up the muscles of the chest, back, shoulders, arms, and core; if you're doing a lower-body workout, warm up the low back, buttocks, hips, and legs. The simplest way to do this is to simulate the exercises you will be doing without using any weights.

You can vary strength-training exercises by how much weight you lift or move, how much resistance you push or pull against, how long you hold a weight up against gravity, and how many times you repeat the exercise in a session. This last variable is usually measured in "reps" and "sets." Rep stands for repetition: lifting a weight or doing an exercise once. A set is a certain number of repetitions. For example, if you were to lift a hand weight 10 times, then rest and repeat, you did two sets of 10 reps.

During your strength-training session, start off doing only as many repetitions (reps) of the exercise as you can do comfortably, eventually working up to a set of 8 to 15 reps (or hold for 10 to 30 seconds, depending on the exercise). If you are unable to do at least 8 repetitions, reduce the weight or resistance. If you can do more than 15 reps, increase the weight or the resistance. As you practice, your body will get stronger to meet the demands you're placing on it. Gradually increase the number of reps, the amount of weight you use, or the number of sets you do, aiming for two to three sets for each exercise.

Do each exercise as slowly as possible and focus your attention on the muscles you're using. Exhale slowly during the part of the exercise that requires the most effort. For example, while you are doing leg lifts, exhale as you raise your leg and inhale as you lower it.

STRATEGIES: SIMPLE STRENGTH TRAINING

There are many ways to build your strength. This simple routine can be done at home, in a hotel room, or even in your office, without any equipment. It utilizes your body weight against the resistance of gravity to help you build muscle. You'll focus on your large muscles so you'll get a great return on your investment.

WALL SQUATS

Muscles: Buttocks and legs

Stand with your back against a wall and your feet one thigh length away from the wall. Bend your knees and lower yourself as if you were going to sit down. Press into the wall with your entire back while squeezing your buttocks and leg muscles. Eventually you'll be able to get your thighs parallel to the ground. Hold as long as you can, aiming for 10 to 30 seconds. Repeat.

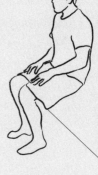

Modifications: Use an exercise ball between your back and the wall for additional support. It's easiest to roll the ball down the wall to get into a sitting position.

SUPERMAN

Muscles: Lower back

Lie face down on the floor with your arms straight out in front of you. Keep your neck in a neutral position by looking down at the floor a few inches ahead of you. Lift your right arm and, if possible, your left leg and hold for 10 to 30 seconds per set. Switch sides. As you get stronger, lift both legs and arms at the same time.

Modification: Position yourself comfortably on your hands and knees with your back level and your neck in neutral position. Start by stretching your right arm out in front of you next to your right ear. If possible, straighten your left leg out behind you at the same time. Hold for 10 to 30 seconds per set. Switch sides.

PUSH-UPS

Muscles: Chest, shoulders, arms, and upper back

At the wall: Place your hands flat on a wall at shoulder height, making sure your hands are wider apart than the width of your shoulders. Place your feet far enough away from the wall so that you can push yourself off the wall. Bend your elbows and slowly bring your body closer to the wall again, keeping your chin lifted off your chest. Repeat 8 to 15 times per set.

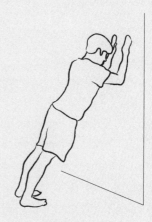

On your knees: While on all fours, with your knees directly under your hips and your hands slightly wider than shoulder width apart, bend your elbows and lower your upper body toward the floor then press yourself back up. As you become stronger, move your knees further behind your hips. Repeat 8 to 15 times per set.

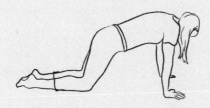

On your toes: Lie down on your stomach. Position your hands under your shoulders, slightly wider than shoulder width apart. Push your entire body off the ground while you're on your toes. Try to maintain a plank position by not allowing your hips to sag down or lift toward the ceiling. Slowly raise and lower your entire body toward the ground. Repeat 8 to 15 times per set. Alternatively, hold the plank position for 10 to 30 seconds.

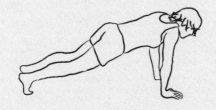

BRIDGE

Muscles: Buttocks, thighs, lower back, and abdominals

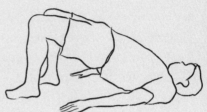

Lie on your back on the floor. Bend your knees and place your feet hip distance apart. Tighten your buttocks and raise your hips off the floor then slowly lower them to the floor. To increase the intensity, do not lower your hips all the way down to the floor. Repeat 8 to 15 times per set. Alternatively, hold for 10 to 30 seconds per set.

SIT-UPS

Muscles: Abdominals

Lie on your back on the floor. Bend your knees and place your feet hip distance apart. Place your hands behind your head or cross your arms across your chest. Keep your neck in neutral position (don't bring your chin toward your chest) and relax your arms and legs. Tighten your abdominal muscles to lift your shoulder blades just off the floor then slowly lower down. Repeat 8 to 15 times per set.

If doing repetitions with your hands across your chest or behind your head is too challenging, bring your hands to the backs of your thighs and gently pull your shoulders off the floor, keeping your chin neutral. Hold for 8 to 15 seconds as you breathe normally (don't hold your breath!). Rest and repeat.

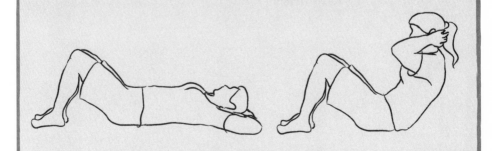

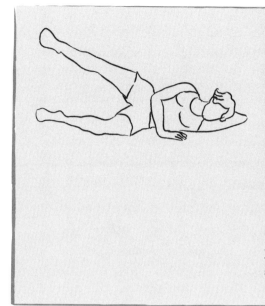

LEG LIFTS

Muscles: Outer and inner thighs and buttocks

Lie on one side on the floor. Bend both legs 45 degrees. Rest your head on your arm. Lift your top leg about halfway as you tighten your muscles in your buttocks and leg. Lift and lower your leg slowly 8 to 15 times per set. For added intensity, do not touch your top leg to your bottom leg. Roll to the other side and repeat.

It takes just two sessions a week to begin to see results. It's important that you rest a muscle group for a minimum of 48 hours between weight-training sessions to allow the muscles to repair and become stronger. People who want to do strength training every day usually alternate between lower- and upper-body exercises, or they work on even smaller groups of muscles. For general health and an increase in muscular strength and endurance, training each muscle group properly even once a week is sufficient.

KEEP IT INTERESTING

- Do resistance exercises at home with weights, cans of food, or milk jugs partially filled with sand or water.

- Consider purchasing other home exercise equipment, such as a weight bench or home gym, if you enjoy the convenience and privacy of working out at home.

- A stability ball—that is, a large rubber exercise ball—is one of the most versatile and affordable pieces of exercise equipment you can own. It's excellent for strength training (especially core strength) and improving flexibility, balance, and coordination. You can do squats, sit-ups, push-ups, and numerous other exercises with the support of the ball.

- If the ball is the most versatile, a rubber exercise band or tubing is the most portable piece of resistance equipment. These long, wide rubber bands can be hooked around your feet or wrists to provide resistance as you do various exercises. You can tighten the band to increase the resistance as needed.

- Exercise in the water. Aquatic exercise enhances your cardio-respiratory fitness while the resistance of the water increases your muscular strength and endurance. Water also provides buoyancy and support for your body, so there is less stress and strain on your joints and muscles.

- Join a fitness center. Choose a place that's convenient and feels comfortable. Most will give you a free pass for a short period of time to try it out and see if it feels right for you. You may also be able to schedule a complimentary session with a fitness professional who will show you how to use the equipment.

- Check your local community center or parks and recreation department for weight training, water aerobics, Pilates, and other classes to help you build your strength.

- Look for Internet-based resources for exercising at home or while traveling.

- Hire a qualified and experienced personal trainer. His or her expertise will help you set up a safe and efficient exercise program and keep you motivated to reach your fitness goals.

- Consider signing up for a "boot camp," an intensive group exercise program designed to rapidly improve your fitness.

- Try yoga. Yoga not only increases your flexibility and calms your mind but also builds muscular strength and endurance with regular practice.

As you build new muscle, you'll find it easier to maintain a healthier weight. As you improve your muscular strength and endurance, you'll increase your metabolism and function more fully in your life. For a limited investment in time, strength training pays big rewards.

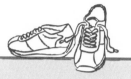

FITNESS Rx
FITT Formula for More Strength

Build your strength by applying the FITT Formula.

- Frequency—Two or more sessions per week

- Intensity—Two to three sets of 8–15 repetitions or 15- to 30-second holds per exercise

- Time—Typically about 20 to 30 minutes per session

- Type—Any activity that works against resistance such as your body weight, rubber tubing, free weights, or exercise equipment

CHAPTER 23

CHALLENGE YOUR BODY

After my son, Tyler, was born, my fit friend Mary offered to walk with me once a week. Although Mary preferred jogging and was in much better shape than I was, she seemed to enjoy our walks. She kept us moving at a decent pace and kept herself challenged by pushing the stroller. I also walked two or three other days each week, and as my fitness level improved, I was able to go faster and farther. I eventually added hills near my home to my route. I would push the stroller up the steep hill then jog down the other side, Tyler giggling all the way.

ESSENTIALS OF OPTIMIZING YOUR FITNESS

As you become accustomed to a more active lifestyle and your body adapts to your new fitness program, you may wonder, "Am I getting the most from my activities?" The answer to this question lies in the "I" of the FITT Formula: intensity, or amount of effort you put into your exercise. After Bridget learned about the importance of intensity, she realized she'd been wasting time doing exactly the same thing for over a year.

> I was just going through the motions, not challenging myself at all. I was fake-exercising! I don't have much free time to be wasting, not getting the full benefit, so I committed myself to putting in the effort my body deserves. I'm already starting to notice an improvement in my fitness level, and I feel great!

WHY BOTHER?

Varying and increasing the intensity of your activity has many benefits for overall health, fitness, and weight loss.

- You'll improve both your fitness level and your cardiovascular health more quickly.
- You'll burn more calories, which will help you lose or maintain weight.
- As your intensity increases, the "aftereffect" on your metabolism increases; in other words, the harder you work, the more calories you burn even *after* you exercise.
- It will keep your exercise sessions interesting and prevent boredom.
- You may increase the "feel good" effect of exercise at higher intensities because of a greater release of endorphins. In addition, you'll experience a greater sense of pride and accomplishment.
- It saves time. When you don't have time for longer bouts of moderate-intensity exercise, you can "trade" for shorter bouts of more intense exercise and still benefit.

> **MINDFUL MOMENT:** For best results, keep your fitness program interesting, challenging, and efficient.

WHAT DO I NEED TO KNOW?

There are many ways to measure the intensity of your exercise. The easiest way is the Talk Test, which allows you to quickly measure your intensity by monitoring your ability to talk during activity. While you're exercising, say a few sentences out loud, like the alphabet or a nursery rhyme. When you're getting started, try to spend the majority of your activity session at an intensity that allows you to speak comfortably. If you feel breathless and have difficulty saying the sentences, decrease your intensity. If you can sing them, you'll want to increase your effort. As your fitness level increases, experiment with occasionally increasing the intensity to the point where it becomes more difficult to speak comfortably.

Two other ways to measure your intensity are the Perceived Exertion Scale and Target Heart Rate.

The Perceived Exertion Scale

You can use a subjective index, called the Perceived Exertion Scale, to assess the level of effort, strain, or discomfort you feel during exercise. When assessing your level of perceived exertion, don't focus on just one factor, such as your breathing; instead, assess your total level of exertion. The number you choose on the Perceived Exertion Scale should reflect the total amount of effort, exertion, stress, and fatigue you are experiencing.

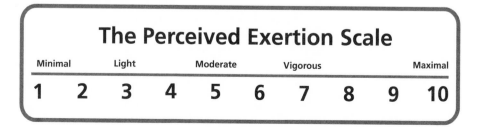

The Perceived Exertion Scale

Minimal	Light		Moderate	Vigorous				Maximal
1	2	3	4	5	6	7	8	9	10

1—Minimal: Barely moving.

2—Very light: No noticeable change in breathing or significant increase in heart rate.

3—Light: You have an awareness of muscles working and slight elevation in breathing and heart rate, but you can easily carry on a conversation or even sing.

4—Moderately light: Feels really manageable; you can comfortably work at this intensity for more than 30 minutes.

5—Moderate: Faster or stronger movement; you are aware of an increase in effort level; heart rate and breathing are up; you can say the alphabet but cannot sing it.

6—Moderate plus: More challenging. You have to maintain focused effort to keep it up.

7—Vigorous: Breathing is becoming heavy; you can say only short sentences before stopping to breathe.

8—Very vigorous: Muscles may be burning; breathing is very heavy and probably open-mouthed; you can only say a few words before having to stop for air.

9—Near maximal: Discomfort verging on pain; breathing is extremely heavy and heart is pounding; muscles are burning. It would be difficult to maintain this intensity for more than a few minutes.

10—Maximal: You are absolutely working as hard as you can. You are able to maintain this intensity for only a few seconds.

Target Heart Rate (THR)

For cardiorespiratory activities, you'll achieve the optimal benefit by keeping your heart rate in your Target Heart Rate (THR) zone. Your THR zone is between 55 and 64 percent of your maximal heart rate (MHR) when you're getting started with exercise. As you become more fit, gradually increase the zone to between 65 and 90 percent of your MHR.

First, practice finding your pulse by gently resting two fingers on the side of your neck (next to your Adam's apple) or on the thumb side of your wrist. To get your 60-second pulse, count your pulse for 10 seconds then multiply that number by six, or count for 15 seconds and multiply by four.

Then while you are exercising, slow down briefly and check your pulse to see if you are in your THR zone. Adjust your intensity up or down to keep yourself in your zone. (If you're on medication that alters your heart rate, such as a beta-blocker, use the Perceived Exertion Scale instead.)

STRATEGIES: INTERVAL WORKOUTS— TAKING IT UP A NOTCH

One of the best and most interesting ways to increase the intensity of your activity is to do "intervals." An interval workout takes your heart rate from the lower end of your THR zone to the upper end several times during the session. Here are two examples of interval workouts; feel free, however, to make up your own.

CARDIO INTERVALS

- Walk at light intensity (perceived exertion of 3) for 5 minutes to warm up.
- Walk for 4 minutes at a moderate intensity (perceived exertion of 5); you can say the alphabet comfortably.
- Walk 1 minute at a vigorous intensity (perceived exertion of 7 or 8); you can still say the alphabet, but it's definitely harder to do so, and you have to stop for breath more frequently while talking.
- Repeat this alternating 4-minute–1-minute pattern four times, for a total of 20 minutes.
- Walk at light intensity for 5 minutes to cool down.

CARDIO AND STRENGTH INTERVALS

EXERCISE	AMOUNT	DESCRIPTION
Wall Squats	Hold for 10–30 seconds	Stand with your back against a wall and your feet one thigh length away from the wall. Bend knees and lower yourself as if you were going to sit. Press into the wall with entire back while squeezing buttocks and leg muscles. Work toward having thighs parallel to the ground. *Modifications:* Use an exercise ball between your back and the wall for additional support. It's easiest to roll the ball down the wall to get into a sitting position.

EXERCISE	AMOUNT	DESCRIPTION
Lateral Steps	Continuously for 30–60 seconds	Pretend you're an Olympic speed skater! Hop from side to side, one leg at a time, staying low to the ground. Make hops as wide as possible. (If you do not want to hop, simply step side to side, using your arms for added intensity.)
Push-ups	8 to 15 reps; when you can do 15 fairly comfortably, challenge yourself with a more advanced position	*At the wall:* Place hands flat on a wall at shoulder height, making sure they are wider than the width of your shoulders. Place feet far enough away from the wall so that you can push yourself off the wall. Bend elbows and slowly bring body closer to the wall again, keeping chin lifted off your chest. *On your knees:* While on all fours with knees directly under hips and hands slightly wider than shoulder width apart, bend elbows and lower upper body toward the floor, and then press back up. As you become stronger, move knees further behind hips. *On your toes:* Lie on stomach with hands positioned under shoulders, slightly wider than shoulders. Push entire body off the ground while on your toes. Try to maintain a plank position by not allowing hips to sag down or lift toward the ceiling. Slowly raise and lower entire body toward the ground.
Soccer Knees	Continuously for 30–60 seconds	Stand upright with feet hip distance apart. Alternate lifting knees as high as you can, keeping torso upright and abdominals engaged, as if you were lightly popping a soccer ball into the air. For added intensity, keep arms overhead and move them in any way that is comfortable.

EXERCISE	AMOUNT	DESCRIPTION
Bridge	8 to 15 reps	Lie on back on floor. Bend knees and place feet hip distance apart. Tighten buttocks and raise hips off the floor then slowly lower them to the floor. To increase the intensity, don't lower your hips all the way down.
Boxer Punches	Continuously for 30–60 seconds	Now you're a boxer. Starting with hands and arms in front of face and chest, punch an imaginary opponent in front of you. Alternate right and left punches as quickly as you can.
Sit-ups	8 to 15 reps	Lie on back on the floor. Bend knees and place feet hip distance apart. Place hands behind head or cross arms across chest. Keep neck in neutral position (don't bring chin toward chest) and relax arms and legs. Tighten your abdominal muscles to lift your shoulder blades just off the floor then slowly lower down. If doing repetitions with hands across your chest or behind your head is too challenging, bring hands to the backs of your thighs and gently pull shoulders off the floor, keeping chin neutral.
March or jog in place	Continuously for 30–60 seconds	March quickly in place, pumping arms for added intensity. Or, if a higher-impact option feels okay, pick it up to a light jog.
Superman	8 to 15 reps	Lie face down on the floor with arms straight out in front of you. Keep neck in a neutral position by looking down at the floor a few inches ahead of you. Slowly lift right arm and left leg off the floor and then slowly lower down. Switch sides. As you get stronger, lift both legs and arms at the same time. *Modification:* Position yourself comfortably on your hands and knees with back level and neck in neutral position. Start by stretching right arm out in front next to right ear. If possible, straighten left leg out behind you at the same time. Alternate sides.

Use the following steps to calculate your THR zone:

1. Calculate your estimated MHR:

   MHR = 220 minus your age

2. Next, calculate your THR zone and write it on an index card.

   Low end of your THR zone = 65% of MHR = 0.65 x MHR

   High end of your THR zone = 90% of MHR = 0.90 x MHR

For example, find the THR zone for a 40-year-old who exercises regularly.

1. MHR = 220 - 40 = 180

2. Low end of her THR zone = 0.65 x 180 = 117

   High end of her THR zone = 0.90 x 180 = 162

   Her THR zone is 117—162.

HOW DO I OPTIMIZE MY FITNESS?

When you first start a fitness program, work your way up gradually by exercising at a perceived exertion level of 5 to 6 (moderate), or at 55 to 64 percent of your MHR.

As you become accustomed to exercising, you'll feel more comfortable at a perceived exertion level of 7 to 8 (vigorous), or in your optimal THR zone of 65 to 90 percent throughout most of your session. As your body becomes more conditioned, exert more effort if you fall below the low end of your target range; slow down if you're above the top end of your range.

Once you're comfortable using one of these methods for monitoring your intensity, you can optimize the benefits of your activity in many different ways.

Cardio: When walking, increase your speed, pump your arms harder or faster, walk uphill, or even pick your pace up to a jog. If you're using a machine such as an elliptical trainer or a bike, you can increase the speed or adjust the resistance, making it harder to maintain the same pace. During a fitness class the instructor will usually offer options for increased intensity, such as making larger motions with your arms and legs.

Strength training: Do additional reps (up to 15) or increase the weight. You can also decrease the time you rest between sets to keep your heart rate elevated. Circuit classes, which alternate strength training with cardio, are great ways to increase your intensity and give you an all-in-one workout.

Flexibility: Stretching should not feel intense, but you can increase the depth of your stretch and the length of time you hold your stretch. You can also increase the intensity by taking Pilates and yoga classes that offer a higher degree of difficulty.

As you experiment with various options, remember to start small and set achievable goals. You may discover, as Bridget did, that you can take your fitness to a whole new level. Keep in mind, however, that you don't always have to focus on increasing your intensity. Sometimes it feels good to just appreciate the movement of your body and fully engage in the experience without trying to achieve something.

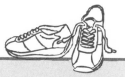

FITNESS Rx
FITT Formula for More of a Challenge

The FITT Formula takes the guesswork out of setting new challenges for yourself.

- Frequency—As always, your body is your best guide.

- Intensity—Use the Talk Test, Perceived Exertion Scale, or Target Heart Rate to monitor your intensity.

- Time—Increase the intensity for all, or part, of your exercise session.

- Type—Increase the intensity of virtually any type of activity by moving faster, using larger movements, and experimenting with intervals.

CHAPTER 24

ON YOUR TERMS

My husband, Owen, completed his first half-marathon in his late forties. I, on the other hand, had signed up to walk it—and didn't even show up!

I've never liked to run and never had the slightest interest in training for an event like that. While I was dieting, I walked regularly and sometimes worked out at the gym, but I've since moved well beyond exercising just to burn calories. For the last eight years or so, I've loved yoga and hiking, and I'm disappointed if I can't fit one or the other in most days of the week.

Why, then, when a friend asked me to walk the half-marathon with her, did I say yes? Because I knew I *could* and I thought I *should*.

It turns out that those reasons weren't good enough because my exercise personality is a poor fit for training for a long-distance event. My travel schedule can be crazy, so I didn't like the pressure of having to train. I hated missing my yoga class when I needed to walk instead. I resented the thought of carving out long periods of time for distance training. As the marathon drew near, I found myself dreading getting up early and dealing with the crowds and the traffic on event day. To be honest, the whole thing reminded me of the times when I was dieting and had to force myself to exercise.

Hate? Resentment? Dread? Enough already! Clearly, training for a half-marathon was not my thing. I had nothing to prove, and it was ruining the joy I find in moving simply for the sake of moving. So I backed out. No guilt, no shame—just an important lesson learned about myself.

Owen reached his goal and rediscovered his love of running. I went back to yoga and hiking and realized how much I love doing things I enjoy and the flexibility of exercising on my own terms.

DO WHAT YOU LOVE, LOVE WHAT YOU DO

Just as it is essential to balance eating for nourishment with eating for enjoyment, you must choose activities that you find both challenging and enjoyable. Moving mindfully—in other words, choosing and doing physical activity with *intention* and *attention*—will help you with this.

Move with intention. Be purposeful when you choose your activities.

- Choose activities that suit your personality and mood.
- Choose activities that meet your body's needs.
- Move with the goal of feeling *better* when you're finished.

Move with attention. Be attentive during your activities.

- Become aware of your surroundings, physical sensations, thoughts, and feelings.
- Listen to your body's cues of intensity, discomfort, and fatigue.
- Appreciate your body's stamina, flexibility, and strength.

When you move with the intention of caring for yourself, you'll choose activities that you find challenging and enjoyable. When you're attentive, you'll appreciate your body's capacity to become stronger and healthier.

MOVING WITH INTENTION

As you learned to be in charge of what you eat, you asked yourself three questions: What do I want? What do I need? and What do I have? These questions can also help you choose the best physical activity at any given time.

- What do I want to do? What do I feel like doing (if anything)? Am I in the mood to be more active or in the mood for structured exercise? Do I want to do housework, work in my garden, walk my

MINDFUL MOMENT: When you discover physical activity you enjoy, exercise will never feel like work again.

dog, or play with my kids? What does my body feel like doing right now—cardio, strength training, or stretching?

- What do I need to do? What have I been doing this week? Am I due for a rest or do I need to get moving somehow today? Have I met the goals I set for my personal fitness prescription? What's missing from my program recently? Does my physical activity reflect balance, variety, and moderation?

- What do I have to do? What are my options for activity? What equipment, classes, or other activities are available to me? What does my time and scheduling allow? What's the weather like? Do I want to go to the gym, be outside, or do something at home? Is there someone I could exercise with?

Your Exercise Personality Quiz

Before you join another gym, drag out your stationary bike, or buy new walking shoes, maximize the likelihood that you're choosing the right activities for your personality. To identify your unique exercise personality traits, circle the answers below that best describe you. This information will help you decide what types of physical activity you're most likely to enjoy and stick with.

Why?

1. My main motivation for exercising is to:
   a. look better
   b. feel better
   c. be healthier
   d. lose weight
   e. other:
2. I am motivated by rewards like:
   a. visual graphs and numbers
   b. money or prizes
   c. intangibles like increased energy or better sleep

It's important to identify your reason(s) for exercising. Write your fitness goals using positive, powerful, measurable terms to keep yourself focused and inspired. Be specific about the results you want and the rewards you'll receive when you achieve your goals. For example, if you're motivated to become healthier and you like to see tangible results, you could make a graph that tracks your resting heart rate and blood pressure. If looking better or losing weight are your goals but take a while to see, you could pay yourself a dollar every time you work out to save up in order to buy yourself a CD or clothing. Even if you enjoy less tangible rewards, be specific about the results you're looking for.

How?

3. Time for exercise:

    a. is not a problem

    b is a challenge but can be arranged when I make it a priority

    c. is last on my list

4. I'd exercise more if it wasn't for:

    a. the time it takes to get to the gym and back

    b. family commitments

    c. work

    d. the cost of a gym membership or equipment

5. I stay on track best when:

    a. I set a goal to work out most days of the week but stay flexible about when

    b. I write my workout schedule in my appointment calendar

    c. I know someone else is expecting me to be there

6. When I decide to do something:

    a. I have a hard time getting started

    b. I stick with it unless it becomes inconvenient

    c. I make it happen no matter what

The reality is that making the commitment to invest time, money, and energy in becoming more active is never easy. When you know what makes it easier for you and anticipate what could get in your way, you can plan to work around those challenges. For example, if you're concerned about taking time away from your family, you could involve them in your workouts, exercise during your workday, or decide that the time it takes will pay off because you're healthier and less stressed.

When?

7. I feel most energetic and alert in the:

    a. morning

    b. afternoon

    c. evening

8. In the past, exercise has worked best:

    a. when I do it early in the day before other things get in my way

    b. when I do it at work during my breaks or lunch hour

    c. when I stop in at the gym on my way home so I don't have to go back out again

    d. when I do it after dinner to unwind or when I have help with the kids

Plan your workouts during your peak energy times when you're most likely to do it. Make it easier on yourself by scheduling a time when it's most convenient.

Where?

9. I love to be:

    a. at home

    b. outdoors

    c. in an exercise environment

10. When people look at me:

    a. I'm self-conscious and embarrassed

    b. I just ignore them

    c. I'm flattered

If you enjoy being at home, use exercise videos or websites, a treadmill, a stationary bike, or a home gym. If you're more of an outdoors type, you'll enjoy walking, hiking, bike riding, or sports. If you need a designated exercise space and don't mind having other people around, join a gym or studio.

Who?

11. I prefer to be:

 a.   by myself

 b.   with a friend or partner

 c   in a group where I know everyone

 d   anonymous in a crowd

12. I need:

 a.   to exercise at my own pace

 b.   the support of a friend or partner

 c.   the accountability of showing up to a class or lesson

 d.   to be pushed by a trainer or teacher

If you prefer to be alone, choose activities like walking, biking, or exercise videos. If you enjoy being with one or two others, invite someone to walk, hike, play tennis, or go to the gym with you. If you enjoy socializing while you exercise, consider joining a sports team, signing up for a class, or arranging classes at church or at work. If you prefer to work out with strangers, join a large gym for weight training, spin classes, or other group exercise. If you need accountability and support, sign up for a class or get a workout buddy or personal trainer to come to your home or meet you at the gym. Mix it up depending on your mood.

What?

13. I am:

 a.   easily bored

 b.   a creature of habit

14. I really like:

 a.   technical gadgets like monitors and tracking programs

b. a really challenging workout so I don't have to think about anything

c. creative or artistic expression

15. When it comes to competition, I

    a feel stressed

    b. like to challenge myself

    c. think a little is healthy and fun

    d. am very competitive

There are many different forms of physical activity, so your challenge is to find several types that suit your preferences. If you're a gadget guru, you might like a fancy pedometer or gyms equipped with high-tech monitors to track your progress on all the machines. If you enjoy artistic expression, you may enjoy dance or yoga. If you thrive on competition, look for team sports or competitive events like races; you can also challenge competitive friends to play racquetball, tennis, or other sports. If you enjoy challenging yourself, set goals and monitor incremental improvements. If you don't like competition, but like to be with others, look for classes and gyms with a supportive environment.

No matter what your personal exercise traits are, get out there and try different activities until you find things that you enjoy.

MOVING WITH ATTENTION

There may be times when you feel like watching television while you do floor exercises or reading a magazine while you work out on a stationary bike. Distracting yourself or multitasking may have its place, but it can also diminish your ability to have a complete mind-body experience. Choosing to move more mindfully increases your awareness of your body, which decreases your risk of injury and boredom and increases your enjoyment and ability to optimize the time you invest. Further, mindfulness during activity has a calming, meditative effect that carries over into other aspects of your life.

STRATEGIES: MINDFUL MOVEMENT

Experiment with the following methods to increase your mindfulness during physical activity:

LIFESTYLE ACTIVITIES

Staying Present: Practice mindfulness during your daily activities like eating, showering, straigtening the house, running errands, and working. When you become distracted, gently remind yourself to breathe and again become aware of your surroundings, sensations, thoughts, and feelings.

CARDIO

Meditative Walking: Inhale slowly for four steps, hold your breath for one step, exhale slowly for four steps, and then hold for one step. Repeat. Experiment with different lengths to see what works best for you.

Environmental Awareness: As you walk, cycle, or jog, be highly aware of the details in your environment: the sights, the sounds, the weather, and so forth. You can even make it part of your training: for example, choose a beautiful tree in the distance and pick up your pace until you reach it.

Technique Focus: When you learn a new activity such as ballroom dancing, tennis, or swimming, you necessarily become more mindful of your body, movements, and technique.

Gratitude Attitude: A powerful technique is to think about everything you're grateful for as you walk. Imagine a ripple that moves outward. Start by expressing gratitude for everything about yourself: your body, your mind, your heart, and your spirit. Then express gratitude for those around you: your family, your friends, your coworkers, and so on. Then move on to other things you are grateful for: where you live, the weather, the cultural events in your city . . . you get the idea.

FLEXIBILITY

Mindful Movement: Yoga and Pilates are usually taught with an emphasis on mindfulness. As you notice your awareness and thoughts drift elsewhere, gently bring your focus back to the present moment.

Centering Breath: Matching your movement to your breath is a powerful centering tool because it requires focus and awareness. Tie slow, deep breaths to your movements so each movement begins and ends precisely with the start and finish of the breath. For example, open your arms slowly overhead as you inhale then lower them back to your sides as you exhale.

Nonjudgmental Awareness: Become curious about your thoughts and feelings as you move into different poses or exercises. Without judgment, notice whether thoughts like "my favorite pose" or "I hate this one" make the activity more or less enjoyable. Practice disconnecting from those habitual thoughts and opinions by focusing on your breath.

Intentional Practice: Before you start, set an intention for your practice that gives you a focus to return to throughout. For example, your intention might be to stay connected to your breath, challenge yourself in some of the poses or exercises, or express gratitude throughout your practice.

STRENGTH TRAINING

Breath Awareness: To ensure both mindfulness and proper movement during strength training, exhale *slowly* as you shorten or contract the muscle (for example, lifting your leg) and inhale slowly as you lengthen or relax the muscle (for example, lowering your leg).

Counting: Count as you do repetitions to ensure slow, steady movement; 1, 2, 3 as you shorten: 1, 2, 3 as you lengthen.

Muscle Focus: Bring your awareness and attention to the muscle group you are working, ensuring that you're doing the exercise primarily with that muscle group. For example, while doing an abdominal crunch, focus on the contraction in the front and center of your abdomen. Be sure you aren't using your hands behind your head to pull you up or that you aren't relying on momentum to swing your body up and down.

> **MINDFUL MOMENT:** Mindful movement increases your appreciation of the present moment.

Mind-Body Scan During Exercise

Focus your attention: Get centered. Tune into the experience and become aware of your body and your surroundings. Pay attention to the sights, sounds, aromas, weather, and other people in your environment.

Focus on your physical sensations: Connect with your body. Tune into your breath, your heart rate, and other sensations. How does your body feel as you move? How do different activities and intensities feel? What do you need to do to make it more comfortable, challenging, or enjoyable?

Focus on your thoughts: What thoughts are running through your mind? What feelings are your thoughts creating? How are your thoughts affecting your experience with this activity?

Focus on your feelings: Become aware of your emotions. What feelings do you have about exercising? Are you having fun or feeling punished? Are you enjoying the atmosphere, the other people, and the experience?

Even Rebecca, a long-time fitness buff, was able to redefine her relationship with exercise by bringing more mindfulness and enjoyment to the experience.

> For fifteen years I'd relied on exercise to keep myself from gaining weight. When I finally disconnected my exercise from my eating, I discovered a sense of freedom I hadn't experienced since I was a child. I realized just how much my attitude had changed while I was walking my four-month-old puppy, Dimetri, on a trail near my house. In the past, I would have been impatient at walking him because my own internal rules dictated that only running was "good enough." However, instead of trying to maximize every single second of exercise for the sake of burning calories, I thoroughly enjoyed my walk. I felt pure joy as I observed Dimetri's goofy little romp

beside me and his curiosity about everything he encountered. I saw the beauty of the huge oak trees along the path and felt the cool breeze on my skin. I was surprised at how great it felt to walk for a change. I was overwhelmed by all the sensations, and I teared up with joy. That was the beginning of my new relationship with exercise—more natural, mindful, and enjoyable.

Becoming more intentional about your thoughts, feelings, and choices of activities will help you discover what inspires, challenges, and rewards you. Becoming more attentive helps you appreciate the privilege of moving your body and allows you to experience the joy of being fully present in the moment. In this way, exercise is no longer a means to an end but an end in and of itself.

PART 4

EAT

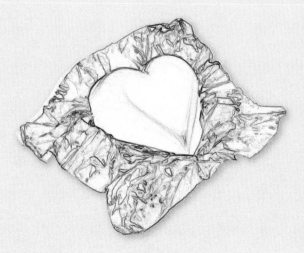

CHAPTER 25

I *AM* HUNGRY!

I am a "foodie." Now, free from a love-hate relationship with food, I enjoy every aspect of eating, from preparation to dining.

I love to leaf through culinary magazines, and I relish the challenge of finding the perfect recipe (sometimes defined by whether we have all of the ingredients on hand) in my files of newspaper clippings. I love farmers markets, import stores, and "big box" stores that offer samples of their featured items. I don't like routine grocery shopping, but fortunately, Owen does. I'm happy to leave that task to him, although I'm never sure what new ingredient he'll come home with. Though he works as a professional spa chef all day, he takes pleasure in preparing food for our family—as long as we clean up. I haven't completely relegated the cooking to him, however. I learned to love to cook from my mother and to bake from my grandmother. Now our children are both wonderful cooks, making them popular with hungry friends.

On Friday or Saturday evenings, Owen and I often open a bottle of wine and make dinner together. He chops while I measure. We both taste and sometimes disagree about how to adjust the seasonings. Together, we divide and conquer a simple salad or the most complicated recipe. We love to entertain family and friends, whether with a gourmet version of a childhood comfort food or a four-course wine pairing. Food brings us together, but our connection is much deeper.

In the following pages, we've shared some of our family's favorite recipes with you. There are suggested menus, or you can try the recipes one at a time if you prefer. We've also included culinary tips in the Chef's Notes, health tips in the Doctor's Notes, and practical tips in the Family Notes. It is our hope that you'll discover (or rediscover) joy in preparing and sharing delicious, nutritious meals with your family and friends. Bon appétit!

SUNDAY BRUNCH
MENU
BRUNCH OVEN EGGS
BROILED GRAPEFRUIT
FRESH FRUIT AND YOGURT PARFAIT

Family meals don't just have to happen at dinner. Plan a leisurely morning meal followed by a trip to the zoo for a little fresh air and exercise.

BRUNCH OVEN EGGS
Serves 4

INGREDIENTS
8 eggs
½ cup light sour cream (not fat-free)
½ cup skim milk (or low-fat)
½ cup shredded sharp cheddar
   cheese
4 green onions thinly sliced (white and
   green parts)
½ cup red or green pepper finely
   chopped
¼ teaspoon salt
⅛ teaspoon pepper

DIRECTIONS
1. Heat oven to 325 degrees and spray
   a 9" round pie pan or 8" square
   baking dish with nonstick spray.
2. Mix all ingredients and pour into the
   baking dish.
3. Bake 25–35 minutes until middle
   is set. Time will vary depending on
   baking dish.

CHEF'S NOTES
Experiment with other ingredients such
as onions, mushrooms, peppers, green
chilies, tomatoes, ham, and different
types of cheese. To make this egg
dish with a crust, line the bottom of the
pan with whole wheat bread then pour
ingredients over the top and bake.

DOCTOR'S NOTES
Cheese is a great source of calcium,
protein, and minerals. It is also high in
saturated fat, so the key is to shred and
sprinkle cheeses for maximal flavor.

FAMILY NOTES:
These reheat pretty well in the
microwave. Make extra on the weekend
for quick high-protein weekday
breakfasts.

NUTRITION ANALYSIS PER SERVING
241 Calories; 15 g Fat; 6 g Saturated fat;
17 g Protein; 9 g Carbohydrate; 1 g Fiber;
392 mg Cholesterol; 377 mg Sodium.

BROILED GRAPEFRUIT
Serves 4

INGREDIENTS

2 grapefruit
4 teaspoons brown sugar

DIRECTIONS

1. Cut each grapefruit in half.
2. With a knife, separate the segments.
3. Sprinkle each half with 1 teaspoon of brown sugar.
4. Set grapefruit in oven and broil until brown sugar starts to bubble.
5. Serve warm and enjoy.

NUTRITION ANALYSIS PER SERVING
49 Calories; trace Fat; 0 g Saturated fat; 1 g Protein;
12 g Carbohydrate; 1 g Fiber; 0 mg Cholesterol;
1 mg Sodium.

CHEF'S NOTES

To section a grapefruit, cut it in half. Use a knife with a sharp tip and cut each section along both sides of the thin membrane.

DOCTOR'S NOTES

Grapefruit and other citrus fruits are a great source of vitamin C. Grapefruit can affect the way your body handles certain medications, so check with your doctor.

FAMILY NOTES

This is a great way to dress up brunch, or you can just serve with whole grain toast and a boiled egg for a workday breakfast. For a cold version, section the grapefruit halves and sprinkle with sugar or honey.

FRESH FRUIT AND YOGURT PARFAIT
Serves 1

INGREDIENTS

1 6- or 8-ounce container nonfat, low-fat, or light yogurt with fruit (choose your favorite flavor)
½ cup high-fiber cereal
½ cup fresh fruit (strawberries, blueberries, raspberries, bananas, peaches)

DIRECTIONS

Layer yogurt, cereal, and fruit in a fancy glass and serve for breakfast, a snack, a light meal, or dessert.

NUTRITION ANALYSIS PER SERVING
Varies depending on brand of yogurt, cereal, and choice
of fruit. This analysis is based on 6 ounces of nonfat
light yogurt: 162 Calories; 1 g Fat; trace Saturated fat;
10 g Protein; 34 g Carbohydrate; 9 g Fiber;
2 mg Cholesterol; 146 mg Sodium.

CHEF'S NOTES

You may also use plain yogurt and sweeten with honey to taste.

DOCTOR'S NOTES

Use whole grain or bran cereal to boost nutrition. You may want to add wheat germ, flax seed, or nuts to make your parfait extra nutrient dense.

FAMILY NOTES

Set up a "parfait bar" with several flavors of yogurt, different types of fruit, and crunchy toppings like cereal, seeds, and nuts.

RUSTIC GRILLED PIZZA PARTY
MENU
WHOLE-WHEAT PIZZA CRUST
ROASTED ROMA TOMATO SAUCE
BASIL PESTO
ASSORTMENT OF TOPPINGS
ANTIPASTI SALAD WITH ITALIAN DRESSING
CINNAMON APPLE PACKETS

Grilling pizzas is a fun, hands-on meal activity to enjoy with your family and friends. Prepare our homemade Whole-Wheat Pizza Crust (or buy pizza dough) and have everyone shape their own unique crusts and go wild with original combinations from a selection of interesting and healthful toppings. We like to give our creations fancy names and slice them up for everyone to try. Serve with Antipasti Salad and finish with Cinnamon Apple Packets. Follow the meal with game night.

RUSTIC GRILLED PIZZA
Serves 6

INGREDIENTS
Pizza dough (one recipe of Whole-wheat Pizza Crust or store bought)
Tomato sauce (one recipe of Roasted Roma Tomato Sauce or store bought)
Pesto (one recipe of Basil Pesto or store bought)

Assortment of Toppings:
Artichoke hearts
Basil leaves (fresh or dried)
Broccoli (lightly steam and pat dry)
Canadian bacon
Cheese (mozzarella, goat, feta, parmesan)
Chicken (precooked and thinly sliced)
Faux pepperoni or sausage
Garlic, fresh or roasted
Ham
Jalapeños
Mushrooms (portobello, button, fresh, or canned, thinly sliced)
Olives (black, green, Mediterranean)
Olive oil
Onions (yellow, red, white, or green; fresh or caramelized)
Pepperoni
Peppers (fresh or roasted)
Pineapple chunks
Peperoncini, sliced
Sausage (precooked crumbles)
Tomato sauce (jarred or Roasted Roma Tomato Sauce)
Tomatoes (fresh, roasted, or sun-dried)

DIRECTIONS

1. Prepare dough ahead of time and divide into individual portions.
2. Set out an assortment of toppings from the list (or divide the ingredient list up and ask your guests to bring them).
3. Allow each guest to prepare their own crust and select their favorite toppings.
4. Have guests name their creations.
5. Share each other's creations—or not!

DOCTOR'S NOTES

Nutritional analysis will vary by topping; for the healthiest pizzas, use loads of veggies but meat and cheese in moderation.

WHOLE-WHEAT PIZZA CRUST
Serves 6

INGREDIENTS

1½ cups warm water, divided
1 envelope dry yeast
2 tablespoons sugar
1½ teaspoons salt
2 tablespoons olive oil
4 cups whole-wheat flour (may substitute white flour but fiber content will be lower)

DIRECTIONS

1. Combine the yeast with ½ cup of warm water and the sugar in a small bowl or measuring cup. Let stand for about 10–15 minutes to ferment.
2. Using your hands, combine the remaining ingredients in a large bowl. Add the dissolved yeast.
3. Turn the mixture out onto a well–flour-dusted surface and begin to knead.
4. Take the heel of your hand and push down on the dough to flatten it out.
5. Fold the dough in half, then half again, and repeat steps 4 and 5 for 5–8 minutes.
6. Once the kneading is done, roll the dough into a ball, coat with oil, and place in a bowl. Cover and allow dough to rise to about twice its original size (about 1 hour).
7. If you want to use the dough the following day, place the dough in the refrigerator instead of allowing it to rise. When ready to use, follow step 6.
8. Once the dough has risen, divide it into six parts. Flatten it into pizza shapes (round or more rustic ovals). Brush one side with olive oil and place on a heated grill oil side down and cook 3–5 minutes until that side is brown.
9. Remove from the grill and brush the uncooked side with olive oil. Turn it over and place your favorite toppings on the grilled side. Place pizza back on the grill, uncooked crust side down. Cover and cook for 3–5 minutes until crust is brown and toppings are heated through.

NUTRITION ANALYSIS PER SERVING OF DOUGH
331 Calories; 6 g Fat; 1 g Saturated fat;
11 g Protein; 63 g Carbohydrate; 10 g Fiber;
0 mg Cholesterol; 539 mg Sodium.

ROASTED ROMA TOMATO SAUCE
Serves 6

INGREDIENTS

10 fresh Roma tomatoes
1 teaspoon dried oregano
1 teaspoon dried basil
Salt and pepper to taste

DIRECTIONS

1. Preheat oven to 400 degrees.
2. Slice tomatoes in half and place on a cookie sheet and bake about 1 hour or until starting to brown.
3. Blend all the ingredients together in a blender or handheld mixer until smooth.
4. Use as pizza sauce or as a simple flavorful pasta sauce.

NUTRITION ANALYSIS PER SERVING OF SAUCE
46 Calories; 1 g Fat; 0 g Saturated fat; 2 g Protein;
10 g Carbohydrate; 2 g Fiber; 0 mg Cholesterol;
19 mg Sodium.

CHEF'S NOTES

Cold temperatures damage tomatoes, so never buy tomatoes that are stored in a cold area. Depending on the variety, ripe tomatoes should be completely red or reddish-orange. Store tomatoes at room temperature (above 55 degrees) out of direct sunlight until they are fully ripened. This allows them to develop nice flavor and aroma. If you must store them for a longer period of time, place them in the refrigerator. Chopped tomatoes can be frozen for use in sauces or other cooked dishes.

DOCTOR'S NOTES

Tomatoes contain large amounts of an antioxidant called lycopene that is released during cooling. Several studies suggest that eating foods rich in lycopene is associated with a lower risk of prostate cancer and cardiovascular disease.

BASIL PESTO
Serves 6

INGREDIENTS

1 cup fresh basil leaves
2 tablespoons olive oil
1 tablespoon Parmesan cheese
1 clove garlic
¼ teaspoon salt

DIRECTIONS

1. Combine all ingredients in a blender and mix until smooth.
2. Chill until ready to use.

CHEF'S NOTES

Pesto is so versatile that you may want to keep a container of it in your refrigerator. To store, place plastic wrap directly on the surface of the pesto or it will turn dark brown. You can also put 1- or 2-tablespoon portions in ice cube trays and freeze. Store the frozen cubes of pesto in an airtight bag in your freezer and use as needed.

NUTRITION ANALYSIS PER SERVING
45 Calories; 5 g Fat; 1 g Saturated fat; trace Protein; trace Carbohydrate; trace Fiber; 1 mg Cholesterol; 96 mg Sodium.

DOCTOR'S NOTES

Basil Pesto is great on pasta, paninis, bruschetta, pizzas, grilled fish, or chicken, as well as in dressings. Blend in walnuts for an additional dose of healthy fats.

FAMILY NOTES

To make an easy pesto pasta dish, prepare your favorite pasta according to package directions. Toss with pesto, chopped walnuts, and sautéed peppers, onions, and fresh spinach leaves.

ANTIPASTI SALAD

Provide a large bowl of salad greens and Italian (regular or light) dressing. While the pizzas are cooking, have people assemble their own Antipasti Salad using leftover pizza toppings. Alternatively, you can make the salad ahead of time with salad greens, artichoke hearts, tomatoes, cucumbers, red onions, olives, and shredded mozzarella.

INGREDIENTS FOR ITALIAN DRESSING

Makes 12 servings
¼ cup red wine vinegar
⅛ teaspoon black pepper
¼ teaspoon thyme
¼ teaspoon basil
¼ teaspoon oregano
1 small clove of garlic, minced
½ teaspoon kosher salt
½ cup extra virgin olive oil

DIRECTIONS

1. Place all dressing ingredients except olive oil in a blender and blend for 10 seconds.
2. Add olive oil to blender in a slow stream until emulsified.
3. Provide a large bowl of salad greens and while the pizzas are cooking have guests assemble their own Antipasti salad using leftover pizza toppings.

CHEF'S NOTES

Use extra virgin olive oil for salads. It's from the first pressing of the olives so the flavor is noticeably better when you're using it in uncooked foods.

NUTRITION ANALYSIS PER TABLESPOON
81 Calories; 9 g Fat; 0 g Saturated fat; trace Protein; trace Carbohydrate; trace Fiber; 0 mg Cholesterol; 80 mg Sodium.

CINNAMON APPLE PACKETS
Serves 6

INGREDIENTS
6 small apples, sliced
6 teaspoons brown sugar
1½ teaspoons cinnamon

DIRECTIONS
1. Preheat grill or oven to 400 degrees.
2. Combine the fruit, brown sugar, and cinnamon in a small bowl.
3. Tear off six 12" × 12" squares of heavy-duty foil and spray with nonstick cooking spray.
4. Divide the fruit mixture evenly among the six foil squares.
5. Fold edges of the foil over or gather and twist foil tightly.
6. Place on rack and cook for about 20 minutes until apples are tender.
7. Serve warm.

NUTRITION ANALYSIS PER SERVING
94 Calories; 1 g Fat; trace Saturated fat; trace Protein; 24 g Carbohydrate; 4 g Fiber; 0 mg Cholesterol; 1 mg Sodium.

CHEF'S NOTES
This easy recipe is also great with peaches, nectarines, blueberries, pears, or bananas—whatever's in season. Cut the fruit ahead of time and allow the kids to prepare the mixture and make the foil packets. When slicing apples or pears, dip the slices into lemon-water to keep them from turning brown. Drain and pat dry before using.

DOCTOR'S NOTES
This is a great way to satisfy your sweet tooth and get more fresh fruit into your diet. You can also add oats and walnuts or pecans for a heartier dessert or snack.

FAMILY NOTES
These packets are perfect for barbeques and camping. Just put them on a rack over hot coals then eat right out of the packet.

FIESTA NIGHT

MENU

VALLE LUNA CHICKEN FAJITAS

UN-REFRIED BEANS

SALSA FRESCA

GUACAMOLE

BAKED TORTILLA CHIPS

The recipe for fajitas was developed by Tia Rita, my grandmother, and is a favorite at my parents' Valle Luna Mexican restaurants in Phoenix, Arizona.

VALLE LUNA CHICKEN FAJITAS

Serves 4

INGREDIENTS

½ cup unsweetened pineapple juice

1 tablespoon garlic powder

1 tablespoon red pepper flakes

2 tablespoons low-sodium soy sauce

1 pound boneless, skinless chicken breasts

½ red bell pepper

½ green bell pepper

½ onion

8 6-inch corn tortillas

DIRECTIONS

1. Prepare the marinade by mixing the first four ingredients in a nonmetallic bowl.
2. Cut chicken lengthwise into ½-inch strips.
3. Place the chicken in the marinade and cover. Marinate in the refrigerator for at least 8 hours or overnight. Drain the chicken to remove the marinade.
4. Cut peppers and onion into ¼-inch slices.
5. Spray a nonstick frying pan with cooking spray and sauté the chicken, bell peppers, and onion until cooked, approximately 8 minutes.
6. Heat the stack of corn tortillas for 1 minute in the microwave.
7. Spread each tortilla with 2 tablespoons of Un-Refried Beans. Top with chicken and veggies, Salsa Fresca, shredded lettuce, diced tomatoes, and Guacamole, then fold or wrap tortilla around the filling.

NUTRITION ANALYSIS PER TWO-FAJITA SERVING
288 Calories; 4 g Fat; 1 g Saturated fat;
29 g Protein; 33 g Carbohydrate; 4 g Fiber;
69 mg Cholesterol; 443 mg Sodium.

CHEF'S NOTES
This recipe is also great with veggies, lean beef, pork, or shrimp.

DOCTOR'S NOTES
Although people think of Mexican food as "fattening," it's very healthy when you emphasize beans, poultry, lean meats, fish, fresh vegetables, and whole grains, and use higher-fat ingredients in moderation.

UN-REFRIED BEANS
Serves 4

INGREDIENTS
1 15-ounce can pinto beans
Optional ingredients: lime juice, salsa, green chilis, jalapeños

DIRECTIONS
1. Drain pinto beans, reserving liquid.
2. Mash the beans with the back of a fork, adding liquid as needed to get a smooth consistency.
3. Heat in a sauce pan and season as desired with lime juice, salsa, green chilis, or jalapeños.

NUTRITION ANALYSIS PER SERVING
83 Calories; trace Fat; 0 g Saturated fat;
5 g Protein; 15 g Carbohydrate; 4 g Dietary Fiber;
0 mg Cholesterol; 442 mg Sodium.

CHEF'S NOTES
Traditional refried beans are made by mashing cooked beans and refrying them with lard. In this easy recipe, the texture is almost identical; give them a boost of flavor using lime juice, salsa, and chilies.

DOCTOR'S NOTES
Beans are an excellent source of fiber, protein, vitamins, and minerals. Use dried beans and cook your own to reduce the sodium content.

FAMILY NOTES
Beans are an inexpensive source of protein; use these in burritos and taco salads too.

SALSA FRESCA
Serves 4

INGREDIENTS
2 cups tomatoes, diced
¼ cup onion, diced
2 tablespoons cilantro, chopped
½ jalapeño, finely diced
1 clove garlic, minced
1 tablespoon lime juice
½ teaspoon salt

DIRECTIONS
Combine all ingredients and refrigerate for 2 hours, if possible, to blend flavors.

NUTRITION ANALYSIS PER SERVING
27 Calories; trace Fat; 0 g Saturated fat;
1 g Protein; 6 g Carbohydrate; 1 g Fiber;
0 mg Cholesterol; 277 mg Sodium.

CHEF'S NOTES
Jalapeños vary in heat intensity. The seeds and white pith are the hottest parts, so adjust according to your preference.

DOCTOR'S NOTES
Salsa is full of healthful ingredients and makes a flavorful condiment in place of higher-fat dips and sauces. Try it with Baked Tortilla Chips.

FAMILY NOTES
Somehow salsa just doesn't seem like vegetables!

GUACAMOLE
Serves 4

INGREDIENTS
1 ripe avocado, diced
1 tablespoon lime juice
½ cup fresh salsa

DIRECTIONS
1. Mash the avocado with the back of a fork.
2. Sprinkle avocado with lime juice to prevent browning.
3. Stir in salsa.
4. Chill until ready to serve.

NUTRITION ANALYSIS PER SERVING
108 Calories; 8 g Fat; 1 g Saturated fat; 2 g Protein; 10 g Carbohydrate; 3 g Fiber; 0 mg Cholesterol; 310 mg Sodium.

CHEF'S NOTES
To cut an avocado, cut it in half lengthwise around the pit, being careful to keep the knife away from your fingers. Twist the two halves in opposite directions to separate. Hold one half in the palm of your hand and tap the pit with a knife, twist, and lift out. Scoop out flesh with a spoon. Before scooping it out, you can make lengthwise cuts for slices or crisscross cuts for cubes.

DOCTOR'S NOTES
Avocados are high in fat—the healthy kind. Use avocados or guacamole in place of other condiments like dips, mayonnaise, and butter that are high in less-healthy fats.

BAKED TORTILLA CHIPS
Serves 4

INGREDIENTS
8 6-inch corn tortillas
2 teaspoons fresh lime juice (optional)
1 teaspoon chili powder (optional)
Vegetable spray
1 teaspoon salt (optional)

DIRECTIONS
Cut each tortilla into 8 wedges and arrange in a single layer on a cookie sheet. Sprinkle with lime juice and chili powder if desired. Spray lightly with vegetable spray and sprinkle with salt. Bake at 350°F until crisp and golden brown, approximately 6–9 minutes. Watch closely so they don't burn!

NUTRITION ANALYSIS
114 Calories; 1 g Fat; trace Saturated fat;
3 g Protein; 24 g Carbohydrate; 3 g Dietary Fiber;
0 mg Cholesterol; 620 mg Sodium.

CHEF'S NOTES
Prepare crisp tortilla strips to garnish the Southwestern Stew (page 340). Cut a tortilla into thin strips instead of wedges and prepare as directed above.

DOCTORS NOTES
These chips are a great alternative to regular chips—but if you prefer regular, just eat them in moderation.

FAMILY NOTES
Use these chip for snacks, salads, and parties.

THE HEALTHY GRILL

MENU

GRILLED SALMON WITH MANGO SALSA
SPINACH SALAD WITH ORANGES
CONFETTI QUINOA
TOASTED ANGEL FOOD CAKE WITH STRAWBERRIES

This colorful summer dinner emphasizes fresh, nutrient-rich ingredients. We serve this meal with chilled Chardonnay.

GRILLED SALMON WITH MANGO SALSA

Serves 4

INGREDIENTS

Salmon
16 ounces salmon fillets
1 teaspoon olive oil
1 teaspoon kosher salt
⅛ teaspoon black pepper

Mango Salsa Ingredients:
½ batch Salsa Fresca (see page 328)
½ mango, diced (see Chef's Notes)

DIRECTIONS

1. Pat salmon dry.
2. Rub with olive oil then season with salt and pepper.
3. Place on hot grill skin side up. Grill about 3 minutes then turn over and grill for about 3 minutes longer.
4. Add one diced mango to fresh salsa.
5. Divide the salmon into four portions; spoon the Mango Salsa over and serve.

CHEF'S NOTES

The easiest way to dice a mango is to slice it lengthwise on either side, close to the large thin pit. Then with the flesh side up, make diagonal cuts both directions, forming a crisscross pattern. Turn the mango half inside out (it will look like a hedgehog). Slice the precut pieces off the skin and add to the salsa.

DOCTOR'S NOTES

Salmon is a wonderful source of important omega-3 fatty acids.

NUTRITION ANALYSIS PER SERVING
172 Calories; 5 g Fat; 1 g Saturated fat; 24 g Protein;
7 g Carbohydrate; 1 g Fiber; 59 mg Cholesterol;
709 mg Sodium.

CONFETTI QUINOA
Serves 4

INGREDIENTS
½ red bell pepper, diced
½ yellow pepper, diced
½ cucumber, diced
½ red onion, diced
1 cup quinoa, cooked as directed
2 tablespoons low sodium soy sauce
1 tablespoon white wine vinegar
3 tablespoons balsamic vinegar

DIRECTIONS
1. Dice the peppers and onion.
2. Peel, cut in half, and remove the seeds from the cucumber, then dice.
3. Cook the quinoa according to the package directions and cool. To cool faster, spread it on a cookie sheet and place it in the refrigerator.
4. Add peppers, cucumber, and onion and gently toss together.
5. Add the soy sauce and vinegars and mix together.

NUTRITION ANALYSIS PER SERVING
189 Calories; 3 g Fat; trace Saturated fat; 7 g Protein; 36 g Carbohydrate; 4 g Fiber; 0 mg Cholesterol; 331 mg Sodium.

CHEF'S NOTES
Make this a main dish by adding feta cheese or tofu.

DOCTOR'S NOTES
Quinoa is one of the few plant sources of complete protein (soybeans are another). It's an interesting grain that can be prepared many different ways.

FAMILY NOTES
As in this recipe for quinoa, adding fresh vegetables to rice, pasta, or other grains maximizes the flavor, texture, color, and nutrients in your dish.

SPINACH SALAD WITH ORANGES
Serves 4

INGREDIENTS

Salad
1 12-ounce bag prewashed spinach
1 medium orange, peeled and chopped
¼ red onion, thinly sliced
1 small can sliced water chestnuts

Dressing
2 tablespoons canola oil
2 tablespoons ketchup
2 tablespoons apple cider vinegar
2 tablespoons Worcestershire sauce
4 tablespoons orange juice
1 tsp of sugar
1 clove garlic, minced

DIRECTIONS
1. Combine dressing ingredients and chill for 1 hour.
2. Toss salad ingredients together in a large salad bowl and drizzle with dressing.

NUTRITION ANALYSIS PER SERVING
121 Calories; 7 g Fat; trace Saturated fat; 3 g Protein; 14 g Carbohydrate; 3 g Fiber; 0 mg Cholesterol; 212 mg Sodium.

DOCTOR'S NOTES
Spinach is another super food, packed with nutrients, phytochemicals, and fiber.

TOASTED ANGEL FOOD CAKE WITH STRAWBERRIES
Serves 4

INGREDIENTS

½ of a store-bought angel food cake (10 inch diameter), cut into eight slices

1 pint fresh strawberries, washed and hulled

4 tablespoons whipped cream (light or regular)

DIRECTIONS

1. Slice the strawberries and place in a bowl in the refrigerator until ready to use. Sweeten with a small amount of sugar or nonnutritive sweetener if needed.
2. Grill the slices of angel food cake over low heat for approximately 30 seconds on each side (until golden brown with light grill marks).
3. Lay one piece of toasted angel food cake on a dessert plate. Lay a second piece so that it is overlapping slightly.
4. Spoon sliced strawberries over the top and top with a spoonful of whipped cream.

CHEF'S NOTES

Grilling the angel food cake makes it crispier so it doesn't get soggy when you put fruit on top.

DOCTOR'S NOTES

Angel food cake is low in fat and calories. Grilling brings out the sweetness; adding fruit is just "icing on the cake."

NUTRITION ANALYSIS PER SERVING
239 Calories; 3 g Fat; 1 g Saturated fat; 5 g Protein; 49 g Carbohydrate; 2 g Fiber; 10 mg Cholesterol; 383 mg Sodium.

FAMILY NIGHT PASTA

MENU

WHOLE-WHEAT PASTA WITH CHERRY TOMATOES
GREEK SALAD
CHOCOLATE CHIP CLOUD COOKIES

My daughter, Elyse, became a vegetarian when she was twelve. She started a cookbook for a class project and eventually published Veggie Teens: A Cookbook and Guide for Vegetarian Teenagers. *These recipes are from* Veggie Teens *(www.VeggieTeensCookbook.com).*

WHOLE-WHEAT PASTA WITH CHERRY TOMATOES
Serves 4

INGREDIENTS

8 ounces whole-wheat pasta (any shape)
1 pint cherry tomatoes, halved (or two medium tomatoes chopped)
2 cloves garlic, minced
2 tablespoons extra virgin olive oil
1 tablespoon balsamic vinegar
6 fresh basil leaves, cut into thin strips
½ teaspoon each, salt and pepper

DIRECTIONS

1. Prepare pasta according to package directions.
2. While the pasta is cooking, sauté tomatoes in 1 tablespoon of the olive oil for 2–3 minutes. Add minced garlic and sauté for about a minute.
3. Drain pasta and return it to the pot.
4. Toss with tomatoes, remaining tablespoon of olive oil, vinegar, and basil.
5. Add the salt and fresh ground pepper or red pepper flakes to taste.

NUTRITION ANALYSIS PER SERVING
276 Calories; 8 g Fat; 1 g Saturated fat; 9 g Protein; 47 g Carbohydrate; 6 g Fiber; 0 mg Cholesterol; 307 mg Sodium.

CHEF'S NOTES

An easy way to cut basil into thin strips is to stack several basil leaves, roll them tightly, and cut into ¼ inch slices. Separate leaves into strips.

DOCTOR'S NOTES

The whole wheat pasta, tomatoes, and monounsaturated olive oil make this a great dish for even the most health-conscious diner.

FAMILY NOTES

Elyse is the only vegetarian in our family; the rest of us love this dish with grilled chicken or salmon.

GREEK SALAD
Serves 4

INGREDIENTS

Salad
2 heads romaine lettuce, chopped
1 cucumber, diced
1 cup grape tomatoes
¼ large red onion, thinly sliced
¼ cup Greek olives
¼ cup feta cheese crumbles

Greek Feta Dressing
1 tablespoon light mayonnaise
1 tablespoon light sour cream
1 tablespoon plain low-fat yogurt
1 teaspoon red wine vinegar
1 tablespoon olive oil
1 tablespoon water
½ teaspoon lemon juice
1 tablespoon feta cheese

DIRECTIONS

1. Place all dressing ingredients except feta cheese into a bowl and blend together with a whisk.
2. Lightly blend in the feta cheese.
3. Toss salad ingredients together and drizzle with Greek Feta Dressing.

NUTRITION ANALYSIS
188 Calories; 12 g Fat; 3 g Saturated fat; 9 g Protein; 17 g Carbohydrate; 8 g Fiber; 12 mg Cholesterol; 281 mg Sodium.

FAMILY NOTES

For a main dish salad, add sliced grilled chicken and serve with pita bread and Red Pepper Hummus. (See page 348)

CHOCOLATE CHIP CLOUD COOKIES

INGREDIENTS
2 egg whites
⅛ teaspoon cream of tartar
½ cup superfine sugar (not powdered)
1 teaspoon vanilla extract
½ cup miniature semisweet chocolate chips (we used the kind with no milk or milk fat)

DIRECTIONS
1. Preheat oven to 275 degrees.
2. Line two cookie sheets with foil and spray with nonstick cooking spray.
3. In a very clean bowl (free of all oil and grease), beat egg whites and cream of tartar on medium speed with a mixer until soft peaks form.
4. Turn mixer to high and gradually beat in sugar until glossy, stiff peaks form.
5. Beat in vanilla. Gently fold in chocolate chips.
6. Drop by teaspoonfuls onto cookie sheets.
7. Bake for 25 minutes at 275 degrees, then reduce heat to 250 degrees and bake for 25 minutes longer. Cookies should be white or just slightly golden.
8. Remove cookies to a rack and cool completely. Store in an airtight container.

NUTRITION ANALYSIS PER COOKIE
23 Calories; 1 g Fat; 1 g Saturated fat; trace Protein; 4 g Carbohydrate; trace Fiber; 0 mg Cholesterol; 4 mg Sodium.

CHEF'S NOTES

When making meringue, any oil, grease, or fat (including egg yolk) will prevent peaks from forming when the egg whites are beaten. Use a very clean bowl and beaters. If any egg yolk gets into the whites, you must discard. For this reason, it is best to separate each egg into a separate bowl. Be careful when working with raw eggs; keep surfaces clean and wash your hands frequently.

DOCTOR'S NOTES

Make ahead and store in an airtight container; two or three of these sweet but light, crispy cookies are a real treat.

FAMILY NOTES

Use miniature chocolate chips or finely chopped regular-sized chocolate chips so they aren't too heavy. You can also experiment with other flavorings and add-ins: peppermint extract and chopped candy canes or almond extract with sliced almonds. These "cloud cookies" are also great to serve or give away during the holidays.

ORIENT EXPRESS
MENU

LETTUCE WRAPS
ORIENTAL NOODLE SALAD
FRUIT KABOBS WITH GINGER YOGURT DIP

Get dinner on the table fast by making the Oriental Noodle Salad the night before. It's better cold anyway.

LETTUCE WRAPS
Serves 4

INGREDIENTS

1 pound ground beef, extra lean
2 tablespoons Hoisin sauce
2 tablespoons peanut butter
1 cucumber, cut in matchstick-sized pieces
2 carrots, cut in matchstick-sized pieces
2 tablespoons mint leaves
8 Boston lettuce leaves

DIRECTIONS

1. Brown ground beef in large nonstick skillet over medium heat 8 to 10 minutes or until beef is no longer pink, breaking up into small crumbles. Drain thoroughly.
2. Stir in Hoisin sauce and peanut butter then heat through. Add cucumber, carrots, and torn mint; toss gently. Serve beef mixture in lettuce leaves. Garnish with mint leaves.

CHEF'S NOTES

This recipe is also good with ground turkey or finely chopped chicken. For a vegetarian version, use a soy-based ground beef substitute.

DOCTOR'S NOTES

Use the leanest ground beef available. Drain thoroughly. You can also rinse excess oil off by placing it in a colander and running very hot water over it.

FAMILY NOTES

Lettuce Wraps are a great example of an appetizer that works well as a light main meal. Keep bottled sauces like Hoisin on hand to make quick versions of your favorite ethnic foods.

NUTRITION ANALYSIS PER SERVING
351 Calories; 24 g Fat; 9 g Saturated fat;
24 g Protein; 9 g Carbohydrate; 2 g Dietary Fiber;
79 mg Cholesterol; 250 mg Sodium.

ORIENTAL NOODLE SALAD
Serves 4

INGREDIENTS

4 ounces whole-wheat spaghetti, cooked according to package directions

1 tablespoon low-sodium soy sauce

2 teaspoons rice vinegar

2 teaspoons lime juice

1 teaspoon sesame oil

1 teaspoon canola oil

½ teaspoon sriracha hot sauce (or other chili sauce to taste), optional

1 teaspoon fresh ginger, grated

½ red pepper, thinly sliced

2 green onions, white and green parts, thinly sliced

½ cup red cabbage, thinly sliced

2 teaspoons toasted sesame seeds

DIRECTIONS

1. While the pasta is cooking, combine the dressing ingredients (soy sauce, rice wine vinegar, lime juice, oil, hot sauce, and ginger).

2. Rinse the pasta in cold water.

3. Toss pasta with dressing, red pepper, onions, and cabbage.

4. Toast the sesame seeds in a dry pan until golden brown (watch carefully!) then sprinkle over the salad.

5. If possible, chill salad for at least an hour before serving.

NUTRITION ANALYSIS PER SERVING

135 Calories; 3 g Fat; trace Saturated fat; 5 g Protein; 23 g Carbohydrate; 3 g Fiber; 0 mg Cholesterol; 156 mg Sodium

FRUIT KABOBS WITH GINGER YOGURT DIP
Serves 4

INGREDIENTS
1 cup nonfat yogurt
2 tablespoons of honey
⅛ teaspoon ground ginger
½ cup each cantaloupe, honeydew, pineapple, and banana, cut into bite sized pieces

DIRECTIONS
1. To make Ginger Yogurt Dip, stir first three ingredients together; chill or serve immediately.
2. Cut fruit into bite-sized chunks.
3. Thread fruit onto toothpicks or wooden skewers.
4. Serve with Ginger Yogurt Dip.

NUTRITION ANALYSIS PER TABLESPOON
115 Calories; trace Fat; 0 g Saturated fat; 4 g Protein; 26 g Carbohydrate; 1 g fiber; 1 mg Cholesterol; 48 mg Sodium.

CHEF'S NOTES
To cut honeydew, cantaloupe, and pineapple, cut about one inch off each end and stand melon up. Cut thick outside skin off by slicing downward in strips. Cut in quarters. Melons: scoop out the seeds. Pineapple: cut out the tough core. Cut into chunks.

DOCTOR'S NOTES
Buy fruit in season for optimal nutrient content and flavor. Try apples, berries, grapes, kiwi fruit, nectarines, oranges, or peaches.

FAMILY NOTES
For variety, make a melon basket instead of skewers. Cut two wedges out of the top of a seedless watermelon, leaving a one inch "handle." Scoop out flesh using a melon-baller or small ice cream scoop—just press the scoop deep into the flesh then twist your wrist to cut all the way around. (Use the leftover "scraps" of watermelon to make Watermelon Ice on page 356). In a separate bowl, combine melon balls and your other choice of fruit then return to basket.

ONE POT SOUTHWESTERN STEW
MENU
SOUTHWESTERN STEW

This one-pot meal is a family favorite because it's easy to put together in just a few minutes from ingredients we usually have in our pantry.

SOUTHWESTERN STEW
Serves 6

INGREDIENTS
1 medium onion, diced
1 medium zucchini, diced
1 medium yellow squash, diced
1½ cups of water
1 16-ounce can beans, drained and rinsed (pinto, black, or kidney beans all work well)
1 16-ounce can corn, low sodium
½ teaspoon ground cumin
2 teaspoons chili powder
1 teaspoon garlic powder
1 16-ounce jar chunky salsa (mild, medium, or hot)
½ cup uncooked instant brown rice

DIRECTIONS
1. Spray the bottom of a large pot with nonstick cooking spray and sauté the onion until it is translucent.
2. Add zucchini and yellow squash and sauté until tender-crisp.
3. Add remaining ingredients and stir.
4. Bring mixture to a boil over medium high heat.
5. Reduce heat to simmer and cook for 15 minutes. Add water as needed.

NUTRITION ANALYSIS PER SERVING
326 Calories; 2 g Fat; trace Saturated fat; 19 g Protein; 63 g Carbohydrate; 22 g Fiber; 0 mg Cholesterol; 367 mg Sodium.

CHEF'S NOTES
For tortilla soup, add 6 cups vegetable, chicken, or beef broth. While soup is cooking, cut 2 corn tortillas into thin strips, toss with 1 tablespoon of lime juice, and sprinkle with chili powder. Place them on a cookie sheet sprayed with nonstick spray and bake at 350 degrees until golden; watch carefully so they don't burn. Spoon soup into bowls then garnish with crisp tortilla strips. For a fancier presentation, put sprigs of cilantro, diced avocado, or a thin slice of lime on top before serving.

DOCTOR'S NOTES
This hearty stew is a quick meal, loaded with fiber. Together, beans and rice have all of the essential amino acids.

FAMILY NOTES
Add browned ground beef or leftover shredded or cubed chicken, turkey, beef, or pork.

LIGHT DINNER BY THE FIRE

MENU

HARVEST VEGETABLE SOUP
OR CHICKEN AND RICE SOUP
WHOLE GRAIN ROLLS
BLUEBERRY PEACH ALMOND CRISP

SIMPLE SOUP BASE

Makes 12 cups of chicken stock or 18 cups of turkey stock

INGREDIENTS

1 leftover chicken carcass (or use
a turkey carcass and double the
following ingredients)
1 onion, quartered
2 carrots, quartered
2 stalks celery, quartered (leaves
removed)
1 bay leaf
Several sprigs fresh herbs, such as
parsley and thyme
Water to cover

DIRECTIONS

1. Place the carcass into a large
stockpot and cover with water
(approximately 14 cups for chicken
and 20 cups for turkey).
2. Place on high heat and bring to a
boil. Reduce heat to medium low
and simmer uncovered for 4 hours.
3. Remove from heat and strain broth
into another pot by pouring it
through cheesecloth or a colander.
4. Refrigerate overnight if possible
then skim off solid fat from the top
and discard.
5. Use within 2 to 3 days or freeze in
6-cup portions.

NUTRITION ANALYSIS PER SERVING
10 Calories; 3 g Fat; 1.5 g Saturated fat; 0 g Protein;
0 g Carbohydrate; 0 g Fiber; 0 mg Cholesterol;
17 mg Sodium.

CHEF'S NOTES

Fresh herbs are best, but dried will do
in a pinch. Dried herbs have a much
stronger flavor, so use about half as
much. In this recipe, use ½ teaspoon
each of parsley and thyme.

DOCTOR'S NOTES

For vegetable broth, leave out the
carcass. Double the amount of
vegetables and sauté them in a
nonstick pan first to boost the flavor.
Cover with 12 cups of water and follow
remainder of directions.

FAMILY NOTES

Homemade soup base is easy and
economical. If you don't have time,
substitute canned or packaged low-
sodium broth in the soup recipes.

HARVEST VEGETABLE SOUP
Serves 4

INGREDIENTS
6 cups broth
1 cup cherry tomatoes, whole
1 cup cabbage, chopped
½ red onion, diced
2 stalks celery, diced
½ pound broccoli florets
¾ cup baby carrots
¾ cup frozen corn kernels
¾ cup frozen peas
¼ teaspoon marjoram (or substitute parsley)
⅛ teaspoon cayenne pepper
¼ teaspoon pepper
1 teaspoon salt

DIRECTIONS
1. Sauté onions, carrots, and celery until soft and fragrant.
2. Add the chicken broth, broccoli, tomatoes, marjoram, and cayenne. Bring to a boil then simmer for 15 minutes
3. Add cabbage, corn, and peas and simmer for 15 minutes more.
4. Season with salt and pepper.

NUTRITION ANALYSIS PER SERVING
146 Calories; 3 g Fat; trace Saturated fat;
11 g Protein; 21 g Carbohydrate; 6 g Fiber;
0 mg Cholesterol; 587 mg Sodium.

CHEF'S NOTES
For a thick chunky vegetable soup, use a slotted spoon to remove 2 cups of vegetables and set aside. Blend remaining ingredients with a hand blender. If you use a regular blender, blend 1 cup of soup at a time to prevent steam from building up in the blender and causing injury. Stir reserved vegetables into blended soup.

DOCTOR'S NOTES
This Harvest Vegetable Soup is nutrient rich, so it's a satisfying way to boost your fluid, veggie, and fiber intake without a lot of calories. Substitute other fresh, frozen, or canned vegetables such as parsley, green beans, cauliflower, zucchini, or spinach leaves.

FAMILY NOTES
When our kids were little we played a game of Guess the Colors; they closed their eyes and took a bite of soup or other veggie-packed food and tried to guess what colors were in their mouth. They enjoyed the game too much to notice that the most colorful foods were vegetables.

CHICKEN AND RICE SOUP
Serves 4

INGREDIENTS
6 cups broth
2 stalks celery, thinly sliced
1 medium carrot, diced
1 medium onion, diced
2 tablespoons parsley, chopped
1 bay leaf
2 cups cooked diced chicken (or 2 cups diced raw chicken breast, but increase cooking time by 15 minutes)
1 cup cooked brown rice (or substitute ½ cup uncooked instant brown rice and ¾ cup of water for the cooked rice)

DIRECTIONS
1. Bring broth, celery, carrot, onion, parsley, and bay leaf to a boil in a large pot.
2. Reduce heat to simmer and add 2 cups of cooked diced chicken and 1 cup of cooked brown rice.
3. Simmer for 15 minutes.

NUTRITION ANALYSIS PER SERVING
281 Calories; 4 g Fat; 1 g Saturated fat; 32 g Protein; 27g Carbohydrate; 2 g Dietary Fiber; 55 mg Cholesterol; 93 mg Sodium.

BLUEBERRY PEACH ALMOND CRISP
Serves 4

INGREDIENTS

Almond Topping:
⅓ cup all-purpose flour
¼ cup packed brown sugar
¼ teaspoon salt
2 tablespoons chilled butter, cut into chunks
⅓ cup oats
3 tablespoons sliced almonds

Blueberry Peach Filling:
2 cups ripe peaches, chopped
2 cups fresh blueberries
2 tablespoons cornstarch
2 tablespoons packed brown sugar
¼ cup orange juice
1 teaspoon ginger

NUTRITION ANALYSIS PER SERVING
339 Calories; 11 g Fat; 4 g Saturated fat; 6 g Protein; 59 g Carbohydrate; 6 g Fiber; 16 mg Cholesterol; 218 mg Sodium.

DIRECTIONS
1. To prepare topping, put the flour, brown sugar, and salt into a medium bowl and stir with a fork. (Note: Topping can also be made by pulsing ingredients in a food processor.)
2. Add chilled butter and press into the mixture with the back of the fork until mixture is coarse.
3. Stir in oats and almonds.
4. Set aside.
5. To prepare filling, combine blueberries and peaches with the other filling ingredients.
6. Spoon into four ramekins or custard cups sprayed with cooking spray.
7. Sprinkle topping over the blueberry peach filling.
8. Bake at 350 degrees for 15 minutes. Serve warm.

MEDITERRANEAN SMALL BITES PARTY
MENU
TUSCAN WHITE BEANS WITH GARLIC
BRUSCHETTA WITH ROASTED GARLIC,
  ROMA TOMATOES, BASIL, AND MOZZARELLA
OLIVE TAPENADE
RED PEPPER HUMMUS
CRISP PITA TRIANGLES
MEDITERRANEAN VEGGIE PLATTER

These recipes make a flavorful, healthful party buffet. If serving wine at your party, offer both a white and a red, such as Pinot Grigio and Chianti from Italy.

TUSCAN WHITE BEANS WITH GARLIC
Serves 4

INGREDIENTS
1 tablespoon olive oil
1 cup onion, diced
⅛ teaspoon crushed red pepper
4 cloves garlic, minced
2 bay leaves
3 16-ounce cans white beans (navy, great northern, or cannelini)
1 tablespoon balsamic vinegar
Salt and pepper to taste

DIRECTIONS
1. Heat oil in large skillet and sauté onion until soft.
2. Add red pepper, garlic, and bay leaves and sauté 3 minutes.
3. Stir in beans (do not drain) and cook for at least 3 more minutes.
4. Stir in vinegar and add salt and pepper to taste.
5. Discard bay leaves and serve in decorative bowls.

NUTRITION ANALYSIS PER SERVING
282 Calories; 3 g Fat; trace Saturated fat; 18 g Protein; 48 g Carbohydrate; 16 g Fiber; 0 mg Cholesterol; 12 mg Sodium.

CHEF'S NOTES
Be careful not to burn the garlic or it will become bitter.

DOCTOR'S NOTES
Beans are really high in fiber and protein. Canned beans usually have a lot of sodium, but you can make your own from dried beans and significantly cut the amount of sodium in this recipe.

FAMILY NOTES
This may not sound like kid food, but you'll probably be surprised how much your family loves these flavorful beans.

BRUSCHETTA WITH ROASTED GARLIC, ROMA TOMATOES, BASIL, AND MOZZARELLA
Serves 8

INGREDIENTS
1 18-inch baguette cut into ¼ inch slices
1 bulb fresh garlic
2½ teaspoons olive oil (divided)
Bunch of fresh basil leaves
4 Roma tomatoes, sliced
8 ounces part-skim mozzarella, thinly sliced

DIRECTIONS
1. Using 2 teaspoons of the olive oil, brush or spray both sides of the bread (you can purchase spray bottles made for oil).
2. Bake at 350 degrees until golden brown. Turn and bake other side.
3. Cool completely and store in airtight container until ready to serve.
4. To make Roasted Garlic, slice the top off the bulb of garlic and place it on the center of a 12" × 12" square of foil.
5. Brush the top of the garlic with ½ teaspoon of olive oil.
6. Gather the foil around the garlic and twist tightly.
7. Bake on the grill or in the oven at 350 degrees until soft, about 20 minutes.
8. Untwist foil and spoon out the soft roasted garlic.
9. Spread roasted garlic on the crisp bread slices.
10. Top each slice with a basil leaf, a slice of mozzarella, and a slice of tomato.

CHEF'S NOTES
Roasted garlic is great in mashed potatoes, in pasta dishes, on grilled pizza, and in dips, and it is delicious spread on panini sandwiches and our Bruschetta.

DOCTOR'S NOTES
Garlic and tomatoes are super foods because they provides important phytochemicals. This snack or appetizer proves that it is possible to combine nutritious with delicious!

FAMILY NOTES
Set up a "Bruschetta bar" and let your family or friends make their own. Offer other toppings like Basil Pesto (page 330), Roasted Red Pepper Hummus (page 348), or chunky Salsa Fresca, well drained.

NUTRITION ANALYSIS PER SERVING
258 Calories; 8 g Fat; trace Saturated fat;
13 g Protein; 33 g Carbohydrate; 2 g Fiber;
15 mg Cholesterol; 500m g Sodium.

OLIVE TAPENADE
Serves 8

INGREDIENTS

⅓ cup Kalamata olives
⅓ cup Greek olives
⅓ cup black olives
2 artichoke hearts (canned, in water)
2 tablespoons capers
2 cloves garlic
2 tablespoons lemon juice

DOCTOR'S NOTES

Olives are rich in healthy monounsaturated fats. They are also relatively high in sodium and calories, so practice moderation.

DIRECTIONS

1. Drain olives and artichoke hearts.
2. Finely chop first six ingredients then combine with lemon juice, or place all ingredients into a food processor and blend until a coarse paste has formed.
3. Place into serving dish and refrigerate until needed.
4. Serve with thinly sliced French bread or our Bruschetta.

NUTRITION ANALYSIS PER SERVING
62 Calories; 6 g Fat; trace Saturated fat; trace Protein; 3 g Carbohydrate; trace Fiber; 0 mg Cholesterol; 303 mg Sodium.

RED PEPPER HUMMUS
Serves 8

INGREDIENTS

2 cans drained garbanzo beans (chickpeas)
1 clove garlic
2 tablespoons olive oil (or tahini paste)
1 teaspoon each lemon and lime juice
1 teaspoon balsamic vinegar
6 ounces roasted peppers, drained
½ teaspoon hot sauce
½ tsp kosher salt

DIRECTIONS

1. Drain and rinse the garbanzo beans and place all the ingredients into a food processor. Process until a coarse paste has formed.
2. Refrigerate until needed then serve with Crisp Pita Triangles.

NUTRITION ANALYSIS PER SERVING OF HUMMUS
108 Calories; 4 g Fat; 1 g Saturated fat; 3 g Protein; 15 g Carbohydrate; 3 g Fiber; 0 mg Cholesterol; 308 mg Sodium.

CHEF'S NOTES

You can make your own roasted peppers by cutting red peppers into quarters, spraying with olive oil then roasting in the oven or on a grill until soft. Peel the skin off the pepper while it is still warm. Hummus often contains tahini, which is sesame paste. You can substitute tahini for the olive oil if you'd like.

DOCTOR'S NOTES

Hummus with Crisp Pita Triangles is a healthy substitute for chips and dip—nobody will miss them!

CRISP PITA TRIANGLES
Serves 8

INGREDIENTS

4 6-inch whole-wheat pita pockets

Vegetable spray

1 teaspoon each paprika and parsley

NUTRITION ANALYSIS PER SERVING OF PITA
TRIANGLES

86 Calories; 1 g Fat; trace Saturated fat;
3 g Protein; 18 g Carbohydrate; 2 g Fiber;
0 mg Cholesterol; 170 mg Sodium.

DIRECTIONS

1. Open each pita pocket and separate the sides. Cut each of the 8 pita halves into 8 wedges and arrange in a single layer on a cookie sheet.
2. Spray lightly with vegetable spray and sprinkle with seasonings.
3. Bake at 350 degrees until crisp and golden brown (watch closely!).

MEDITERRANEAN VEGGIE PLATTER

Arrange artichoke hearts, grape tomatoes, thickly sliced cucumbers, red onions cut into wedges and separated, several different types of olives, and roasted red peppers (see Chef's Notes on page 346) on a platter and drizzle with Italian Dressing (see page 325). Place toothpicks nearby.

MEDITERRANEAN PLATE

Assemble a beautiful light meal by piling Greek Salad (see page 335) or baby greens and grape tomatoes drizzled with olive oil and balsamic vinegar on one side of a large plate. Fan the pita triangles along the other edge of the plate and arrange mounds of Olive Tapenade and Red Pepper Hummus in the middle.

CELEBRATION DINNER
MENU

DRIED CHERRY AND PEAR SAUCE OVER
HERB-RUBBED PORK TENDERLOIN
LEMONY GREEN BEANS WITH ALMONDS
ROASTED ROOTS
BITTERSWEET CHOCOLATE SOUFFLÉS

*This menu is great for special occasions like birthdays, anniversaries,
and Valentine's Day. Pinot Noir pairs beautifully with the pork.*

DRIED CHERRY AND PEAR SAUCE
Serves 6

INGREDIENTS
2 cups diced Bosc pears
½ cup dried cherries
1 teaspoon butter
2 tablespoons brown sugar
1 cup apple cider

DIRECTIONS
1. Dice pears and cook in a saucepan over medium heat.
2. Add dried cherries and stir to heat.
3. Add cider and sugar then simmer until the volume of liquid has been reduced by half.
4. Add salt and pepper to taste.
5. Spoon warm sauce over sliced Pork Tenderloin.

NUTRITION ANALYSIS PER SERVING
164 Calories; 2 g Fat; 1 g Saturated fat; 1 g Protein;
39 g Carbohydrate; 3 g Fiber; 3 mg Cholesterol;
16 mg Sodium.

CHEF'S NOTES
You can substitute apples for pears, dried cranberries for cherries, or Bourbon for apple cider. If using Bourbon, carefully light it on fire at the end of cooking to burn off any remaining alcohol (and impress your guests!).

DOCTOR'S NOTES
Using fruit in your main dish meals, like the pears and dried cherries in this recipe, is a flavorful way to provide additional vitamins, fiber, and phytochemicals.

FAMILY NOTES
Pork Tenderloin with Pear and Dried Cherry Sauce is a relatively simple but elegant dish. Overlap slices of pork on a serving platter and drizzle with the sauce; spoon the Roasted Roots around the pork before serving your family and guests.

HERB-RUBBED PORK TENDERLOIN
Serves 6

INGREDIENTS

2 pork tenderloins (approximately 1½ pounds total weight)
1 tablespoon dried chives
1 tablespoon dried parsley
1 tablespoon dried thyme
1 tablespoon vegetable oil

DIRECTIONS

1. Preheat oven to 400 degrees.
2. Remove silver skin from pork if necessary (see Chef's Notes).
3. Mix the herbs (chives, parsley, and thyme) in a large plastic bag.
4. Rub pork with the oil then place into the plastic bag to coat evenly with herbs.
5. Heat heavy skillet on the stove on high until smoking.
6. Place pork in the skillet and sear it, turning until all sides are browned (see Chef's Notes).
7. Once pork is seared, place it in a pan in a 400-degree oven (if your skillet is oven safe, you may place it directly into the oven from the stove).
8. Bake pork for 9–13 minutes or until desired tenderness. Do not overcook; it should still be moist inside.
9. After baking, let the pork rest for 10 minutes.
10. Slice into ½-inch thick slices and serve with Dried Cherry and Pear Sauce.

CHEF'S NOTES

Pork tenderloin can be found in the meat department of most grocery stores. They are usually sold in packs of two. This recipe calls for a total weight of 1½ pounds. "Silver skin" is the shiny silvery membrane sometimes left on the pork tenderloin after the fat has been removed. It is very tough and will cause the meat to curl if left on. To remove the silver skin, slip the tip of a sharp knife between the skin and the meat; lift slightly as you slice it off. To keep the tenderloin moist, sear it by placing it in an extremely hot pan. Brown all sides quickly to seal in the juices.

DOCTOR'S NOTES

Pork is a good source of protein, iron, B-vitamins (B_{12}, B_6, thiamin, niacin, and riboflavin), zinc, phosphorous, potassium, and magnesium. When the external visible fat on pork is removed before cooking, the result is a cut of meat that compares to chicken in calories, cholesterol, and fat content. Pork tenderloin is the leanest, but any cuts from the loin are good selections.

FAMILY NOTES

Leftover pork tenderloin is great on a salad, in fajitas, in Southwestern Stew (see page 340) or with an Asian-inspired sauce and stir-fried vegetables for a quick second meal.

NUTRITION ANALYSIS PER 4-OUNCE SERVING
161 Calories; 6 g Fat; 2 g Saturated fat; 24 g Protein;
1 g Carbohydrate; 1 g Fiber; 74 mg Cholesterol;
59 mg Sodium.

LEMONY GREEN BEANS WITH ALMONDS
Serves 6

INGREDIENTS
1 pound fresh green beans
1 tablespoon butter
1 tablespoon fresh lemon juice
2 tablespoons slivered almonds
½ teaspoon salt

DIRECTIONS
1. Trim the ends off the green beans and "string" them by pulling the tough string from the edge of each bean.
2. Put green beans and 1 cup of water in a large pot. Cook on medium high for 10–15 minutes until beans are bright green and tender crisp.
3. Drain off any remaining water and add butter, stirring to melt and coat the beans. Sprinkle with lemon juice, salt, and toasted almonds (see Chef's Notes).

NUTRITION ANALYSIS PER SERVING
56 Calories; 4 g Fat; 1 g Saturated fat; 2 g Protein;
6 g Carbohydrate; 3 g Fiber; 5 mg Cholesterol;
221 mg Sodium.

CHEF'S NOTES
To toast nuts or seeds, place them in a dry nonstick pan. Shake or stir frequently until they start to turn golden. Remove from hot pan immediately to cool.

DOCTOR'S NOTES
Lemon juice is a flavor brightener, so you don't need loads of butter and salt to make your vegetables taste great.

FAMILY NOTES
For maximum nutrition, the fresher, the better. If fresh vegetables aren't available, frozen vegetables are a close second because they are frozen at their peak. To help retain their vitamins and minerals, don't overcook them.

ROASTED ROOTS
Serves 6

INGREDIENTS
3 medium baking potatoes, peels left on, cut into ½-inch cubes
2 medium sweet potatoes, peels left on, cut into ½-inch cubes
2 yellow onions cut in eighths
½ pound baby carrots
2 tablespoons olive oil
1 tablespoon dried parsley
1½ teaspoons kosher salt
½ teaspoon black pepper

CHEF'S NOTES
Make sure potatoes are cut the same size so they'll cook evenly.

DOCTOR'S NOTES
Sweet potatoes have been ranked number one in nutrition because they are high in vitamins A and C and beta-carotene. We leave the potato peels on for extra fiber.

DIRECTIONS
1. Preheat oven to 450 degrees.
2. Wash and cut up baking potatoes.
3. Trim any tough pieces off the sweet potatoes and cut up.
4. Cut off each end of the onion then peel. Cut the onion in half then cut each half into quarters to make eight pieces.
5. Put potatoes, onions, and baby carrots in a large plastic bag.
6. Add olive oil, parsley, salt, and pepper to the vegetables in the bag. Seal the bag and shake until all the vegetables are coated.
7. Spread vegetables evenly onto a large cookie sheet and roast for 40–60 minutes, turning once or twice. Cook until vegetables are tender on the inside and potatoes are slightly crispy on the outside.

NUTRITION ANALYSIS PER SERVING
163 Calories; 5 g Fat; 1 g Saturated fat; 3 g Protein; 28 g Carbohydrate; 4 g Fiber; 0 mg Cholesterol; 495 mg Sodium.

FAMILY NOTES
These are as good as French fries or mashed potatoes, but healthier.

BITTERSWEET CHOCOLATE SOUFFLÉS
Serves 4

INGREDIENTS
Cooking spray
½ cup sugar, divided
¼ cup cocoa powder
1 tablespoon all-purpose flour
Pinch of salt
¼ cup skim milk
½ teaspoon vanilla extract
2 large egg yolks
2 large egg whites
⅛ teaspoon cream of tartar
2 ounces bittersweet chocolate, finely chopped

CHEF'S NOTES
Soufflés have more steps than most of the recipes we've given you, but the elegant presentation and fantastic flavors are well worth it. By knowing a couple of simple tips, you'll get great results every time. To make sure your egg whites form nice peaks, be sure there is no yolk in them and that the bowl is perfectly clean (no fat or grease on it). Stop mixing when the stiff peaks form or you'll "break" them and the egg whites will start to liquefy again. To keep the egg whites fluffy, fold the chocolate in by picking up the mixture and gently turning it over. Don't overmix, or you'll lose the air.

DIRECTIONS

1. Preheat oven to 350 degrees.
2. Coat 4 (4-ounce) ramekins with cooking spray then sprinkle with 1 tablespoon of the sugar.
3. Combine 4 tablespoons sugar, cocoa, flour, and salt in a small saucepan. Gradually add milk while whisking until blended.
4. Bring to a boil over medium heat and cook until thick while stirring constantly (about 3 minutes).
5. Remove from heat and let cool for 3 minutes.
6. Gradually stir in egg yolks and vanilla.
7. Spoon chocolate mixture into a large bowl and allow to cool.
8. Place egg whites in a large, very clean bowl. Beat with a mixer on high until foamy.
9. Gradually add remaining sugar (3 tablespoons) and cream of tartar, beating mixture until shiny stiff peaks form.
10. Gently stir one-fourth of egg white mixture into chocolate mixture.
11. Gently fold in remaining egg white mixture and the chopped chocolate.
12. Spoon into prepared ramekins.
13. Bake at 350 degrees for 15 minutes or until puffy and set. Sprinkle with powdered sugar.

NUTRITION ANALYSIS PER SERVING
230 Calories; 11 g Fat; 6 g Saturated fat; 6 g Protein; 35 g Carbohydrate; 4 g Fiber; 94 mg Cholesterol; 39 mg Sodium.

DOCTOR'S NOTES

One of my favorite foods is chocolate. It used to be a real trigger food for me, but now it's simply one of my life's many pleasures.

Chocolate may have some health benefits due to the antioxidants it contains and its positive effects on your brain chemistry. Those benefits come from the cocoa itself; consequently, these soufflés emphasize those ingredients while keeping the sugar and fat to a minimum. Keep in mind that most chocolate candy is high in sugar and saturated fat, so moderation is the key.

FAMILY NOTES

Both kids love these—especially Elyse (like mother, like daughter I guess)!

BETTER THAN FAST FOOD
MENU
PORTOBELLO MUSHROOM BURGERS
WITH CHIPOTLE AIOLI
CRISPY OVEN FRIES WITH SPICY KETCHUP
BROCCOLI AND ALMOND SALAD
WATERMELON ICE OR FRESH FRUIT SMOOTHIES

*It's not as fast as fast food, but it tastes a lot better! Invite
your neighbors over to slow down for a while. We love a
spicy red Zinfandel (or a cold beer!) with this meal.*

PORTOBELLO MUSHROOM BURGERS
WITH CHIPOTLE AIOLI
Serves 4

INGREDIENTS
1 pound ground beef, 95 percent lean
1 egg
1 tablespoon steak seasoning
4 red onion slices
2 portobello mushroom caps
4 lettuce leaves
4 tomato slices
2 tablespoons chipotle aioli (see Chef's
Notes)
4 hamburger buns

DIRECTIONS
1. Heat grill to medium.
2. Combine ground beef, egg, and
steak seasoning. Form four patties.
Refrigerate or grill immediately.
3. Place patties, mushroom caps, and
onions on the grill.
4. Grill burgers until they reach an
internal temperature of 160 degrees.
5. Grill mushrooms and onions for
approximately 3 minutes on each side
until soft. Remove from the grill.

6. Separate onion into rings and slice
each mushroom cap into six strips.
7. Lightly toast buns on the grill, cut
side down.
8. Spread ½ tablespoon of the
Chipotle Aioli on each of the bottom
buns and set a grilled patty on top.
9. Top each burger with grilled onion
rings and three strips of mushroom.
Top with lettuce and tomato.

NUTRITION ANALYSIS PER SERVING
456 Calories; 7 g Fat; 2 g Saturated fat; 17 g Protein;
27 g Carbohydrate; 2 g Fiber; 78 mg Cholesterol;
878 mg Sodium.

CHEF'S NOTES
Make Chipotle Aioli puree by stirring
½ teaspoon of chipotle puree into 2
tablespoons of mayonnaise. (Chipotle
puree is made by blending a 7-ounce
can of chipotle chiles in adobo sauce
in a blender or food processor into a
thick paste. Store remaining puree in the
refrigerator for spicy pastas and sauces.)

CRISPY OVEN FRIES WITH SPICY KETCHUP
Serves 4

INGREDIENTS

For Fries:
1 pound russet or sweet potatoes,
thinly sliced
2 tablespoons canola oil
1 teaspoon parsley
½ teaspoon salt
½ teaspoon garlic powder

For Spicy Ketchup:
4 tablespoons ketchup
1 tablespoon Worcestershire sauce
2–4 drops hot pepper sauce, to taste
1 teaspoon brown sugar
Ground pepper, to taste

DIRECTIONS
1. Scrub potatoes and pat dry.
2. Using a mandolin, slice unpeeled potatoes into ⅛-inch thick chips.
3. Place potatoes into a large bowl and coat with oil.
4. Sprinkle seasonings over potatoes and stir with a large spoon.
5. Place potatoes on a large baking sheet in a single layer. If using both russet and sweet potatoes, put them on separate baking sheets since required cooking time may be different.
6. Place in an oven preheated to 450 degrees and bake for 30–45 minutes. Turn potatoes every 5–10 minutes, until they are golden brown and crispy.
7. Meanwhile, stir ketchup ingredients together.

NUTRITION ANALYSIS PER SERVING OF FRIES
151 Calories; 7 g Fat; 2 g Protein;
21 g Carbohydrate; 2 g Fiber; 0 mg Cholesterol;
302 mg Sodium.

NUTRITION ANALYSIS PER SERVING OF KETCHUP
21 Calories; trace Fat; trace Saturated fat; trace
Protein; 5 g Carbohydrate; trace Fiber; 0 mg
Cholesterol; 215 mg Sodium.

CHEF'S NOTES
For prettiest presentation, serve both russet and sweet potato fries in a fancy martini glass lined with a cone made from a paper circle.

DOCTOR'S NOTES
Sweet potatoes are ranked number one in nutrition for vegetables!

BROCCOLI AND ALMOND SALAD
Serves 4

INGREDIENTS

For Salad:
2 tablespoons dried cranberries
2 cups raw broccoli florets
1 tablespoon slivered almonds
1 tablespoon onions, finely diced

For Broccoli Dressing:
1 tablespoon light mayonnaise
½ tablespoon red wine vinegar
½ tablespoon sugar
¼ teaspoon salt
⅛ teaspoon ground black pepper

DIRECTIONS

1. Mix dressing ingredients in a medium-sized bowl until creamy.
2. Add salad ingredients to the dressing and stir until well coated.

NUTRITION ANALYSIS PER SERVING
41 Calories; 2 g Fat; trace Saturated fat;
2 g Protein; 5 g Carbohydrate; 2 g Fiber;
1 mg Cholesterol; 176 mg Sodium.

CHEF'S NOTES
Substitute cauliflower or chopped cabbage for the broccoli, or sunflower seeds for the almonds if desired.

DOCTOR'S NOTES
Broccoli is a super food because it is loaded with vitamins and fiber.

FAMILY NOTES
This has become one of our family's signature dishes for potlucks.

WATERMELON ICE
Serves 4

INGREDIENTS
6 cups watermelon (or other melon) chunks, seeds removed
1 tablespoon lemon juice
2 tablespoons sugar (if needed)

DIRECTIONS
1. Place about half the watermelon chunks, lemon juice, and sugar (if needed) in a blender.
2. Blend to combine.
3. Add remaining watermelon and blend until smooth.
4. Pour watermelon mixture in a shallow baking dish and place in the freezer.
5. If possible, stir every 30 minutes. Freeze until icy, approximately 2–3 hours.
6. Remove and scrape or scoop into a decorative glass to serve. Garnish with mint.

NUTRITION ANALYSIS PER SERVING
99 Calories; 1 g Fat; 0 g Saturated fat; 1 g Protein; 23 g Carbohydrate; 1 g Fiber; 0 mg Cholesterol; 5 mg Sodium.

CHEF'S NOTES
Just about any fruit can be frozen then blended into a fruit ice.

DOCTOR'S NOTES
Frozen fruit is a great snack or dessert.

FAMILY NOTES
This is a sweet treat for a hot day. Put some miniature chocolate chips in to look like watermelon seeds.

FRESH FRUIT SMOOTHIES
Serves 2

INGREDIENTS
1 cup skim milk
1 cup non-fat fruit flavored yogurt (any flavor)
1 cup chopped fresh or frozen fruit (such as strawberries, bananas, blueberries, raspberries or peaches)
Ice if needed

DIRECTIONS
1. Place all ingredients into a blender and blend until smooth.
2. Pour into tall glasses.

NUTRITION ANALYSIS PER SERVING
172 Calories; 1 g Fat; 0 g Sat Fat; 10 g Protein; 33 g Carbohydrate; 2 g Fiber; 4 mg Cholesterol; 130 mg Sodium.

CHEF'S NOTES
Freeze fresh fruit by placing berries or chunks of bananas or peaches on a cookie sheet and freeze until firm. Store frozen fruit in an airtight container

DOCTOR'S NOTES
Smoothies make a great breakfast, light lunch, after school snack or dessert.

FAMILY NOTES
You can make frozen fruit pops too. Freeze smoothies in ice cube trays, popsicle molds, or paper cups. Insert a wooden stick when they are partially frozen.

MAIN DISH SALADS

GARDEN SALAD WITH GRILLED CHICKEN,
CRANBERRIES, AND WALNUTS
WRITE-YOUR-OWN-RECIPE SALAD BAR

Main dish salads made with interesting greens, fresh produce, protein, and a great dressing are the perfect way to balance eating for nourishment with eating for enjoyment!

GARDEN SALAD WITH GRILLED CHICKEN, CRANBERRIES, AND WALNUTS
Serves 6

INGREDIENTS

For Balsamic Vinaigrette dressing:
½ cup olive oil
¼ cup balsamic vinegar
1 clove garlic
1 teaspoon sugar
Salt and pepper to taste

For salad:
12 cups mixed greens
16 ounces of grilled chicken breast, thinly sliced
6 tablespoons dried cranberries
6 tablespoons chopped walnuts

DIRECTIONS
1. Place all dressing ingredients in a blender and blend for 30 seconds until emulsified; chill.
2. Arrange mixed greens on a plate. Arrange sliced chicken breast on top and sprinkle with cranberries and walnuts.
3. Drizzle dressing over top.

NUTRITION ANALYSIS
330 Calories; 25 g Fat; 3 g Saturated fat; 22 g Protein; 8 g Carbohydrate; 4 g Fiber; 46 mg Cholesterol; 68 mg Sodium.

CHEF'S NOTES
Using this basic combination as an example, try other items from the Write-Your-Own-Recipe Salad Bar on the next page. Some examples: replace the chicken with salmon, feta, or blue cheese; replace the dried cranberries with dried cherries, mandarin oranges, pears, strawberries, or grilled beets; replace the walnuts with almonds or sunflower seeds.

DOCTOR'S NOTES
Emulsifying an oil-based dressing gives it a creamy texture without adding saturated fat.

FAMILY NOTES
Make a wrap by folding a serving of salad into a tortilla or thin, soft flatbread, or make a pita pocket by filling half of a pita with salad.

WRITE-YOUR-OWN-RECIPE SALAD BAR

Create great salads by selecting one or more items from each column. Start with greens then add your favorite veggies and/or fruit. Be sure to add protein if you're making a main dish salad. Use bottled dressing or make your own.

GREENS	VEGGIES	FRUIT	PROTEIN	DRESSINGS
Arugula	Artichokes	Apples	Beans	Balsamic
Baby greens	Asparagus	Bananas	Black	Reduction
Basil	Avocado	Blackberries	Garbanzo	Balsamic
Bok choy	Baby corn	Blueberries	Navy	Vinaigrette
Cabbage	Bean sprouts	Boysenberries	Kidney	(p. 357)
Green	Beets	Cantaloupe	Pinto	Greek (p. 335)
Napa	Bell peppers	Cherries	Cheeses	Italian (p. 325)
Red	Broccoli	(dried)	Blue	Lemon Herb
Cilantro	Capers	Coconut	Cheddar	Vinaigrette
Chard	Carrots	Cranberries	Feta	Oriental
Endive	Cauliflower	(dried)	Goat	Ranch
Fennel	Celery	Grapefruit	Mozzarella	Salsa
Lettuce	Chives	Grapes	Parmesan	Spinach
Butter	Corn	Honeydew	Chicken	Vinegar and Oil
Green leaf	Cucumbers	Kiwi	Eggs	Yogurt (p. 338)
Iceberg	Garlic	Mandarin	Meats	
Romaine	Green beans	oranges	Nuts	
Kale	Eggplant	Mangoes	Almonds	
Leeks	Jalapeño	Oranges	Cashews	
Mint	Jicama	Papaya	Hazelnuts	
Parsley	Mushrooms	Pomegranates	Peanuts	
Spinach	Olives	Peaches	Pecans	
Watercress	Onions	Pears	Pine	
	Peas	Pineapple	Walnuts	
	Peperoncini	Raisins	Salmon	
	Potatoes	Raspberries	Seeds	
	Radishes	Strawberries	Flax	
	Snap peas	Watermelon	Poppy	
	Snow peas		Pumpkin	
	Tomatoes		Sesame	
	Water		Sunflower	
	chestnuts		Soybeans	
	Zucchini		Tofu	
			Tuna	
			Turkey	

HEALTH NOTES

DEPRESSION AND ANXIETY

Depression and anxiety are serious medical problems often caused by imbalances in brain chemistry.

Depression can cause symptoms such as

- Persistent sadness or hopelessness
- Loss of interest in enjoyable activities
- Loss of appetite or eating too much
- Sleeping too much or not enough
- Feeling tired
- Feeling unworthy or guilty
- Difficulty concentrating, remembering, or making decisions
- Thinking about death or suicide (Important! If you have thoughts of suicide, seek help immediately.)

Anxiety can cause symptoms that include

- Restlessness, irritability, or feeling edgy
- Excessive worrying

- Fearing that something bad is going to happen, a sense of impending doom
- Difficulty concentrating
- Trembling, twitching, or shaking
- Feeling of fullness in the throat or chest
- Breathlessness or rapid heartbeat
- Lightheadedness or dizziness
- Sweating or cold, clammy hands
- Excessive startle reflex
- Muscle tension, aches, or soreness
- Fatigue
- Sleep problems such as trouble falling asleep or staying asleep

It's very important to be evaluated by your doctor or therapist if you have symptoms of depression or anxiety lasting for two weeks or more. Though the symptoms can seem overwhelming, depression and anxiety can and should be treated.

EATING DISORDERS

Eating disorders arise from a variety of physical, emotional, social, and familial issues, all of which need to be addressed for effective prevention and treatment. The most effective and long-lasting treatment for an eating disorder is some form of psychotherapy or counseling, coupled with careful attention to medical and nutritional needs. Ideally, this treatment should be tailored to the individual and will vary according to both the severity of the disorder and the patient's individual problems, needs, and strengths.

Anorexia Nervosa Anorexia nervosa is a serious, potentially life-threatening eating disorder characterized by self-starvation and excessive weight loss.

The criteria for anorexia nervosa are found in the American Psychiatric Association's *Diagnostic and Statistical Manual of Mental Disorders,* 4th edition (DSM-IV). There are four basic criteria for the diagnosis of anorexia nervosa:

1. The refusal to maintain body weight at or above a minimally normal weight for age and height. Body weight less than 85 percent of the expected weight is considered minimal.
2. An intense fear of gaining weight or becoming fat, even though the person is underweight.
3. Self-perception that is grossly distorted and weight loss that is not acknowledged.
4. In women who have already begun their menstrual cycle, at least three consecutive periods are missed (amenorrhea), or menstrual periods occur only after a hormone is administered.

The DSM-IV further identifies two subtypes of anorexia nervosa. In the binge-eating/purging type, the individual regularly engages in binge eating or purging behavior, which involves self-induced vomiting or the misuse of laxatives, diuretics, or enemas during the current episode of anorexia. In the restricting type, the individual severely restricts food intake but does not engage in the behaviors seen in the binge-eating type.

Bulimia Nervosa Bulimia nervosa is a serious, potentially life-threatening eating disorder characterized by a cycle of bingeing and compensatory behaviors such as self-induced vomiting designed to undo or compensate for the effects of binge eating.

The criteria for bulimia nervosa are found in the American Psychiatric Association's *Diagnostic and Statistical Manual of Mental Disorders,* 4th edition (DSM-IV). There are five basic criteria in the diagnosis of bulimia:

1. Recurrent episodes of binge eating. This is characterized by eating within a two-hour period an amount of food that is definitely larger than most people would eat during a similar period of time and under similar circumstances.

2. A sense of lack of control over the eating during the episode, or a feeling that one cannot stop eating.

3. In addition to the binge eating, there is an inappropriate compensatory behavior in order to prevent weight gain. These behaviors can include self-induced vomiting, misuse of laxatives, diuretics, enemas or other medications, fasting, or excessive exercise.

4. Both the binge eating and the compensatory behaviors must occur at least two times per week for three months and must not occur exclusively during episodes of anorexia.

5. Finally, there is dissatisfaction with body shape and/or weight.

The DSM-IV also identifies two subtypes of bulimia nervosa. The purging type regularly engages in self-induced vomiting or the misuse of laxatives, diuretics, or enemas. The non-purging type engages in other inappropriate compensatory behaviors, such as fasting or excessive exercise, rather than purging methods.

Eating Disorder Not Otherwise Specified, or EDNOS Disordered eating that does not meet the criteria for anorexia nervosa or bulimia nervosa.

Binge-Eating Disorder (BED) Binge-eating disorder is a type of eating disorder not otherwise specified and is characterized by recurrent binge eating without the regular use of compensatory measures to counter the binge eating.

Someone with BED has frequent episodes of binge eating, occurring at least two days a week for six months. Binge-eating episodes are associated with at least three of the following symptoms.

- Eating rapidly
- Eating until feeling uncomfortably full
- Eating when not hungry
- Eating alone because of embarrassment
- Feeling disgusted, depressed, or guilty after overeating

It's very important to be evaluated by your doctor or therapist if you have symptoms of an eating disorder.

METABOLIC SYNDROME

Many overweight individuals develop insulin resistance: their tissues ignore insulin signals. Insulin resistance allows the blood glucose levels to remain too high. The body tries to compensate by producing even more insulin, resulting in hyperinsulinemia. These high insulin levels promote fat storage and inhibit fat burning.

Hyperinsulinemia contributes to the development of Metabolic Syndrome, which increases the risk of developing diabetes and heart disease. It is characterized by

- A waist that measures more than 40 inches in men or 35 inches in women
- High blood pressure
- High triglyceride levels
- Low HDL ("good" cholesterol)
- High fasting blood sugars

Diabetes is a disease in which the blood glucose levels are too high, either because there isn't enough insulin (called Type I) or because the body isn't using insulin properly (called Type II, the most common type). Diabetes causes damage to important tissues, potentially leading to heart disease, kidney failure, blindness, and amputations. Many overweight people develop Type II diabetes and nearly four out of five diabetics are overweight or obese.

There is ongoing research into the relationship between diet and Metabolic Syndrome; here are a few irrefutable facts when it comes to managing insulin and blood sugar levels.

- When you consume more calories than your body needs, you'll increase your fat stores, which increases your risk of Metabolic Syndrome.
- Exercise decreases insulin resistance.
- Weight loss is the most effective way of improving insulin resistance. When you lose weight, your blood sugar and insulin levels decrease, decreasing your risk of diabetes, high cholesterol, high blood pressure, and heart disease.

CHOLESTEROL AND HEART DISEASE

There are many known risk factors for heart disease: these include smoking, high blood pressure, diabetes, family history, obesity, physical inactivity, and high cholesterol. Your liver manufactures cholesterol because it's necessary for building cell membranes and nerve tissue, helping produce necessary hormones for body regulation, and producing bile acids for digestion. Other animals manufacture cholesterol for these same reasons; therefore, dietary cholesterol is found in the animal products you may eat, such as meat, poultry, egg yolks, cheese, whole milk, and other whole-milk dairy products.

For some people, high cholesterol levels and heart disease run in their families; their bodies may be genetically programmed to manufacture too much cholesterol. Others manufacture the right amount of cholesterol but eat too much cholesterol and saturated fat in their diets, raising their blood cholesterol levels and putting themselves at increased risk of heart disease.

Knowing your cholesterol level is important for determining whether you are at increased risk of heart disease. However, the total cholesterol doesn't tell the whole story. Cholesterol is transported in different forms, which have different effects.

LDL: Low-density lipoproteins (LDL) are considered "bad" because they are sticky and likely to form fatty deposits and plaque on the walls of your arteries, which leads to blockage. A healthy person's LDL level should be less than 130 mg/dl. A person with other risk factors, such as a history of heart disease or diabetes, should maintain an LDL level of less than 100 mg/dl. Eating polyunsaturated and monounsaturated fats (olive, peanut, and canola oils) may help lower your LDL levels. Remember:

LDL = Lousy Cholesterol = The Lower the better.

HDL: High-density lipoproteins (HDL) are considered "good" because they help carry away cholesterol stuck to the walls of the arteries. A high level of HDL is associated with a lower incidence of heart disease. An HDL level of more than 40 mg/dl is optimal. Regular physical activity and exercise can raise your levels of this "good" cholesterol. Remember:

HDL = Happy Cholesterol = The Higher the better.

Triglycerides: Triglycerides are another form in which fat is transported through the blood. Triglyceride levels below 150 mg/dl are considered normal according to the National Heart, Lung and Blood Institute. Higher levels can be the result of eating high-fat foods, drinking alcohol in excess, diabetes, inherited disorders, and pancreatic disorders. Very high levels can have serious medical complications.

If you have a personal or family history of elevated cholesterol levels, heart disease, or diabetes, you'll want to be even more cautious about eating high-cholesterol foods and saturated fats. If necessary, consult a dietitian to help you determine how to change your diet. If your cholesterol remains high despite regular exercise and a diet low in cholesterol and saturated fat, medications may be necessary to lower your cholesterol to safe levels. Discuss this with your health care professional.

VITAMINS AND MINERALS AT A GLANCE

VITAMINS MINERALS	SIGNIFICANT SOURCES	MAJOR FUNCTIONS	RECOMMENDED DAILY INTAKE
Vitamin A (retinol, retinal, carotene)	Yellow/orange fruits and vegetables: carrots, sweet potatoes, canta-loupe; watermelon, dark green leafy vegetables, spinach, tomatoes, broccoli, liver, milk, margarine	Promotes eye health and protection against night blindness; helps keep skin healthy; helps body resist infection, building strong bones and teeth	Women, 14 yrs and up: 700 mcg Men, 14 yrs and up: 900 mcg
Vitamin D	Exposure to sun, forti-fied milk, small amounts of butter, liver, egg yolk, salmon, sardines, fish-liver oils	Increases calcium and phosphorous absorption and utilization; helps bones and teeth harden	Up to 50 yrs: 5 mcg (200 IU), 51–70 yrs: 10 mcg (400 IU), >70 yrs: 15 mcg (600 IU); or approx. 15 mins in the sun. Note: Many experts are calling for a significant increase in the recom-mended daily intake. Talk to your health care professional.
Vitamin E	Vegetable oils, marga-rine, butter, eggs, whole grains, wheat germ, liver, leafy greens	Works as antioxidant preventing destruc-tion of vitamins A, C, fatty acids, and cell membranes	14 yrs and up: 15 mg
Vitamin K	Leafy green vegetables, milk, soybean oil, egg yolks (Intestinal bacteria synthesizes most of the vitamin K the body needs.)	Helps the clotting action of blood in wounds	19 yrs and up: 90 mcg

VITAMINS MINERALS	SIGNIFICANT SOURCES	MAJOR FUNCTIONS	RECOMMENDED DAILY INTAKE
Vitamin C	All citrus fruits and juices, strawberries, mango, cantaloupe, papaya, brussels sprouts, tomatoes, green/red peppers, cabbage, spinach, broccoli, kale and turnip greens, potatoes, mustard greens	Forms glue that holds body cells together; strengthens blood vessels; promotes iron absorption; speeds healing; boosts immune system	Women, 19 yrs and up: 75 mg Men, 19 yrs and up: 90 mg
Folate, Folic Acid	Legumes, oranges, strawberries, green leafy vegetables, asparagus, whole grains, sunflower seeds, liver	Promotes red blood cell formation; greatly reduces birth defects of brain and spine; recent evidence shows reduces risk of heart disease	14 yrs and up: 400 mcg Pregnant/Lactating: 600/500 mcg
Vitamin B_{12}	Animal products: meat, fish, poultry, eggs, milk, and milk products	Assists in maintenance of nerve tissue and normal blood cell formation	14 years and up: 2.4 mcg
Vitamin B_6, Pyridoxine	Poultry, fish, pork, unprocessed whole grains, legumes, potatoes, sweet potatoes, nuts, avocados, bananas, brewer's yeast	Necessary for metabolism of protein; needed to build certain amino acids and turn others into hormones; helps build red blood cells and maintain nerve tissue; metabolizes polyunsaturated fats	19–50 yrs: 1.3 mg Women, 51 yrs and up: 1.5 mg Men, 51 yrs and up: 1.7 mg
Niacin (B_3)	Meat, poultry, fish, liver, peanuts, legumes, whole grain or enriched cereals and breads	Helps the body produce energy from carbohydrate and fat; plays a role in maintaining healthy skin, nerves, and digestive system	Women, 14 yrs and up: 14 mg Men, 14 yrs and up: 16 mg

VITAMINS MINERALS	SIGNIFICANT SOURCES	MAJOR FUNCTIONS	RECOMMENDED DAILY INTAKE
Riboflavin (B$_2$)	Meat, liver, fish, milk, yogurt, cheese, eggs, dark green leafy vegetables, enriched breads and cereals	Plays a role in healthy skin and eyes; is a part of enzymes that cells use to produce energy	Women, 19 yrs and up: 1.1 mg Men, 19 yrs and up: 1.3 mg
Thiamin (B$_1$)	Legumes, whole grains, cereals, sunflower seeds, nuts, pork, liver, other meats	Is a key part of enzymes that are needed to turn carbohydrate into energy; promotes normal appetite and nerve function	Women, 19 yrs and up: 1.1 mg Men, 19 yrs and up: 1.2 mg
Calcium	Milk, yogurt, cheese, collard greens, fortified orange juice and other products, salmon, and sardines with bones	Builds and maintains strong bones and teeth; helps muscles contract and relax normally	19–50 yrs: 1000 mg > 51 yrs: 1200 mg
Iron	Meat (especially beef), seafood, legumes, dried fruits, fortified cereals	Builds red blood cells to maintain healthy blood and transport oxygen in body	Women, 19–50 yrs: 18 mg Women, 51 and up: 8 mg Men, 19 and up: 8 mg
Magnesium	Unprocessed foods, whole seeds such as nuts, legumes, and unmilled grains; green vegetables, bananas	Numerous biochemical and physiological processes require or are modulated by magnesium; critical to the transmission of impulses and electrical potentials of nerves and muscle membranes	Women, 19–30 yrs: 310 mg Women, 31 and up: 320 mg Men, 19–30 yrs: 400 mg Men, 31 and up: 420 mg
Potassium	Vegetables, milk, yogurt, meat, poultry, fish, and fruits	Helps the body maintain normal blood pressure and cell functions	14 yrs and up: 4700 mg

VITAMINS MINERALS	SIGNIFICANT SOURCES	MAJOR FUNCTIONS	RECOMMENDED DAILY INTAKE
Sodium	Table salt (¼ tsp = 2400 mg), most prepared foods	Used by the body to control blood pressure and blood volume	< 2300 mg (approximately 1 tsp. of salt)
Zinc	Meat, liver, eggs, seafood, cereals	No single enzyme function has been determined; however, a deficiency of zinc may cause loss of appetite, growth retardation, skin changes, and immunologic abnormalities	Women, 19 yrs and up: 8 mg Men, 19 yrs and up: 11 mg

UNDERSTANDING NUTRITION LABELS

Food labels are informative and can ultimately improve your health and well-being if you understand how to interpret them. Remember, though, not to use nutrition information to deprive yourself or ignore your body's signals about what it wants and needs.

Ingredient List

The ingredient lists tell you what was used to prepare the food. Ingredients are listed in order from the most to the least based on weight. This list is really helpful for getting the specifics, particularly if you have allergies, prefer to avoid eating certain ingredients (high-fructose corn syrup or hydrogenated and partially hydrogenated oils, for instance), or want information about additives and preservatives.

Nutrition Facts

Use the Nutrition Facts to educate yourself about the nutrient content of food, but not to label food as "good" or "bad." Here is a brief overview with helpful tips for interpretation.

Nutrition Facts

Serving Size 1 cup (228g)
Serving Per Container 2

Amount Per Serving		
Calories 260	Calories from Fat 120	
		% Daily Value*
Total Fat 13g		20%
Saturated Fat 5g		25%
Cholesterol 30mg		10%
Sodium 660mg		28%
Total Carbohydrate 31g		10%
Dietary Fiber 0g		
Sugars 5g		
Protein 5g		
Vitamin A 4%		Vitamin C 2%
Calcium 15%		Iron 4%

*Percent Daily Values are based on a 2,000 calorie diet. Your daily values may be higher or lower depending on your calorie needs.

	Calories	2,000	2,500
Total Fat	Less than	65g	80g
Saturated Fat	Less than	20g	25g
Cholesterol	Less than	300mg	300mg
Sodium	Less than	2,400mg	2,400mg
Total Carbohydrate		300g	375g
Dietary Fiber		25g	30g

Calories per gram:
Fat 9 • Carbohydrate 4 • Protein 4

Serving Size Always check the listed serving size first. For example, one package may actually contain four servings. The portions listed are not necessarily recommended amounts, and they may not represent what most people eat. If it's inconvenient to measure your serving, use the Servings Per Container to estimate one serving (for example, one-fourth of the container). Don't forget, hunger and fullness levels should be determining how much you eat, not just the amount listed on the food label.

The nutrient information and Percent Daily Values listed on the food label are based on one serving. If the serving size is one cup and you consume two cups, multiply all numbers by two.

Calories Calories (total) and calories (from fat) are listed under the Amount Per Serving information. Total calories include calories from fat. Calories give you energy, but remember, if you consume more than you need, they're stored as fat. Looking at calories may help you determine if certain food items are upsetting your balance between calories in and calories out and preventing you from reaching a healthier weight.

Percent Daily Value (%DV) Keeping track of your daily intake can be time-consuming, tedious, and in most cases, unnecessary. However, knowing how much you're getting of a certain nutrient can be beneficial. Percent Daily Values (%DV) were designed to help consumers quickly see how much of their daily needs are being met through the selected food item. In an ideal situation where you had a food label for everything you ate, adding up each nutrient's %DV would indicate how well you're meeting your nutrient needs. Being close to 100 percent of the daily value for each item would indicate a well-balanced daily intake.

Located on the right side of the label, %DVs are reference numbers based on a person who consumes 2,000 calories a day. This may be more or less than what your body needs. Although not exactly individualized, %DV can be used to evaluate the food in hand. For nutrients you want to eat more of, like fiber and calcium, you want to see higher %DVs. For those nutrients you want to eat less of, like fat, cholesterol, and sodium, look for lower %DVs.

Fat On the label, total fat, saturated fat, and trans fat are listed in grams (g) and as a %DV. The %DV is based on 65 g of total fat (30 percent of a 2,000-calorie diet) and 20 g of saturated fat (10 percent of a 2,000-calorie diet). That doesn't mean you shouldn't eat a food with a high %DV; it simply means you'll want to balance it by selecting other lower-fat foods. For example, you may select cheese (a higher-fat food) but accompany it with wheat crackers or fruit (lower-fat foods).

Cholesterol Due to the prevalence of heart disease, cholesterol is listed on the label. It's listed in milligrams (mg) and as a %DV. The %DV is based on 300 mg of cholesterol. If your doctor has provided stricter guidelines for heart health, you may find it easier to track your cholesterol intake in milligrams.

Sodium Sodium is a mineral used by the body to control blood pressure and blood volume. Most nutrition experts recommend a daily maximum of less than 2,400 milligrams of sodium. The amount of sodium in a serving of food is listed in milligrams (mg) and as a %DV.

Carbohydrates These are listed as Total (in grams and %DV), Dietary Fiber (in grams and %DV based on 25 grams per day), and Sugars (in grams only). If you subtract Dietary Fiber and Sugars from the Total grams, the remaining number is the grams of starch. A food with 5 grams or more of fiber is considered high fiber.

Protein Protein is listed in grams per serving. Compare this with the personal daily protein needs you calculated for yourself previously in chapter 14.

Vitamins The food label also lists %DV for Vitamin A, Vitamin C, calcium, and iron. Others may be listed; only these four are required. This information will help you target nutrient-rich foods, but the best way to ensure that you get all the vitamins and minerals you need is by eating a wide variety. (For more details, read the section on micronutrients in chapter 15.)

Nutrition Claims

You'll also sometimes find nutrition claims listed on the front of a package, describing various nutritional qualities. These descriptors can be helpful if you know what they mean (and sometimes misleading if you don't).

Basic Terminology

Free:

- Calorie-free: 5 calories or less per serving
- Fat-free: less than 0.5 grams of fat (or 0.5 grams of saturated fat) per serving
- Cholesterol-free: less than 2 mg of cholesterol per serving
- Sugar-free: less than 0.5 grams of sugar per serving

Low:

- Low Calorie: 40 calories or less per serving
- Low Fat: 3 grams or less of fat (or 1 gram of saturated fat) per serving
- Low Cholesterol: 20 mg or less of cholesterol per serving
- Low Sodium: 140 mg or less of sodium per serving
- Low Carb: There are currently no guidelines for the use of this term.

Reduced, Less, Fewer (such as Reduced Calories or Less Fat): at least 25 percent less (calories, sugar, or fat) than a similar product

Light: One-third fewer calories, half the fat, or half the sodium of a similar food. Caution: light can also describe the texture and the color of the product.

Lean: A serving of meat, poultry, or seafood that contains less than 10 grams of fat, 4.5 grams of saturated fat, and 95 grams of cholesterol.

Extra Lean: Less than 5 grams of fat, 2 grams of saturated fat, and 95 mg of cholesterol

Health Claims

Health claims on food labels are claims by manufacturers of food products that their food will reduce the risk of developing a disease or condition. However, not all health claims are equal.

Solid These claims are based on reliable evidence and are approved by the FDA. A specific disease will be stated, such as "A diet low in total fat may reduce the risk of heart disease."

Preliminary These are based on incomplete or unreliable evidence and will include a disclaimer like "The FDA has determined the evidence is inconclusive."

Structure/Function These unreliable claims do not require any evidence. Look for words like "maintains" (as in maintains bone health) and "supports" (as in supports the immune system). These are found on food and supplements and require no approval by the FDA.

Nutrition Labels in the Real World

- Nutrition labels are also available for fresh meats, seafood, and produce; just ask your grocer.
- Don't forget to check the label on your vitamin/mineral supplements; remember, more of a good thing is not necessarily better.
- Many fast-food and chain restaurants make nutrition information available to their customers. This information is often available on the Internet.
- Many foods that claim "reduced fat" or "low carb" have substituted other ingredients and may have as many calories as the original. If you're going to read the claims on the front of the label, you have to pay attention to the Nutrition Facts on the back, too.
- Products with labels like "reduced," "light," or "low" can help you reach your health goals, but if such products don't taste good to you,

you won't feel satisfied when you eat them. In that case, it's better to stick with the original version and eat it less often or in smaller amounts. Remember, no food is forbidden.

- To evaluate for vitamin or mineral content, consider the following when looking at the %DVs:

    > 20%   = Excellent source

    10–19% = Good source

EXERCISE CLEARANCE

Play it safe by considering a visit to your doctor to get medical clearance before starting an exercise program. Your doctor will help you determine if you have any underlying medical problems that need to be addressed to be sure exercise is safe for you. You can use the "Physical Activity Readiness Questionnaire (PAR-Q) and You" on the next page to help you determine whether you should see your doctor before you start an exercise program.

If indicated, you and your doctor will explore your family history and personal cardiovascular risk factors such as age, current level of fitness, smoking history, blood pressure, cholesterol levels, diabetes, and other markers for heart disease. You'll also want to discuss any musculoskeletal problems and other medical issues that may affect your exercise program.

It's also very important to seek immediate medical attention if you have symptoms of chest pain, shortness of breath, dizziness, lightheadedness, or loss of consciousness, or if you develop those symptoms while exercising.

THE PHYSICAL ACTIVITY READINESS QUESTIONNAIRE (PAR-Q) AND YOU: A QUESTIONNAIRE FOR PEOPLE AGED 15 TO 69

(Physical Activity Readiness Questionnaire [PAR-Q] © 2002. Used with permission from the Canadian Society for Exercise Physiology, www.csep.ca.)

Regular physical activity is fun and healthy, and increasingly more people are starting to become more active every day. Being more active is very safe for most people. However, some people should check with their doctor before they start becoming much more physically active.

If you are planning to become much more physically active than you are now, start by answering the seven questions in the box below. If you are between the ages of 15 and 69, the PAR-Q will tell you if you should check with your doctor before you start. If you are over 69 years of age, and you are not used to being very active, check with your doctor.

Common sense is your best guide when you answer these questions. Please read the yes-no questions carefully and answer each one honestly.

1. Has your doctor ever said that you have a heart condition and that you should only do physical activity recommended by a doctor?

2. Do you feel pain in your chest when you do physical activity?

3. In the past month, have you had chest pain when you were not doing physical activity?

4. Do you lose your balance because of dizziness or do you ever lose consciousness?

5. Do you have a bone or joint problem (for example, back, knee or hip) that could be made worse by a change in your physical activity?

6. Is your doctor currently prescribing drugs (for example, water pills) for your blood pressure or heart condition?

7. Do you know of any other reason why you should not do physical activity?

If you answered YES to one or more questions, talk with your doctor by phone or in person BEFORE you start becoming much more physically active or BEFORE you have a fitness appraisal. Tell your doctor about the PAR-Q and which questions you answered YES.

- You may be able to do any activity you want—as long as you start slowly and build up gradually. Or, you may need to restrict your activities to those which are safe for you. Talk with your doctor about the kinds of activities you wish to participate in and follow his or her advice.

- Find out which community programs are safe and helpful for you.

If you answered NO honestly to all PAR-Q questions, you can be reasonably sure that you can:

- Start becoming much more physically active, but begin slowly and build up gradually. This is the safest and easiest way to go.

- Take part in a fitness appraisal. This is an excellent way to determine your basic fitness so that you can plan the best way for you to live actively. It is also highly recommended that you have your blood pressure evaluated. If your reading is over 144/94, talk with your doctor before you start becoming much more physically active.

Delay becoming much more active:

- If you are not feeling well because of a temporary illness such as a cold or a fever, wait until you feel better; or

- If you are or may be pregnant, talk to your doctor before you start becoming more active.

PLEASE NOTE: If your health changes so that you then answer YES to any of the above questions, tell your fitness or health professional. Ask whether you should change your physical activity plan.

Informed Use of the PAR-Q: The Canadian Society for Exercise Physiology, Health Canada, and their agents assume no liability for persons who undertake physical activity, and if in doubt after completing this questionnaire, consult your doctor prior to physical activity.

REFERENCES

Adam, T. C., and E. S. Epel. 2007. Stress, eating, and the reward system. *Physiology & Behavior* 91 (4): 449–58.

Aikman, S. N., K. E. Min, and D. Graham. 2006. Food attitudes, eating behavior, and the information underlying food attitudes. *Appetite* 47 (1): 111–14.

Allan, J. L., M. Johnston, and N. Campbell. 2008. Why do people fail to turn good intentions into action? The role of executive control processes in the translation of healthy eating intentions into action in young Scottish adults. *BMC Public Health* 8:123.

American College of Sports Medicine. 2000. *ACSM's guidelines for exercise testing and prescription* (6th ed.). Baltimore: Lippincott Williams & Wilkins.

American College of Sports Medicine. 2001. *ACSM's resource manual for guidelines for exercise testing and prescription* (4th ed.). Baltimore: Lippincott, Williams, & Wilkins.

American College of Sports Medicine. 2006. *ACSM's resource manual for guidelines for exercise testing and prescription* (5th ed.). Baltimore: Lippincott Williams & Wilkins.

American Dietetic Association. 2009. Non-nutritive sweeteners and adverse effects. http://www.adaevidencelibrary.com/evidence.cfm?evidence_summary_id=250283.

American Dietetic Association. 2007. Food nutrient data for Choose Your Foods: Exchange lists for diabetes. http://www.eatright.org/cps/rde/xchg/ada/hs.xsl/nutrition_13961_ENU_HTML.htm.

American Dietetic Association, and Dietitians of Canada. 2003. Position of the American Dietetic Association and Dietitians of Canada: Vegetarian diets. *Journal of the American Dietetic Association* 103 (6): 748–65.

American Heart Association. 2009. Make healthy food choices. http://www.americanheart.org/presenter.jhtml?identifier=537

American Heart Association Nutrition Committee. A. H. Lichtenstein, et al. 2006. Diet and lifestyle recommendations revision 2006: A scientific statement from the American Heart Association Nutrition Committee. *Circulation* 114 (1): 82–96.

American Psychiatric Association. 1994. *DSM-IV: Diagnostic and statistical manual of mental disorders* (4th ed.). Washington, D.C.: American Psychiatric Association.

Anderson, J. W. 2003. Whole grains protect against atherosclerotic cardiovascular disease. *The Proceedings of the Nutrition Society* 62 (1): 135–42.

Andlauer, W., P. Stehle, and P. Furst. 1998. Chemoprevention—A novel approach in dietetics. *Current Opinion in Clinical Nutrition and Metabolic Care* 1 (6): 539–47.

Andrade, A. M., G. W. Greene, and K. J. Melanson. 2008. Eating slowly led to decreases in energy intake within meals in healthy women. *Journal of the American Dietetic Association* 108 (7): 1186–91.

Apfeldorfer, G., and J. P. Zermati. 2001. Cognitive restraint in obesity. history of ideas, clinical description. [La restriction cognitive face a l'obesite. Histoire des idees, description clinique]. *Presse Medicale* 30 (32): 1575–80.

Avalos, L. C., and T. L. Tylka. 2006. Exploring a model of intuitive eating with college women. *Journal of Counseling Psychology* 53 (4): 486–97.

Bacon, L., Keim, et al. 2002. Evaluating a 'non-diet' wellness intervention for improvement of metabolic fitness, psychological well-being, and eating and activity behaviors. *International Journal of Obesity and Related Metabolic Disorders: Journal of the International Association for the Study of Obesity* 26 (6): 854–65.

Bacon, L., J., S. Stern, M. D. Van Loan, and N. L. Keim. 2005. Size acceptance and intuitive eating improve health for obese, female chronic dieters. *Journal of the American Dietetic Association* 105 (6): 929–36.

Balkin, T. J., T. Rupp, D. Picchioni, and N. J. Wesensten. 2008. Sleep loss and sleepiness: Current issues. *Chest* 134 (3): 653–60.

Barlow, C. E., H. W. Kohl III, L. W. Gibbons, and S. N. Blair. 1995. Physical fitness, mortality, and obesity. *International Journal of Obesity and Related Metabolic Disorders: Journal of the International Association for the Study of Obesity* 19 (suppl 4): S41–44.

Barnes, P. M., and C. A. Schoenborn. 2003. *Physical activity among adults: United States, 2000: Advanced data from vital and health statistics.* Hyattsville, MD: National Center for Health Statistics.

Bazzano, L. A., et al. 2002. Fruit and vegetable intake and risk of cardiovascular disease in U.S. adults: The first National Health and Nutrition Examination Survey epidemiologic follow-up study. *The American Journal of Clinical Nutrition* 76 (1): 93–99.

Bellisle, F., and A. M. Dalix. 2001. Cognitive restraint can be offset by distraction, leading to increased meal intake in women. *The American Journal of Clinical Nutrition* 74 (2): 197–200.

Bellisle, F., and A. M. Dalix, and G. Slama. 2004. Non food-related environmental stimuli induce increased meal intake in healthy women: Comparison of television viewing versus listening to a recorded story in laboratory settings. *Appetite* 43 (2): 175–80.

Berrett, M. E., R. K. Hardman, K. A. O'Grady, and P. S. Richards. 2007. The role of spirituality in the treatment of trauma and eating disorders: Recommendations for clinical practice. *Eating Disorders* 15 (4): 373–89.

Berthoud, H. R., and C. Morrison. 2008. The brain, appetite, and obesity. *Annual Review of Psychology* 59:55–92.

Birch, L. L., S. L. Johnson, G. Andresen, J. C. Peters, and M. C. Schulte. 1991. The variability of young children's energy intake. *New England Journal of Medicine* 324:232.

Bish, C. L., H. M. Blanck, M. K. Serdula, M. Marcus, H. W. Kohl III, and L. K. Khan. 2005. Diet and physical activity behaviors among Americans trying to lose weight: 2000 Behavioral Risk Factor Surveillance System. *Obesity Research* 13 (3): 596–607.

Bisogni, C. A., M. Connors, C. M. Devine, and J. Sobal. 2002. Who we are and how we eat: A qualitative study of identities in food choice. *Journal of Nutrition Education and Behavior* 34 (3): 128–39.

Bisogni, C. A., et al. 2007. Dimensions of everyday eating and drinking episodes. *Appetite* 48 (2): 218–31.

Bisogni, C. A., M. Jastran, L. Shen, and C. M. Devine. 2005. A biographical study of food choice capacity: Standards, circumstances, and food management skills. *Journal of Nutrition Education and Behavior* 37 (6): 284–91.

Blass, E. M., D. R. Anderson, H. L. Kirkorian, T. A. Pempek, I. Price, and M. F. Koleini. 2006. On the road to obesity: Television viewing increases intake of high-density foods. *Physiology & Behavior* 88 (4–5): 597–604.

Blundell, J. E., and J. Cooling. 2000. Routes to obesity: Phenotypes, food choices and activity. *The British Journal of Nutrition* 83 (suppl 1): S33–38.

Blundell, J. E., and A. Gillett. 2001. Control of food intake in the obese. *Obesity Research* 9 (suppl 4): S263–70.

Blundell, J. E., C. L. Lawton, J. R. Cotton, and J. I. Macdiarmid. 1996. Control of human appetite: Implications for the intake of dietary fat. *Annual Review of Nutrition* 16:285–319.

Bongaard, B. S. 2008. Mind over cupcake. *Explore* 4 (4): 267–72.

Bray, G. A. 1969. Effect of caloric restriction on energy expenditure in obese patients. *Lancet* 2 (7617): 397–98.

Brouwer, I. A., et al. 2006. Effect of fish oil on ventricular tachyarrhythmia and death in patients with implantable cardioverter defibrillators: The study on omega-3 fatty acids and ventricular arrhythmia (SOFA) randomized trial. *The Journal of the American Medical Association* 295 (22): 2613–19.

Brown, R., J. Ogden. 2004. Children's eating attitudes and behaviour: A study of the modelling and control theories of parental influence. *Health Education Research* 19 (3): 261–71.

Brunstrom, J. M., and G. I. Mitchell. 2006. Effects of distraction on the development of satiety. *The British Journal of Nutrition* 96 (4): 761–69.

Canadian Society for Exercise Physiology. 2002. Physical Activity Readiness Questionnaire (PAR-Q). Retrieved January 19, 2009, from http://www.csep.ca/main.cfm?cid=574&nid=5110 and used with permission.

Canetti, L., E. Bachar, and E. M. Berry. 2002. Food and emotion. *Behavioural Processes* 60 (2): 157–64.

Carnethon, M. R., S. S. Gidding, R. Nehgme, S. Sidney, D. R. Jacobs Jr., and K. Liu. 2003. Cardiorespiratory fitness in young adulthood and the development of cardiovascular disease risk factors. *The Journal of the American Medical Association* 290 (23): 3092–3100.

Carper, J. L., J. Orlet Fisher, and L. L. Birch. 2000. Young girls' emerging dietary restraint and disinhibition are related to parental control in child feeding. *Appetite* 35 (2): 121–29.

Carroll, S., E. Borkoles, and R. Polman. 2007. Short-term effects of a non-dieting lifestyle intervention program on weight management, fitness, metabolic risk, and psychological well-being in obese premenopausal females with the metabolic syndrome. *Applied Physiology, Nutrition, and Metabolism [Physiologie Appliquee, Nutrition et Metabolisme]* 32 (1): 125–42.

Center for Mindful Eating. The principles of mindful eating. Retrieved December 4, 2008, from http://tcme.org/principles.htm.

Centers for Disease Control and Prevention. Physical activity for a healthy weight. Retrieved December 23, 2008, from http://www.cdc.gov/nccdphp/dnpa/healthyweight/physical_activity/index.htm/.

Cochrane, G. 2008. Role for a sense of self-worth in weight-loss treatments: Helping patients develop self-efficacy. *Canadian Family Physician Medecin De Famille Canadien* 54 (4): 543–47.

Coelho, J. S., J. Polivy, C. P. Herman, and P. Pliner. 2008. Effects of food-cue exposure on dieting-related goals: A limitation to counteractive-control theory. *Appetite* 51 (2): 347–49.

Colditz, G. A. 1992. Economic costs of obesity. *American Journal of Clinical Nutrition* 55:S503–7.

Cooling, J., J. Barth, and J. Blundell. 1998. The high-fat phenotype: Is leptin involved in the adaptive response to a high fat (high energy) diet? *International Journal of Obesity and Related Metabolic Disorders: Journal of the International Association for the Study of Obesity* 22 (11): 1132–35.

Cornier, M. A., S. S. Von Kaenel, D. H. Bessesen, and J. R. Tregellas. 2007. Effects of over-feeding on the neuronal response to visual food cues. *The American Journal of Clinical Nutrition* 86 (4): 965–71.

Craig, W., and L. Beck. 1999. Phytochemicals: Health protective effects. *Canadian Journal of Dietetic Practice and Research: A Publication of Dietitians of Canada [Revue Canadienne de la Pratique et de la Recherche en Dietetique: Une Publication des Dietetistes du Canada]* 60 (2): 78–84.

Cummings, S., E. S. Parham, G. W. Strain, and the American Dietetic Association. 2002. Position of the American Dietetic Association: Weight management. *Journal of the American Dietetic Association* 102 (8): 1145–55.

Dansinger, M. L., J. A. Gleason, J. L. Griffith, H. P. Selker, and E. J. Schaefer. 2005. Comparison of the Atkins, Ornish, Weight Watchers, and Zone diets for weight loss and heart disease risk reduction: A randomized trial. *The Journal of the American Medical Association* 293 (1): 43–53.

Davies, K. M., et al. 2000. Calcium intake and body weight. *The Journal of Clinical Endocrinology and Metabolism* 85 (12): 4635–38.

de Nooijer, J., E. de Vet, J. Brug, and N. K. de Vries. 2006. Do implementation intentions help to turn good intentions into higher fruit intakes? *Journal of Nutrition Education and Behavior* 38 (1): 25–29.

Desmet, P. M., and H. N. Schifferstein. 2008. Sources of positive and negative emotions in food experience. *Appetite* 50 (2–3): 290–301.

Diliberti, N., P. L. Bordi, M. T. Conklin, L. S. Roe, and B. J. Rolls. 2004. Increased portion size leads to increased energy intake in a restaurant meal. *Obesity Research* 12 (3): 562–68.

Dischman, R. K., R. A. Washburn, and G. W. Heath. 2003. *Physical activity epidemiology.* Champaign, IL: Human Kinetics Publishers.

Dohm, F. A., J. A. Beattie, C. Aibel, and R. H. Striegel-Moore. 2001. Factors differentiating women and men who successfully maintain weight loss from women and men who do not. *Journal of Clinical Psychology* 57 (1): 105–17.

Donatelle, R., C. Snow, and A. Wilcox. 1999. *Wellness: Choices for health and fitness* (2nd ed.). Belmont, CA: Wadsworth Publishing Company.

Drewnowski, A., C. Kurth, J. Holden-Wiltse, and J. Saari. 1992. Food preferences in human obesity: Carbohydrates versus fats. *Appetite* 18 (3): 207–21.

Drewnowski, A., and V. Fulgoni 3rd. 2008. Nutrient profiling of foods: creating a nutrient-rich food index. *Nutr Rev* 66(1): 21–2.

Duyff, R. L. 1996. The American Dietetic Association's Complete Food & Nutrition Guide. Minneapolis: Chrominized Publishing.

Dye, L., and J. E. Blundell. 1997. Menstrual cycle and appetite control: Implications for weight regulation. *Human Reproduction* (Oxford, England) 12 (6): 1142–51.

Dykes, J., E. J. Brunner, P. T. Martikainen, and J. Wardle, J. 2004. Socioeconomic gradient in body size and obesity among women: The role of dietary restraint, disinhibition and hunger in the Whitehall II study. *International Journal of Obesity and Related Metabolic Disorders: Journal of the International Association for the Study of Obesity* 28 (2): 262–68.

Eneli, I. U., P. A. Crum, and T. L. Tylka. 2008. The trust model: A different feeding paradigm for managing childhood obesity. *Obesity* (Silver Spring, Md.) 16 (10): 2197–2204.

Epel, E. S., et al. 2000. Stress and body shape: Stress-induced cortisol secretion is consistently greater among women with central fat. *Psychosomatic Medicine* 62 (5): 623–32.

Erkkila, A. T., A. H. Lichtenstein, D. Mozaffarian, and D. M. Herrington. 2004. Fish intake is associated with a reduced progression of coronary artery atherosclerosis in postmenopausal women with coronary artery disease. *The American Journal of Clinical Nutrition* 80 (3): 626–32.

Esch, T., J. W. Kim, and G. B. Stefano 2006. Neurobiological implications of eating healthy. *Neuro Endocrinology Letters* 27 (1–2): 21–33.

Esch, T., and G. B. Stefano. 2004. The neurobiology of pleasure, reward processes, addiction and their health implications. *Neuro Endocrinology Letters* 25 (4): 235–51.

Expert Panel on Detection, Evaluation, and Treatment of High Blood Cholesterol in Adults. 2001. Executive summary of the third report of the National Cholesterol Education Program (NCEP) expert panel on detection, evaluation, and treatment of high blood cholesterol in adults (adult treatment panel III). *The Journal of the American Medical Association* 285 (19): 2486–97.

Farshchi, H. R., M. A. Taylor, and I. A. Macdonald. 2004. Decreased thermic effect of food after an irregular compared with a regular meal pattern in healthy lean women. *International Journal of Obesity and Related Metabolic Disorders: Journal of the International Association for the Study of Obesity* 28 (5): 653–60.

Fedoroff, I., J. Polivy, and C. P. Herman, C. P. 2003. The specificity of restrained versus unrestrained eaters' responses to food cues: General desire to eat, or craving for the cued food? *Appetite* 41 (1): 7–13.

Fedoroff, I., J. Polivy, and C. P. Herman, C. P. 1997. The effect of pre-exposure to food cues on the eating behavior of restrained and unrestrained eaters. *Appetite* 28 (1): 33–47.

Fernstrom, J. D., and G. D. Miller, (eds.). 1994. *Appetite and body of weight regulation: Sugar, fat, and macronutrient substitutes.* Boca Raton: CRC Press.

Field, A. E., et al. 2003. Relation between dieting and weight change among preadolescents and adolescents. *Pediatrics* 112 (4): 900–906.

Field, A. E., et al, R. R. Wing, J. E. Manson, D. L. Spiegelman, and W. C. Willett. 2001. Relationship of a large weight loss to long-term weight change among young and middle-aged U.S. women. *International Journal of Obesity and Related Metabolic Disorders: Journal of the International Association for the Study of Obesity* 25 (8): 1113–21.

Fisher, J. O., and L. L. Birch. 2000. Parents' restrictive feeding practices are associated with young girls' negative self-evaluation of eating. *Journal of the American Dietetic Association* 100 (11): 1341–46.

Fisher, J. O., Y. Liu, L. L. Birch, and B. J. Rolls. 2007. Effects of portion size and energy density on young children's intake at a meal. *The American Journal of Clinical Nutrition* 86 (1): 174–79.

Fletcher, B., et al. 2005. Managing abnormal blood lipids: A collaborative approach. *Circulation* 112 (20): 3184–3209.

Ford, E. S., A. H. Mokdad, W. H. Giles, and D. W. Brown. 2003. The metabolic syndrome and antioxidant concentrations: Findings from the third National Health and Nutrition Examination Survey. *Diabetes* 52 (9): 2346–52.

Fox, C. S., et al. 2008. Relations of thyroid function to body weight: Cross-sectional and longitudinal observations in a community-based sample. *Archives of Internal Medicine* 168 (6): 587–92.

Fox, M. K., B. Devaney, K. Reidy, C. Razafindrakoto, and P. Ziegler. 2006. Relationship between portion size and energy intake among infants and toddlers: Evidence of self-regulation. *Journal of the American Dietetic Association* 106 (suppl 1): S77–83.

Gaesser, G. 2002. *Big Fat Lies*. Carlsbad, CA: Gurze Books.

Gast, J., and S. R. Hawks. 1998. Weight loss education: The challenge of a new paradigm. *Health Education & Behavior: The Official Publication of the Society for Public Health Education* 25 (4): 464–73.

Gerstein, D. E., G. Woodward-Lopez, A. E. Evans, K. Kelsey, and A. Drewnowski. 2004. Clarifying concepts about macronutrients' effects on satiation and satiety. *Journal of the American Dietetic Association* 104 (7): 1151–53.

Gibson, E. L. 2006. Emotional influences on food choice: Sensory, physiological and psychological pathways. *Physiology & Behavior* 89 (1): 53–61.

Goldfarb, A. H., and A. Z. Jamurtas. 1997. Beta-endorphin response to exercise: An update. *Sports Medicine* (Auckland, N.Z.) 24 (1): 8–16.

Goldfield, G. S., K. B. Adamo, J. Rutherford, and C. Legg. 2008. Stress and the relative reinforcing value of food in female binge eaters. *Physiology & Behavior* 93 (3): 579–87.

Guyton, A. C., and J. E. Hall. 2000. *Textbook of medical physiology* (10th ed). Philadelphia: W. B. Saunders Company.

Hardman, A. E. 2001. Issues of fractionization of exercise (short vs. long bouts). *Medicine and Science in Sports and Exercise* 33 (suppl 6): S421–27; discussion S452–53.

Hasler, C. M., A. S. Bloch, C. A. Thomson, E. Enrione, and C. Manning. 2004. Position of the American Dietetic Association: Functional foods. *Journal of the American Dietetic Association* 104 (5): 814–26.

Hawks, S. R., H. Madanat, T. Smith, and N. De La Cruz. 2008. Classroom approach for managing dietary restraint, negative eating styles, and body image concerns among college women. *Journal of American College Health* 56 (4): 359–66.

Hays, N. P., and S. B. Roberts. 2008. Aspects of eating behaviors "disinhibition" and "restraint" are related to weight gain and BMI in women. *Obesity* (Silver Spring, Md.) 16 (1): 52–58.

Heber, D. 2004. Vegetables, fruits and phytoestrogens in the prevention of diseases. *Journal of Postgraduate Medicine* 50 (2): 145–49.

Herman, C. P. 2005. Lessons from the bottomless bowl. *Obesity Research* 13 (1): 2.

Herman, C. P., and J. Polivy. 2005. Normative influences on food intake. *Physiology & Behavior* 86 (5): 762–72.

Herman, C. P., and J. Polivy. 2008. External cues in the control of food intake in humans: The sensory-normative distinction. *Physiology & Behavior* 94 (5): 722–28.

Herman, C. P., T. van Strien, and J. Polivy. 2008. Undereating or eliminating overeating? *American Psychologist* 63 (3): 202–3.

Hetherington, M. M. 2007. Cues to overeat: Psychological factors influencing overconsumption. *The Proceedings of the Nutrition Society* 66 (1): 113–23.

Hetherington, M. M., A. S. Anderson, G. N. Norton, and L. Newson. 2006. Situational effects on meal intake: A comparison of eating alone and eating with others. *Physiology & Behavior* 88 (4–5): 498–505.

Hetherington, M. M., R. Foster, T. Newman, A. S. Anderson, and G. N. Norton. 2006. Understanding variety: Tasting different foods delays satiation. *Physiology & Behavior* 87 (2): 263–71.

Institute of Medicine. 2006. *Dietary Reference Intakes: The Essential Guide to Nutrient Requirements*. Washington, D.C.: The National Academies Press.

Jacqmain, M., E. Doucet, J. P. Despres, C. Bouchard, and A. Tremblay. 2003. Calcium intake, body composition, and lipoprotein-lipid concentrations in adults. *The American Journal of Clinical Nutrition* 77 (6): 1448–52.

Jakicic, J. M., B. H. Marcus, K. I. Gallagher, M. Napolitano, W. Lang. 2003. Effect of exercise duration and intensity on weight loss in overweight, sedentary women: A randomized trial. *The Journal of the American Medical Association* 290 (10): 1323–30.

Jastran, M. M., C. A. Bisogni, J. Sobal, C. Blake, and C. M. Devine. 2009. Eating routines: Embedded, value based, modifiable, and reflective. *Appetite* 52 (1): 127–36.

Jenkins, D. J., et al. 2008. Fish-oil supplementation in patients with implantable cardioverter defibrillators: A meta-analysis. *Canadian Medical Association Journal [Journal de l'Association Medicale Canadienne]* 178 (2): 157–64.

Jequier, E. 2002. Leptin signaling, adiposity, and energy balance. *Annals of the New York Academy of Sciences* 967:379–88.

Jinks, C., K. Jordan, and P. Croft. 2006. Disabling knee pain—another consequence of obesity: Results from a prospective cohort study. *BMC Public Health* 6:58.

Johnston, L., H. R. Reynolds, M. Patz, D. B. Hunningshake, K. Schultz, and B. Westereng. 1998. Cholesterol-lowering benefits of a whole grain oat ready-to-eat cereal. *Nutrition in Clinical Care* 1:6–12.

Joshipura, K. J., et al. 2001. The effect of fruit and vegetable intake on risk for coronary heart disease. *Annals of Internal Medicine* 134 (12): 1106–14.

Katzer, L., A. J. Bradshaw, C. C. Horwath, A. R. Gray, S. O'Brien, and J. Joyce. 2008. Evaluation of a "nondieting" stress reduction program for overweight women: A randomized trial. *American Journal of Health Promotion* 22 (4): 264–74.

Kesaniemi, Y. K., E. Danforth Jr., M. D. Jensen, P. G. Kopelman, P. Lefebvre, and B. A. Reeder. 2001. Dose-response issues concerning physical activity and health: An evidence-based symposium. *Medicine and Science in Sports and Exercise* 33 (suppl 6): S351–58.

Keys, A. 1950. *The biology of human starvation.* Minneapolis: University of Minnesota Press.

King, G. A., C. P. Herman, and J. Polivy. 1987. Food perception in dieters and non-dieters. *Appetite* 8 (2): 147–58.

Kleiner, S. M. 1999. Water: An essential but overlooked nutrient. *Journal of the American Dietetic Association* 99 (2): 200–206.

Knutson, K. L., K. Spiegel, P. Penev, and E. Van Cauter. 2007. The metabolic consequences of sleep deprivation. *Sleep Medicine Reviews* 11 (3): 163–78.

Kraemer, W. J., and S. J. Fleck. 1987. *Designing resistance training programs* (2nd ed.). Champaign, IL: Human Kinetics.

Krauss, R. M., et al. 2000. AHA dietary guidelines: Revision 2000: A statement for healthcare professionals from the nutrition committee of the American Heart Association. *Circulation* 102 (18): 2284–99.

Kris-Etherton, P. M., W. S. Harris, L. J. Appel, and the American Heart Association Nutrition Committee. 2002. Fish consumption, fish oil, omega-3 fatty acids, and cardiovascular disease. *Circulation* 106 (21): 2747–57.

Kris-Etherton, P. M., K. D. Hecker, and A. E. Binkoski. 2004. Polyunsaturated fatty acids and cardiovascular health. *Nutrition Reviews* 62 (11): 414–26.

Kris-Etherton, P. M., K. D. Hecker, and A. E. Binkoski, et al. 2002. Bioactive compounds in foods: Their role in the prevention of cardiovascular disease and cancer. *The American Journal of Medicine* 113 (suppl 9B): S71–88.

LaForge, R. 1995. Exercise-associated mood alterations: A review of interactive neurobiologic mechanisms. *Medicine, Exercise, Nutrition and Health* 4 (1): 17–32.

Lebel, J. L., J. Lu, and L. Dube. 2008. Weakened biological signals: Highly developed eating schemas amongst women are associated with maladaptive patterns of comfort food consumption. *Physiology & Behavior* 94 (3): 384–92.

Lefevre, M., P. M. Kris-Etherton, G. Zhao, and R. P. Tracy. 2004. Dietary fatty acids, hemostasis, and cardiovascular disease risk. *Journal of the American Dietetic Association* 104 (3): 410–19; quiz 492.

Leinonen, K. S., K. S. Poutanen, and H. M. Mykkanen. 2000. Rye bread decreases serum total and LDL cholesterol in men with moderately elevated serum cholesterol. *The Journal of Nutrition* 130 (2): 164–70.

Leslie, W. S., C. R. Hankey, and M. E. Lean. 2007. Weight gain as an adverse effect of some commonly prescribed drugs: A systematic review. *QJM: Monthly Journal of the Association of Physicians* 100 (7): 395–404.

Lichtenstein, A. H., et al. 2006. Diet and lifestyle recommendations revision 2006: A scientific statement from the American Heart Association Nutrition Committee. *Circulation* 114 (1): 82–96.

Lin, Y. C., R. M. Lyle, L. D. McCabe, G. P. McCabe, C. M. Weaver, and D. Teegarden. 2000. Dairy calcium is related to changes in body composition during a two-year exercise intervention in young women. *Journal of the American College of Nutrition* 19 (6): 754–60.

Liu, R. H. 2003. Health benefits of fruit and vegetables are from additive and synergistic combinations of phytochemicals. *The American Journal of Clinical Nutrition* 78 (suppl 3): S517–20.

Liu, R. H. 2004. Potential synergy of phytochemicals in cancer prevention: Mechanism of action. *The Journal of Nutrition* 134 (suppl 12): S3479–85.

Liu, S., et al. 2000. Fruit and vegetable intake and risk of cardiovascular disease: The Women's Health Study. *The American Journal of Clinical Nutrition* 72 (4): 922–28.

Loos, R. J., and T. Rankinen. 2005. Gene-diet interactions on body weight changes. *Journal of the American Dietetic Association* 105 (suppl 5): S29–34.

Lowe, M. R., G. D. Foster, I. Kerzhnerma, R. M. Swain, and T. A. Wadden. 2001. Restrictive dieting vs. "undieting" effects on eating regulation in obese clinic attenders. *Addictive Behaviors* 26 (2): 253–66.

Lowe, M. R., and T. V. Kral. 2006. Stress-induced eating in restrained eaters may not be caused by stress or restraint. *Appetite* 46 (1): 16–21.

Ma, Y., et al. 2003. Association between eating patterns and obesity in a free-living U.S. adult population. *American Journal of Epidemiology* 158 (1): 85–92.

Macdiarmid, J. I., A. Vail, J. E. Cade, and J. E. Blundell. 1998. The sugar-fat relationship revisited: Differences in consumption between men and women of varying BMI. *International Journal of Obesity and Related Metabolic Disorders: Journal of the International Association for the Study of Obesity* 22 (11): 1053–61.

Macht, M. 1999. Characteristics of eating in anger, fear, sadness and joy. *Appetite* 33 (1): 129–39.

Macht, M. 2008. How emotions affect eating: A five-way model. *Appetite* 50 (1): 1–11.

Macht, M., J. Gerer, and H. Ellgring. 2003. Emotions in overweight and normal-weight women immediately after eating foods differing in energy. *Physiology & Behavior* 80 (2–3): 367–74.

Macht, M., and G. Simons. 2000. Emotions and eating in everyday life. *Appetite* 35 (1): 65–71.

Mann, T. et al. 2007. Medicare's search for effective obesity treatments: diets are not the answer. *American Psychologist* 62(3): 220–233.

Mann, T., and A. Ward. 2001. Forbidden fruit: Does thinking about a prohibited food lead to its consumption? *The International Journal of Eating Disorders* 29 (3): 319–27.

May, E. L., M. I. May, and O. R. May. 2008. *Veggie Teens: A cookbook and guide for teenage vegetarians.* Phoenix: Am I Hungry? Publishing.

McInnis, K. J., B. A. Franklin, and J. M. Rippe. 2003. Counseling for physical activity in overweight and obese patients. *American Family Physician* 67 (6): 1249–56.

Mela, D. J. 2001. Determinants of food choice: Relationships with obesity and weight control. *Obesity Research* 9 (suppl 4): S249–55.

Mela, D. J. 2006. Eating for pleasure or just wanting to eat? Reconsidering sensory hedonic responses as a driver of obesity. *Appetite* 47 (1): 10–17.

Mela, D. J, and P. J. Rogers. 1998. *Food, eating and obesity: The psychobiological basis of appetite and weight control.* London: Chapman and Hall.

Melanson, E. L., T. A. Sharp, J. Schneider, W. T. Donahoo, G. K. Grunwald, and J. O. Hill. 2003. Relation between calcium intake and fat oxidation in adult humans. *International Journal of Obesity and Related Metabolic Disorders: Journal of the International Association for the Study of Obesity* 27 (2): 196–203.

Mellin, L. 1997. *The solution.* New York: HarperCollins Publishers.

Mensink, R. P., P. L. Zock, A. D. Kester, and M. B. Katan. 2003. Effects of dietary fatty acids and carbohydrates on the ratio of serum total to HDL cholesterol and on serum lipids and apolipoproteins: A meta-analysis of 60 controlled trials. *The American Journal of Clinical Nutrition* 77 (5): 1146–55.

Miller, G. D., J. K. Jarvis, and L. D. McBean. 2000. *Handbook of dairy foods and nutrition* (2nd ed.) (especially pages 319, 332–40). Boca Raton: CRC Press.

Mokdad, A. H., et al. 2003. Prevalence of obesity, diabetes, and obesity-related health risk factors, 2001. *The Journal of the American Medical Association* 289 (1): 76–79.

Monteiro, C. A., W. L. Conde, and B. M. Popkin. 2007. Income-specific trends in obesity in Brazil: 1975–2003. *American Journal of Public Health* 97 (10): 1808–12.

Muller, H., A. S. Lindman, A. L. Brantsaeter, and J. I. Pedersen. 2003. The serum LDL/ HDL cholesterol ratio is influenced more favorably by exchanging saturated with unsaturated fat than by reducing saturated fat in the diet of women. *The Journal of Nutrition* 133 (1): 78–83.

National Alliance for Nutrition and Activity. June 2002. From wallet to waistline: The hidden costs of super sizing. Washington, D. C.: NANA.

National Eating Disorders Association. General information. Retrieved January 19, 2009, from http://www.nationaleatingdisorders.org.

National Heart, Lung, and Blood Institute. 2001. Expert panel on detection, evaluation, and treatment of high blood cholesterol in adults (Adult Treatment Panel III): Executive summary of the third report of the National Cholesterol Education Program (NCEP). *Journal of the American Medical Association* 285 (19): 2486–97.

National Heart, Lung, and Blood Institute. Therapeutic Lifestyle Changes Diet. Retrieved December 22, 2008, from http://www.nhilbi.nih.gov/cgi-bin/chd/step2intro.cgi.

The National Weight Control Registry. Research findings. Retrieved December 23, 2008, from http://www.nwcr.ws/Research/default.htm.

Newman, E., D. B. O'Connor, and M. Conner. 2008. Attentional biases for food stimuli in external eaters: Possible mechanism for stress-induced eating? *Appetite* 51 (2): 339–42.

Nitzke, S., J. Freeland-Graves, and the American Dietetic Association. 2007. Position of the American Dietetic Association: Total diet approach to communicating food and nutrition information. *Journal of the American Dietetic Association* 107 (7): 1224–32.

Orrell-Valente, J. K., L. G. Hill, W. A. Brechwald, K. A. Dodge, G. S. Pettit, and J. E. Bates. 2007. "Just three more bites": An observational analysis of parents' socialization of children's eating at mealtime. *Appetite* 48 (1): 37–45.

Ouwehand, C., and D. T. de Ridder. 2008. Effects of temptation and weight on hedonics and motivation to eat in women. *Obesity* (Silver Spring, Md.) 16 (8): 1788–93.

Ozier, A. D., O. W. Kendrick, J. D. Leeper, L. L. Knol, M. Perko, and J. Burnham. 2008. Overweight and obesity are associated with emotion- and stress-related eating as measured by the eating and appraisal due to emotions and stress questionnaire. *Journal of the American Dietetic Association* 108 (1): 49–56.

Painter, J. E., B. Wansink, and J. B. Hieggelk. 2002. How visibility and convenience influence candy consumption. *Appetite* 38 (3): 237–38.

Parker, B. A., K. Sturm, C. G. MacIntosh, C. Feinle, M. Horowitz, and I. M. Chapman. 2004. Relation between food intake and visual analogue scale ratings of appetite and other sensations in healthy older and young subjects. *European Journal of Clinical Nutrition* 58 (2): 212–18.

Patel, S. R., A. Malhotra, D. P. White, D. J. Gottlieb, and F. B. Hu. 2006. Association between reduced sleep and weight gain in women. *American Journal of Epidemiology* 164 (10): 947–54.

Poehlman, E. T. 1989. A review: Exercise and its influence on resting energy metabolism in man. *Medicine and Science in Sports and Exercise* 21 (5): 515–25.

Polivy, J. 1996. Psychological consequences of food restriction. *Journal of the American Dietetic Association* 96 (6): 589–92; quiz 593–94.

Polivy, J., Coleman, J., and C. P. Herman. 2005. The effect of deprivation on food cravings and eating behavior in restrained and unrestrained eaters. *The International Journal of Eating Disorders* 38 (4): 301–9.

Polivy, J., and C. P. Herman. 1999. Distress and eating: Why do dieters overeat? *The International Journal of Eating Disorders* 26 (2): 153–64.

Polivy, J., C. P. Herman, R. Hackett, and I. Kuleshnyk. 1986. The effects of self-attention and public attention on eating in restrained and unrestrained subjects. *Journal of Personality and Social Psychology* 50 (6): 1253–60.

Pollan, M. 2008. *In defense of food: An eater's manifesto*. New York: The Penguin's Press.

Pollock, M. L., et al. 1998. ACSM position stand: The recommended quantity and quality of exercise for developing and maintaining cardiorespiratory and muscular fitness, and flexibility in healthy adults. *Medicine & Science in Sports & Exercise* 30 (6): 975–91.

Price, C. J., and E. A. Thompson. 2007. Measuring dimensions of body connection: Body awareness and bodily dissociation. *Journal of Alternative and Complementary Medicine* (New York, N.Y.) 13 (9): 945–53.

Proulx, K. 2008. Experiences of women with bulimia nervosa in a mindfulness-based eating disorder treatment group. *Eating Disorders* 16 (1): 52–72.

Provencher, V., et al. 2007. Defined weight expectations in overweight women: Anthropometrical, psychological and eating behavioral correlates. *International Journal of Obesity* 31 (11): 1731–38.

Provencher, V., C. Begin, M. P. Gagnon-Girouard, A. Tremblay, S. Boivin, and S. Lemieux. 2008. Personality traits in overweight and obese women: Associations with BMI and eating behaviors. *Eating Behaviors* 9 (3): 294–302.

Provencher, V., C. Begin, M. P. Gagnon-Girouard, A. Tremblay, S. Boivin, and S. Lemieux, C. Begin, A. Tremblay, L. Mongeau, S. Boivin, and S. Lemieux. 2007. Short-term effects of a "health-at-every-size" approach on eating behaviors and appetite ratings. *Obesity* (Silver Spring, Md.) 15 (4): 957–66.

Rakel, D. P., and J. Hedgecock. 2008. Healing the healer: A tool to encourage student reflection towards health. *Medical Teacher* 30 (6): 633–35.

Reicks, M., J. Mills, and H. Henry. 2004. Qualitative study of spirituality in a weight loss program: Contribution to self-efficacy and locus of control. *Journal of Nutrition Education and Behavior* 36 (1): 13–15.

Richards, P. S., M. E. Berrett, R. K. Hardman, and D. I. Eggett. 2006. Comparative efficacy of spirituality, cognitive, and emotional support groups for treating eating disorder in patients. *Eating Disorder,* 14 (5): 401–15.

Richardson, D. P. 2003. Wholegrain health claims in Europe. *The Proceedings of the Nutrition Society* 62 (1): 161–69.

Ripsin, C. M., et al. 1992. Oat products and lipid lowering. A meta-analysis. *The Journal of the American Medical Association* 267 (24): 3317–25.

Rissanen, T. H., et al. 2003. Low intake of fruits, berries and vegetables is associated with excess mortality in men: The Kuopio Ischaemic Heart Disease risk factor (KIHD) study. *The Journal of Nutrition* 133 (1): 199–204.

Riva, G., M. Manzoni, D. Villani, A. Gaggioli, and E. Molinari. 2008. Why you really eat: Virtual reality in the treatment of obese emotional eaters. *Studies in Health Technology and Informatics* 132:417–19.

Robert McComb, J. J., A. Tacon, P. Randolph, and Y. Caldera. 2004. A pilot study to examine the effects of a mindfulness-based stress-reduction and relaxation program on levels of stress hormones, physical functioning, and submaximal exercise responses. *Journal of Alternative and Complementary Medicine* (New York, N.Y.) 10 (5): 819–27.

Rogers, P. J. 1999. Eating habits and appetite control: A psychobiological perspective. *The Proceedings of the Nutrition Society* 58 (1): 59–67.

Rolls, B. J. 2003. The supersizing of America: Portion size and the obesity epidemic. *Nutrition Today* 38 (2): 42–53.

Rolls, B. J, L. S. Roe, and J. S. Meengs. 2006. Larger portion sizes lead to a sustained increase in energy intake over 2 days. *Journal of the American Dietetic Association* 106 (4): 543–49.

Roth, G. 2004. *Breaking free from emotional eating.* New York: Plume.

Saylor, C. 2004. The circle of health: A health definition model. *Journal of Holistic Nursing: Official Journal of the American Holistic Nurses' Association* 22 (2): 97–115.

Scherwitz, L., and D. Kesten. 2005. Seven eating styles linked to overeating, overweight, and obesity. *Explore* (New York, N.Y.) 1 (5): 342–59.

Schwartz, B. 2002. *Diets don't work.* Houston: Breakthru Publishing.

Selby, E. A., M. D. Anestis, and T. E. Joiner. 2008. Understanding the relationship between emotional and behavioral dysregulation: Emotional cascades. *Behaviour Research and Therapy* 46 (5): 593–611.

Siep, N., A. Roefs, A. Roebroeck, R. Havermans, M. L. Bonte, and A. Jansen. 2009. Hunger is the best spice: An MRI study of the effects of attention, hunger and calorie content on food reward processing in the amygdala and orbitofrontal cortex. *Behavioural Brain Research* 198 (1): 149–58.

Skinner, J. D., W. Bounds, B. R. Carruth, and P. Ziegler. 2003. Longitudinal calcium intake is negatively related to children's body fat indexes. *Journal of the American Dietetic Association* 103 (12): 1626–31.

Slavin, J. 2003. Why whole grains are protective: Biological mechanisms. *The Proceedings of the Nutrition Society* 62 (1): 129–34.

Slavin, J. L. 2008. Position of the American Dietetic Association: Health implications of dietary fiber. *Journal of the American Dietetic Association* 108 (10): 1716–31.

Smeets, A. J., and M. S. Westerterp-Plantenga. 2008. Acute effects on metabolism and appetite profile of one meal difference in the lower range of meal frequency. *The British Journal of Nutrition* 99 (6): 1316–21.

Smith, B. W., B. M. Shelley, J. Dalen, K. Wiggins, E. Tooley, and J. Bernard. 2008. A pilot study comparing the effects of mindfulness-based and cognitive-behavioral stress reduction. *Journal of Alternative and Complementary Medicine* (New York, N.Y.) 14 (3): 251–58.

Soetens, B., C. Braet, and E. Moens. 2008. Thought suppression in obese and non-obese restrained eaters: Piece of cake or forbidden fruit? *European Eating Disorders Review: The Journal of the Eating Disorders Association* 16 (1): 67–76.

Spoor, S. T., M. H. Bekker, T. Van Strien, and G. I. van Heck. 2007. Relations between negative affect, coping, and emotional eating. *Appetite* 48 (3): 368–76.

Stroebele, N., and J. M. De Castro. 2004. Effect of ambience on food intake and food choice. *Nutrition* (Burbank, Calif.) 20 (9): 821–38.

Stroebele, N., and J. M. De Castro. 2004. Television viewing is associated with an increase in meal frequency in humans. *Appetite* 42 (1): 111–13.

Stroebele, N., and J. M. De Castro. 2006. Influence of physiological and subjective arousal on food intake in humans. *Nutrition* (Burbank, Calif.) 22 (10): 996–1004.

Stroebele, N., and J. M. De Castro. 2006. Listening to music while eating is related to increases in people's food intake and meal duration. *Appetite* 47 (3): 285–89.

Sullivan, H. W., and A. J. Rothman. 2008. When planning is needed: Implementation intentions and attainment of approach versus avoidance health goals. *Health Psychology: Official Journal of the Division of Health Psychology, American Psychological Association* 27 (4): 438–44.

Thirlby, R. C., F. Bahiraei, J. Randall, and A. Drewnoski. 2006. Effect of roux-en-Y gastric bypass on satiety and food likes: The role of genetics. *Journal of Gastrointestinal Surgery: Official Journal of the Society for Surgery of the Alimentary Tract* 10 (2): 270–77.

Thomson, M., J. C. Spence, K. Raine, and L. Laing. 2008. The association of television viewing with snacking behavior and body weight of young adults. *American Journal of Health Promotion* 22 (5): 329–35.

Tomiyama, A. J., T. Mann, and L. Comer. 2009. Triggers of eating in everyday life. *Appetite* 52 (1): 72–82.

Torres, S. J., and C. A. Nowson. 2007. Relationship between stress, eating behavior, and obesity. *Nutrition* (Burbank, Calif.) 23 (11–12): 887–94.

Tribole, E., and E. Resch. 2003. *Intuitive eating: A revolutionary program that works*. New York: St. Martin's Griffin.

Tylka, T. L. 2006. Development and psychometric evaluation of a measure of intuitive eating. *Journal of Counseling Psychology* 53 (2): 226–40.

Urbszat, D., C. P. Herman, and J. Polivy. 2002. Eat, drink, and be merry, for tomorrow we diet: Effects of anticipated deprivation on food intake in restrained and unrestrained eaters. *Journal of Abnormal Psychology* 111 (2): 396–401.

U. S. Department of Agriculture, Agricultural Research Service. 2007. USDA National Nutrient Database for Standard Reference, Release 21. Nutrient Data Laboratory Home Page, http://www.ars.usda.gov/nutrientdata.

U. S. Department of Health and Human Services. 2006. DASH eating plan: Lower your blood pressure. Retrieved December 22, 2008, from http://www.nhlbi.nih.gov/health/public/heart/hbp/dash/new_dash.pdf.

U. S. Department of Health and Human Services. Physical activity guidelines for Americans 2008. Retrieved December 23, 2008, from http://www.health.gov/PAGuidelines/guidelines/default.aspx/.

U. S. Department of Health and Human Services, and U. S. Department of Agriculture. 2005. Dietary guidelines for Americans 2005. Retrieved December 21, 2008, from http://www.health.gov/dietaryguidelines/dga2005/document/pdf/DGA2005.pdf.

U. S. National Library of Medicine, and the National Institutes of Health. Caffeine in the diet. Retrieved January 18, 2009, from http://www.nlm.nih.gov/medlineplus/ency/article/002445.htm.

Van Horn, L., et al. 2008. The evidence for dietary prevention and treatment of cardiovascular disease. *Journal of the American Dietetic Association* 108 (2): 287–331.

Van Strien, T., M. A. Rookus, G. P. Bergers, J. E. Frijters, and P. B. Defares. 1986. Life events, emotional eating and change in body mass index. *International Journal of Obesity* 10 (1): 29–35.

Vartanian, L. R., C. P. Herman, and J. Polivy. 2008. Judgments of body weight based on food intake: A pervasive cognitive bias among restrained eaters. *The International Journal of Eating Disorders* 41 (1): 64–71.

Vartanian, L. R., C. P. Herman, and B. Wansink. 2008. Are we aware of the external factors that influence our food intake? *Health Psychology: Official Journal of the Division of Health Psychology, American Psychological Association* 27 (5): 533–38.

Vieth, R., et al. 2007. The urgent need to recommend an intake of vitamin D that is effective. *Am J Clin Nutr* (85): 649–650.

Wallis, D. J., and M. M. Hetherington. 2004. Stress and eating: The effects of ego-threat and cognitive demand on food intake in restrained and emotional eaters. *Appetite* 43 (1): 39–46.

Wansink, B. 2004. Environmental factors that increase the food intake and consumption volume of unknowing consumers. *Annual Review of Nutrition* 24:455–79.

Wansink, B. 2006. *Mindless eating: Why we eat more than we think.* New York: Bantam Books.

Wansink, B. 2006. What really determines what we eat: The hidden truth. *Diabetes Self-Management* 23 (6): 44, 47–48, 51.

Wansink, B., and J. Kim. 2005. Bad popcorn in big buckets: Portion size can influence intake as much as taste. *Journal of Nutrition Education and Behavior* 37 (5): 242–45.

Wansink, B., J. E. Painter, and Y. K. Lee. 2006. The office candy dish: Proximity's influence on estimated and actual consumption. *International Journal of Obesity* 30 (5): 871–75.

Wansink, B., J. E. Painter, and J. North. 2005. Bottomless bowls: Why visual cues of portion size may influence intake. *Obesity Research* 13 (1): 93–100.

Wansink, B., C. Payne, and C. Werle. 2008. Consequences of belonging to the "clean plate club." *Archives of Pediatrics & Adolescent Medicine* 162 (10): 994–95.

Wansink, B., and C. R. Payne. 2008. Eating behavior and obesity at Chinese buffets. *Obesity* (Silver Spring, Md.) 16 (8): 1957–60.

Wansink, B., and K. van Ittersum. 2007. Portion size me: Downsizing our consumption norms. *Journal of the American Dietetic Association* 107 (7): 1103–06.

Wansink, B., K. van Ittersum, and J. E. Painter. 2006. Ice cream illusions bowls, spoons, and self-served portion sizes. *American Journal of Preventive Medicine* 31 (3): 240–43.

Wargovich, M. J. 1999. Nutrition and cancer: The herbal revolution. *Current Opinion in Clinical Nutrition and Metabolic Care* 2 (5): 421–24.

Westenhoefer, J. 2005. Age and gender dependent profile of food choice. *Forum of Nutrition* 57:44–51.

Wheeler, M. L. 2003. Nutrient database for the 2003 exchange lists for meal planning. *Journal of the American Dietetic Association* 103 (7): 894–920.

Whitney, E. N., and S. R. Rolfes. 2008. Understanding nutrition (11th ed.). Belmont, CA: Wadsworth Group.

Williams, J. M., et al. 2002. Mood, eating behaviour and attention. *Psychological Medicine* 32 (3): 469–81.

Wing, R. R. 1999. Physical activity in the treatment of the adulthood overweight and obesity: Current evidence and research issues. *Medicine and Science in Sports and Exercise* 31 (suppl) 11: S547–52.

Woods, S. C., R. J. Seeley, D. Porte Jr., and M. W. Schwartz. 1998. Signals that regulate food intake and energy homeostasis. *Science* (New York, N.Y.) 280 (5368): 1378–83.

World Health Organization. 2009. Global database on body mass index. Retrieved January 18, 2009, from http://www.who.int/bmi/index.jsp.

Wray, S., and R. Deery. 2008. The medicalization of body size and women's healthcare. *Health Care for Women International* 29 (3): 227–43.

Yeomans, M. R. 2006. Olfactory influences on appetite and satiety in humans. *Physiology & Behavior* 87 (4): 800–804.

Young, L. R., and M. Nestle. 2002. The contribution of expanding portion sizes to the U.S. obesity epidemic. *American Journal of Public Health* 92 (2): 246–49.

Young, L. R., and M. Nestle. 2007. Portion sizes and obesity: Responses of fast-food companies. *Journal of Public Health Policy* 28 (2): 238–48.

Zellner, D. A., et al. 2006. Food selection changes under stress. *Physiology & Behavior* 87 (4): 789–93.

Zemel, M. B., W. Thompson, A. Milstead, K. Morris, and P. Campbell. 2004. Calcium and dairy acceleration of weight and fat loss during energy restriction in obese adults. *Obesity Research* 12 (4): 582–90.

ABOUT THE AUTHOR

Michelle May, M.D., a physician and recovered yo-yo dieter, empowers individuals to take charge of their lives and eat mindfully without deprivation and guilt. As a physician, speaker, writer, workshop facilitator, and consultant, Michelle delivers her crucial and timely message with passion, energy, humor, and insight that transforms the way people view weight management.

Her interest in healthy lifestyles stems from her own personal struggle with food and weight. After years of chronic dieting, she resolved her own weight issues by developing a healthy, balanced relationship with food. Her primary goal has been to inspire others to improve their health with her compassionate and constructive approach.

Michelle is the founder and CEO of the Am I Hungry?® Workshops that guide participants to eat instinctively again, live a more active lifestyle, and balance eating for enjoyment with eating for health. Am I Hungry?® received the Excellence in Patient Education Innovation Award and is available through corporate wellness programs, medical offices, hospitals, fitness centers, and insurance companies. She has trained and licensed Am I Hungry?® facilitators around the world.

Michelle is the award-winning author of *Am I Hungry? What to Do When Diets Don't Work. Am I Hungry?* is the basis for the American Academy of Family Physicians' national health and fitness campaign, Americans in

Motion. Michelle is also the author of *"H" is for Healthy: Weight Management for Kids* written to encourage healthy attitudes and behaviors in young children.

Dr. May is a board-certified family physician who had fourteen years of clinical experience in Phoenix, Arizona, before leaving private practice to devote her time fully to Am I Hungry?® She received her bachelor's degree in psychology from Arizona State University and her medical degree from the University of Arizona College of Medicine. She completed a three-year family medicine residency at Good Samaritan Medical Center in Phoenix, where she served as chief resident.

She is well-respected by her physician colleagues, who elected her to serve as president of the Arizona Academy of Family Physicians. She was the chairperson for the Subcommittee on Women of the 93,000-member American Academy of Family Physicians (AAFP) and was elected to serve in the AAFP Congress of Delegates, the policy-forming body of the organization, for eight years. She served on the AAFP Commission on the Health of the Public and as the chair of the Americans in Motion Advisory Panel. She was also chair of the AAFP Women's Health and Physician Wellness Conference and a member of the American Medical Association's Healthy Lifestyles' Advisory Panel. She is also a recognized leader in many other professional and community organizations promoting healthy lifestyles.

Michelle must practice what she preaches in order to balance her personal and professional life while maintaining her own optimal health. She cherishes her relationships with her husband, Owen, and her two children, Tyler and Elyse. She enjoys hiking near her home in Phoenix, Arizona, and recently became a certified yoga instructor. She and Owen, a professional chef, share a passion for gourmet and healthful cooking, recipe development, wine tasting, and traveling.

INDEX

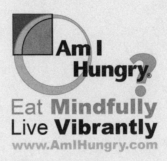

Eat Mindfully
Live Vibrantly
www.AmIHungry.com

Please visit www.AmIHungry.com

- Download free motivational posters and register to receive a complimentary subscription to our Am I Hungry? e-newsletter.
- Find an Am I Hungry?® program in your area (or start one!).
- Download discussion questions for your book club.
- Browse our other books, workbooks, DVDs, and other resources.
- Buy an "Am I Hungry?" bracelet to help you increase your awareness.
- Try more delicious healthy recipes (with photos).
- Comment on Dr. May's Eat What You Love blog.
- Play the Eat What You Love video game.
- Read motivational articles and inspiring stories.
- Download free patient education materials.
- Register for Am I Hungry?® programs and special events.
- Arrange to have Michelle May, M.D. present at your conference or event.
- Request private Am I Hungry?® coaching.
- Set up worksite Am I Hungry?® workshops.
- Become a trained and licensed Am I Hungry?® facilitator.
- Purchase this book at special quantity discounts for promotions, fund-raising, book clubs, or educational use.